The Australian Family
—— Guide to ——
Natural Therapies

Nancy Beckham was born in New Zealand, but has lived in Australia since 1971. She is a professionally qualified teacher, company secretary, horticulturist, herbalist, naturopath, homoeopath and yoga teacher, and runs her own naturopathic clinic in Oatley, New South Wales. She regularly contributes articles to magazines dealing with alternative health care. Her interests include Vedantic philosophy.

The
Australian Family
— Guide to —
Natural
Therapies

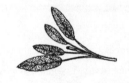

NANCY BECKHAM

VIKING

While every care has been taken in compiling the information in this book, it is in no way intended to replace or supersede professional medical advice. Neither the author nor the publisher may be held responsible for any action or claim resulting from the use of this book or any information contained in it.

Viking
Penguin Books Australia Ltd
487 Maroondah Highway, PO Box 257
Ringwood, Victoria 3134, Australia
Penguin Books Ltd
Harmondsworth, Middlesex, England
Penguin Putnam Inc.
375 Hudson Street, New York, New York 10014, USA
Penguin Books Canada Limited
10 Alcorn Avenue, Toronto, Ontario, Canada M4V 3B2
Penguin Books (N.Z.) Ltd
Cnr Rosedale and Airborne Roads, Albany, Auckland, New Zealand
Penguin Books (South Africa) (Pty) Ltd
4 Pallinghurst Road, Parktown 2193, South Africa

Parts of this book appeared in *The Family Guide to Natural Therapies* published by Greenhouse Publications, 1988.
First published as a completely revised and expanded edition by Penguin Books Australia Ltd, 1994.
This new and updated edition published by Penguin Books Australia Ltd, 1999.

10 9 8 7 6 5 4 3

Typeset in Bembo condensed by Midland Typesetters, Maryborough
Design by Leonie Stott, Penguin Design Studio
Printed and bound in Australia by Australian Print Group, Maryborough

National Library of Australia
Cataloguing-in-Publication data:
Beckham, Nancy.
    The Australian family guide to natural therapies.
    Rev. ed.
    Includes index.
    ISBN 0 670 90668 9.
    1. Naturopathy. I. Title
615.535

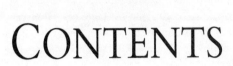

CONTENTS

INTRODUCTION

I wrote the first edition of this book in 1986–87. Over ten more years of research and seeing patients has given me much new information and we now have diseases that were not named when this book was originally published. Consequently, this new edition has been extensively revised and many topics rewritten. A chapter has been added on Common Childhood Ailments, as well as a segment on nutritional strategies for babies and infants.

Health care is changing rapidly. For various reasons, some natural remedies have been taken off the market or lost their popularity since the first edition. Others were not previously available to the general public – *Ginkgo biloba* and *Silybum marianum* (milk thistle) are two examples. Particular remedies are now used for different purposes, such as hot chilli externally for pain relief.

There are many out-of-date books on natural remedies in homes and libraries. Although much of the information may be interesting or useful, some may be inappropriate. Fortunately, most people are not game enough to try old, heroic treatments. You should always use judgement about what advice is consistent with common sense and when you need to get practitioner help.

An example of what not to do is the story of one young man who turned up at my clinic with his favourite, well-worn health book under his arm. It was written in 1957. Some years earlier he had fractured his ankle and it hadn't healed to his satisfaction. What he wanted me to do was create an ulcer in the lower leg to produce a counter-irritant or draining effect. Momentarily speechless, I read the instructions in the book. I explained that I wouldn't aggravate his leg in this way and that leg ulcers were extremely difficult to heal so he might end up with two chronic complaints. Instead, I offered to show him how to apply a mustard plaster. He accepted, went off happily with a bag of black mustard seeds and months later rang to say that his ankle was much better.

The main purposes of this new edition, however, remain unaltered:
• to give practical information for self treatment
• to encourage people with health problems to try new approaches, for even a little improvement is better than none
• to show the preventive value of improving your diet and lifestyle.

You should apply the advice for simple or professionally diagnosed conditions, or ask your practitioner if you can use any of the remedies as support therapy.

I hope that the information in the book will provide a greater understanding of the causes and complexities of ill health and will encourage you to take an active interest in your own wellbeing.

In the context of this book, health treatments could be placed into the following four categories.

1 Self treatments

These treatments cover many common and mild conditions, and while some say that many complaints get better by themselves, my own view is that it is better to treat them because minor problems can often develop into more serious ones. Also, seemingly minor irritations may indicate a basic weakness or an aggravating factor. Sometimes problems may be treated by eliminating something or making lifestyle adjustments rather than taking remedies.

The treatments suggested in this book are generally safe when used in the manner suggested but you should, firstly, read the segment entitled 'How to Use This Book' on pages 1–2. Interactions of drugs and natural remedies are a possibility and it is necessary to get specific practitioner advice about this.

2 Adjunct therapies

Not only support treatments but also certain dietary and lifestyle changes could be classified under this heading. In treating high blood pressure, for example, it would be wise to reduce fat and salt intake, exercise regularly and so on, irrespective of whether pharmaceutical drugs or natural remedies are prescribed.

3 Treatments by natural therapists

Many naturopaths now receive four years of full-time training, so they are competent to carry out basic physical examinations, take blood pressure and similar procedures. They are also trained to refer patients for medical diagnosis and treatment where this is appropriate, the prime consideration being the welfare of the patient. The advantage of seeing a naturopath or herbalist is that you will be advised of preventive measures. In addition, many remedies and formulae that may be effective for a particular condition are not available at retail outlets but only through qualified natural therapists.

Herbal and other natural remedies are usually slow-acting and rely on a gradual build-up; the more deeply ingrained the condition, the more difficult it is to treat. As a rough guide, I usually warn patients that a month of treatment is required for every year the problem has existed. Even where there is a hereditary predisposition to some condition there are steps people can take to prevent the deterioration of their health and it is in this area that I find iris analysis particularly useful.

4 Medical/pharmaceutical treatments

Generally speaking, medical practitioners are the most competent people to evaluate symptoms and diagnose disorders. Unless you get a professional diagnosis, in the first instance, you may not know for certain whether you have, for example, a cardiac condition or nervous palpitations or whether your exhaustion or depression is due to poor handling of stress or anaemia. However, orthodox treatments do not usually concentrate on preventive measures. Many of the drugs used by doctors are not 'cures' but work on symptoms; this may be at some cost to the patient as most drugs have side effects in the short and long term.

With all drug therapy, and most medical interventions, there are potential dangers. Obviously, in life-threatening conditions and serious trauma, it may not be feasible for a doctor to explain all the possibilities to you. However, in the majority of circumstances, you should ask questions and perhaps find out if there would be any harm done by postponing a decision while you weigh up the risks and benefits or get a second opinion.

Natural therapies

The brief comments I have made about the cultivation of herbs, in Chapter 16, relate to temperate conditions. In most cases, fresh herbs make better remedies than do dried, but not everyone is able to grow or buy them in this form.

There is merit in encouraging people to be actively involved in improving their health but there are also some problems. For instance, there is a current trend that people collect wild plants and weeds for use as medicines and foods. However, if you collect plants in built-up areas they may contain very high levels of industrial pollutants such as lead. As well as this, many councils spray with weedicides, and often use large quantities of agricultural pesticides and other chemicals on their road verges. The main danger, however, relates to the difficulty of identification of the plants, for there is not one text that supplies adequate pictures and comparisons to make definite field identification possible, especially for untrained people. Another problem is the question of plant names: this is why professionals use the Latin version for identification purposes, but even this is being complicated by international reclassification and renaming. Herbal preparations can be bought ready-made from retail stores or obtained from herbal practitioners.

Most natural therapy treatments are long term because they work to restore correct functioning; in other words, through stimulation, strengthening or some other process, they provide the means whereby you get yourself well. This is why our treatments do not lend themselves to the standard, scientific, double-blind clinical studies.

I make no apology for suggesting things people can do to improve their health. Many of the old-fashioned 'cures' were effected by a combination of remedies including diet, herbs, water therapy, linaments, rest and kindness. There is a definite need for practical information about self treatment, general health and prevention, for if everyone went to the doctor for every trivial ailment, the medical system couldn't cope, and not everyone can afford to see a natural therapist for general advice and minor problems.

Causes of health problems

Throughout the book I have endeavoured to give a simple but comprehensible explanation of the known or suspected causes of common health problems. The difficulty is that there are so many different possibilities. It is also impossible to make a clear distinction between causes of conditions and contributing factors. If the fundamental nature of disease was a simple problem, there would be no sick people. I don't have a single explanation so I have adopted a practical approach somewhere between the 'cosmics' and the scientists.

It is well known that we can inherit certain diseases and predispositions, that excess alcohol damages your liver, cigarette smoking may lead to lung cancer and that dietary and environmental toxins can cause diseases. As well as the known medical or scientific reasons, there are various theories that illness relates to birth trauma, undiagnosed flaws in the structure of the spine, electromagnetic forces, your past life, how you think and so on. For the most part we usually can't pin down one cause. I might say that an infection or stress are possible causes of rheumatoid arthritis but these don't cause a joint problem in the majority of people. All I can say is that life isn't always fair.

At a different level, it's hard to believe that a perfect, silent, unseen, guiding power would be giving us these sorts of punishments – or lessons. A 'perfect power' would be forgiving. Why didn't IT make us perfect?

Sooner or later everyone will be sick for at least a portion of their lives. When you're restricted by illness or injury, there's usually time to think. Presumably, if you think long enough and deep enough, you will eventually come to a greater understanding of life. There's more to it than caring for your body and worrying about diseases. What about spiritual nourishment, relationships or leading a good and worthy life?

In our everyday material world, common sense and scientific knowledge indicate that in the long run the average person will have improved wellbeing and longevity if he or she eats wholesome food, gets sufficient sleep, has adequate exercise and avoids known hazards. There are harmful things in the world but this doesn't mean we should knowingly add to the burden.

Being healthy and noble are both worthwhile goals. You should take care of both your body and mind because they are your means of experience and progress.

CHAPTER 1

USING NATURAL REMEDIES

HOW TO USE THIS BOOK

1 Read the Introduction as well as Chapters 1 and 2 to get an understanding of the recommended treatments and the cautions associated with them.

2 The Contents page of the book has a full list of the conditions you can treat. For your particular problem, read the description and causes first, then decide if you need practitioner diagnosis.

3 For each problem I have given a number of different remedies. You should not take all of these. I have tried to give a number of remedies for each condition because, depending where you live, it may not be possible to obtain some of the suggested products. In order to select the herb or herbs most suited to you and your condition, I suggest you read the description given in Chapter 16.

Some remedies can be made at home –

infusions of culinary herbs, for example – but many herbal preparations have to be professionally produced. Good combination remedies are also available at health food stores and pharmacies and you will be able to check most of the herbal ingredients in Chapter 16.

4 If a herbal remedy is to be applied externally this information is given; otherwise assume recommended herbs are to be taken internally.

5 To a large extent, dietary supplements depend on your diet and your biochemistry. For instance, if you eat at least five cups of fruit and vegetables a day you are unlikely to need a vitamin C supplement. If your diet is generally poor, a combined multi-vitamin and mineral may be most appropriate. You may need to consult a health practitioner to help identify your individual nutrient requirements.

6 As far as practicable, recommended

foods should be included in your meals regularly in normal dietary quantities.

7 The items suggested under the heading 'From the Kitchen' should be included as part of your normal diet. Dried or fresh thyme, for example, may be used in garlic bread, salads, casseroles and added to home-made scones, or a few leaves can be added to a herbal tea. Herbalists also prescribe it as a fluid extract. The distinction between a medicinal and a culinary herb is not always precise.

8 The herbs and other remedies suggested in this book are safe for general use if they are used as directed by the manufacturer. Naturopathic and herbal practitioners will advise doses for the products they supply. I have given herbal doses in Chapter 16 as a guide and because some people have access to home-grown herbs.

9 As a general rule, I recommend that herbal extracts and nutritional supplements be taken in about 100 ml of water after meals, except for herbal bitters – used for weak digestion – which are more effective if taken about thirty minutes before meals.

HOW TO USE HERBS

Decoctions

Decoctions are the most suitable way of using barks and roots.

The herb is cut as small as possible, or powdered, then covered in a saucepan with cold fresh water, preferably filtered. The usual amounts of the types of herbs covered in this book are 10–20 g herb to 500 ml water. If you add a tablespoon of vinegar to the water, this helps to extract the plant's constituents and functions as a preservative.

Bring water to the boil, cover with lid and simmer for at least 30 minutes. Then let cool, strain and store resultant liquid in the refrigerator in a sealed jar or bottle. I prefer to make decoctions fresh every second day, but they will keep for 5 days.

A common dose is 50 ml three times daily. Barks and roots often taste bitter so you may need to add honey to them, or take them with fruit juice. If you are using something like dandelion root powder as a coffee substitute 1 teaspoon per mug is plenty.

NOTE *Do not use an aluminium saucepan for making decoctions.*

Infusions (teas)

Infusions are made with dried and fresh leaves or flowers. Pour boiling water over the herb, let it stand for 2–3 minutes, strain then drink without the addition of milk. Some herbal teas are improved in flavour by the addition of a little ginger root, cinnamon, a slice of lemon or a little honey. You can use them as iced teas, in combinations, or cold with fruit juices.

For the herbs covered in this book, a common therapeutic dose would be 10 g of dried herb per cup of boiling water, with 2–4 cups daily. Use less if the herbs are powdered, and double if using fresh plants. If you are using herbs as a tea rather than a medicine a teaspoon per cup is sufficient, or according to your taste.

NOTE *Do not use an aluminium teapot.*

Tinctures and fluid extracts

These are liquid, concentrated herbal preparations that are commonly used by professional herbalists. They are also known as herbal extracts. Herbs prepared in this way have daily doses varying from a few drops to 30 ml which is why they are not usually part of self treatments. Some are available to the general public and when using these, as well as products from a herbalist, follow the instructions on the label and do not use more than one herb or one compound at a time when self treating, unless you average the total doses. Tinctures and fluid extracts are preserved with alcohol. Tinctures are weaker than fluid extracts and contain more alcohol.

Tablets and capsules

The doses vary. Follow the instructions on the label and, as a general rule, use one herb or formula at a time.

Compresses

A small towel or heavy bandage is saturated with a strained, cooled infusion or decoction, and placed over the affected area. Hot compresses are usually called fomentations.

Mouthwashes and gargles

These can be made from infusions or decoctions prepared in the usual way and allowed to cool to blood heat; or 2–3 drops of essential oil such as aniseed added to half a glass of tepid water; or a fluid extract or tincture diluted in water. It is better to spit out the gargle otherwise you swallow the infected mucus.

Half to one teaspoon of glycerine may be added to a gargle to make it more palatable, soothing and more effective. This is particularly recommended when using herbs such as sage, which have a high tannin content and which may dry the throat linings.

Washes and baths

These also use strained, cooled infusions or decoctions and essential oils. The amounts need to be varied depending on the area of the body.

For a full bath, you could use about 2 cups of fresh herbs in a stocking (with the top tied). Let the hot water run on it and then allow the water to cool. Before using a full body bath, try a foot bath first to test for sensitivity.

If you're using aromatic oils, only about 10 drops are required in the bath.

Herbal ointments

Here are a few examples of herbs and oils that can be used in this way.

Itchiness	Finely powdered liquorice or chickweed.
Dry, ageing skin	Calendula fluid extract with vitamin E oil (break open 5 capsules).
Infections	Echinacea fluid extract with 10 drops tea tree oil.

A simple way of making your own is to stir dried, finely powdered or liquid herbs into a plain base, such as an aqueous cream that you can buy from a pharmacy.

As a guide, use approximately 1 dessertspoon of herbs to 100 g of aqueous cream or other base. Another option is to add about 10 drops of an essential oil to 100 g of the base. Non-aromatic oils, such as almond oil, can also be included, especially for dry skins.

There's no reason why you can't

combine the various ingredients as long as you test them individually on the skin before making up the ointments. In case you have an allergic reaction, I suggest the testing be done on a small area.

Inhalations

These give quick relief to blocked nasal passages and sore throats. A chamomile inhalation is often useful for inflamed and congested airways' passages and for young asthmatics. Simply make a strong tea and hold the face over the steam (this also helps to clear the skin).

Most herbal inhalations use essential oils such as aniseed, lemon, peppermint and eucalyptus. The easiest way to have an inhalation is to put 3–6 drops of essential oil (less for children) into a cup, pour over hot water and then place a towel around the cup and over your nose, while you breathe in the fumes. Some people put a paper bag over the cup and cut a hole in one corner. There does not seem to be any purpose in using a large bowl and placing a towel over the whole head because you will need to use more oil and water and you don't need the steam in your eyes and hair.

NOTE *Hot water and children are a dangerous combination so you will need to hold the cup.*

An even simpler variation is to use a few drops of oil on a handkerchief under your pillow or in a vaporiser. Tea tree oil is quite antiseptic so it may help prevent other members of the family catching the infection.

Herbal pillows

These contain dried crushed herbs that commonly function as mild sedatives. They are surprisingly effective due to the particular aromas of the herbs used. Catnip, hops and lavender are often used for insomnia, while aromas such as aniseed, thyme and lemon are suggested for respiratory problems. Various types of herbal pillows can be purchased from gift shops or you can make your own.

A simple method of making a herbal pillow is to grind dried herbs as finely as possible, add a little powdered orris root, and put this into a small pillow case that is then stitched together at the open end. This flattish pillow can be placed at the bottom of the normal pillow. It is usually necessary to remove some of the filling from a standard pillow, otherwise it will be too high.

Hot foot baths (or hand baths)

The common way of preparing these is to make a very strong decoction (or an infusion in a pot), leave it to stand for 10 minutes, then strain into a bowl, adding sufficient hot water to cover the feet. Soak feet in it for about 5 minutes once or twice a day. This preparation may be reheated and used several times. A number of herbs can be used, including chamomile, lemon balm and rosemary. A simpler option for hand and foot baths is to use a few drops of an aromatic oil in the water.

For a stimulating effect, baths can be made using mustard or chilli powder. A teaspoon of either is sufficient for most people. Mix it to a paste first, then add hot water. Hot foot baths can give relief to headaches, coughs and colds as well as stimulating the circulation in the feet.

Alternating hot and cold baths stimulate local circulation, although these are difficult to organise. There are various timings for these – I suggest 4 minutes in hot water, 1 minute in cold, finishing with cold. The recommended therapeutic time for this whole procedure is up to 30 minutes. Depending on the area of the body, this timing can also be used for compresses, to speed the healing of sprains and strains.

If you are using a foot bath for an arthritic or joint problem, particularly where the problem is in the lower limbs, it is not a good idea to do this in a sitting position because the circulation 'pools' in the area of the feet; however, with a little planning beforehand, you can lie on your back on a soft rug, with your knees bent and the foot bath at a comfortable distance for your feet.

Maurice Mességué, a French herbalist, used hand and foot baths and, rather unethically, wrote gossipy things about some of his famous patients. His two main books, *Health Secrets of Plants and Herbs* and *Of Men and Plants*, are not readily available but you could get them through your library.

Poultices

These are 'drawing' and soothing and usually applied hot. They are helpful for healing bruises, breaking up congestion, withdrawing pus or embedded particles from the skin.

Starchy substances are commonly used. A very thick, porridge-like consistency is required, and this is applied warm over gauze or hot inside a towel. Poultices may be thickened with bran if necessary. Always test the heat on the inside of your arm before applying the poultice.

Hot chest poultices feel wonderfully soothing, particularly for an irritating cough. It is not a good idea to apply a chest poultice if you are living alone because if you fall asleep, when you wake up, what was a hot, soothing remedy will be a cold, soggy mass on your chest.

For coughs, I like to use some crushed aniseed and thyme; bring these to the boil in water and thicken the mixture with linseed meal. This is wrapped in a towel and placed over the chest, on top of another folded towel. Leave on for about 15–20 minutes. As it cools down, remove the towel under the poultice. Some people place a partially filled hot water bottle on top, or plastic wrap, to retain the heat. It helps to use an essential oil as a chest rub before applying the poultice. Obviously it works better if you are in bed and covered with blankets.

In the old days, people used clay, bread, cooked figs and even hot, baked potatoes wrapped in towels as poultices. Another traditional remedy was mustard, but this may be too strong for some people.

Hot poultices are also helpful for relieving joint and muscle pain and the result is improved if a warming substance is rubbed in first, such as wintergreen oil.

NOTE *In all cases, care needs to be taken not to burn the patient.*

During acute, highly painful or inflamed phases of joint problems, added heat may aggravate. In these cases, rest, moist warmth or cold poultice applications are usually more appropriate. Effective cold poultices for reducing inflammation can be made from bruised or chopped washed cabbage, comfrey or plantain leaves. Grated raw potato and carrot pulp are helpful for swellings. Crushed, fresh garlic mixed with a little flour and water is suggested for sores and minor injuries that are slow to heal.

Plasters

These may be used instead of some of the heroic 'counter-irritants' which are described in old medical and naturopathic books. Counter irritation is where you bring about an irritation of the skin to relieve an underlying problem. Plasters are suggested remedies for long-standing joint problems.

The quantities of ingredients used to make a plaster will vary according to the area to be covered, but a basic recipe is:

> 2 teaspoons mustard powder (the powder derived from black mustard seeds is stronger than that of other mustard species, although all produce a yellow, hot-tasting powder)
>
> 2 teaspoons hot chilli powder
>
> 2 teaspoons linseed meal
>
> 1 teaspoon wintergreen oil (or any linament-type oil or ointment)

Mix together over a low heat with sufficient castor oil to make a thick paste. Apply over affected area, cover with plastic wrap and then bandage firmly with a heavy elastic bandage.

Leave plasters on overnight or, alternatively, don't bandage and lie under an infra-red lamp for about 30 minutes, making sure that your skin is not burnt. Protect the surrounding areas with a towel.

A simpler version of the above is to simmer the ground mustard seeds in water, strain and then – as hot as your hands can tolerate – make into flat patties,

---

CAUTION *Try a small test area of skin first. The idea of the plaster is to make the skin red but not to cause blisters. The redness usually disappears in a few days, at which time a moisturiser should be rubbed into the skin to prevent dryness.*

---

applying them over the affected area.

Some people are allergic or sensitive to both chilli and mustard and, naturally, should not use these plasters.

Plasters may be varied for individual needs, but they are never used immediately following an injury, on broken skin surfaces or where a chronic joint problem is an acute inflammatory phase.

I have had success with plasters for old sporting injuries, for limbs that have not fully recovered from fractures, for chest muscle pain where medical diagnosis has not traced a cause and in various types of arthritis.

As a general guideline, a plaster may be applied once or twice a week for several months but it is somewhat drying to the skin.

Herbal vinegars

The easiest way to make herb vinegar is to put some dried or fresh herbs into a bottle, then completely cover them with vinegar. I prefer balsamic or rice vinegar but apple cider vinegar is also recommended.

All edible herbs and spices may be added to vinegar. A digestive herbal vinegar may be made as follows. For each 500 ml of vinegar, add about 4 teaspoons of dried herbs, choosing from ginger, turmeric, hops, chicory, hot chilli, cinnamon, cloves, mustard, fenugreek, and a handful of fresh herbs such as rosemary, peppermint, tarragon, fennel, basil, oregano.

The dosage is 2–4 teaspoons a day on vegetables or savoury dishes. As a salad dressing, I combine it with equal quantities of salt-reduced Tamari.

Vinegar acts as a preservative and has the capacity to extract plant components. The herbs must be covered with vinegar otherwise they might go mouldy. I suggest you strain out the vinegar and use it by itself when you have used about half the vinegar.

CAUTION Only small quantities of cinnamon, cloves, hot chilli and mustard should be added. Do not use nutmeg. People with gastric ulcers or inflammatory intestinal conditions should not ingest vinegar.

Herbal honeys

Any fresh or dried herbs may be used. There are a number of ways to make herb honey but the easiest method is to melt a pure honey over low heat, together with the finely cut dried herb. Do not boil the honey. Pour the mixture into a clean jar; when cool, cover and leave to stand for a week in a warm place. If you use a plant with very hard leaves, such as rosemary, it is preferable to remelt the honey and strain it.

You may also make a 'sedative honey' by combining, say, catnip, chamomile and wood betony and using it as required. I suggest a dose of 1 teaspoon of the honey to avert an anxiety attack or about ½ teaspoon three or four times daily for general nervousness.

I like to make herb honeys with the fresh, tiny, new growth tips of lemon balm and sage and you will get more ideas of which herbs to use in the later chapters of this book.

Barley or rice malt are honey alternatives.

Powdered herbs

Much as I love herbs, I have to admit that some of them have a frightful taste. However, I sometimes prescribe them in powdered form. These are then mixed into a small portion of food or taken with juice or honey. The doses should be on the labels, otherwise take the quantity given in the individual entries in Chapter 16, 'Recommended Herbs' – substituting grams for millilitres.

CAUTIONS

• Professional herbalists commonly use herbal extracts or tinctures in combinations. For home treatments, it may be wise to use one of the recommended herbs at a time; if you want to combine a few herbs, then you should average the dose. My experience is that combinations are stronger than single herbs so if one herb has a 2 ml dose and the other 3 ml, your combined dose would be 2.5 ml.

• Keep herbal extracts, tablets and oils out of the reach of children.

• Whether you are dedicated to the use of natural therapies or newly seeking alternative remedies, it is important to ensure that you have correctly identified the problem, and for this reason I would recommend that people seek the services of a qualified practitioner for diagnosis and intital treatment advice. For serious conditions, the treatments in this book could be considered more in the nature of adjunct therapies. Discuss this with your practitioner.

• Do not eat plants that you cannot positively identify.

• **Volatile oils** (also known as essential or aromatic oils)

In the herbal system practised by most professional herbalists in Australia, an important distinction is made between pharmaceutical drugs and herbal medicine. Herbalism uses the whole leaf, root or other usable part, while drugs derived from plants utilise one constituent extracted from the plant. When you consider that most plants have over a hundred known constituents, you can appreciate that herbalism is based on historical experience to a large extent because no one knows the detailed pharmacology of all the hundreds of constituents nor how they all work together. Herbalists know how remedies made from whole plants will perform from experience passed on over the centuries, together with their own clinical experience and some scientific trials.

The volatile oils are the exception to the herbal rule of using the whole plant. They are extracted from plants such as eucalyptus and peppermint. As a rough guide, the volatile oil content is about 1 per cent of the plant. The combination of these volatile oils in a plant gives it a characteristic odour, such as thyme and lavender. It is important to remember that, although many of these oils are pleasantly fragrant and some are quite palatable, such as aniseed, they are more in the nature of drugs than other herbal remedies and need to be used with care.

1 Unless specifically directed, do not use them internally.
2 Inhalations and gargles are usually recommended at a strength of a few drops per ½ cup of warm water.
3 Keep these oils away from the eyes.
4 Do not use them on babies under three months.
5 Large amounts externally may irritate and dry the skin.
6 Occasionally people have dramatic allergic reactions to aromatic substances.

A brief outline of Aromatherapy, which uses volatile oils extensively, is given in the next chapter.

• In some cases, fasting, juice diets or special diets may be appropriate but these must always be supervised by a qualified practitioner.

• Haemorrhages (bleeding) must always be checked by a medical practitioner.

• The vitamins and minerals recommended should be taken according to the manufacturer's instructions. If you are self treating, then I recommend that you discontinue after about three months if no improvement is effected. If your condition has improved, then reduce the dose as low as possible to maintain your health or, better still, seek professional advice for an appropriate maintenance programme.

• While I recommend that people take steps to improve their health, I am not suggesting that they self treat with some of the heroic treatments written up in old natural therapy and medical texts – treatments which, for example, cause violent vomiting or purging.

• If you have an allergic-type reaction to a food or herb, then the only sensible action is to discontinue taking it; it is clearly an aggravation for you even though it may help others.

When introducing new substances, I suggest a two-day trial for each item as sometimes there are delayed reactions. If you are aggravated by a particular product, try having a break from it for, say, seven days and then retest it. The problem may have been mild food poisoning, a viral attack or something unrelated to the particular product.

• If you are taking pharmaceutical drugs, never stop these suddenly unless instructed by your medical practitioner because you may get a 'rebound' effect, that is, the condition may dramatically worsen.

While taking pharmaceutical drugs, be careful about taking herbs without advice from your practitioner.

• Charcoal has the ability to absorb a number of chemicals, toxins and minerals so do not take charcoal tablets if you are taking prescribed pharmaceutical drugs as there is a possibility that the effectiveness of the medicine will be reduced. Charcoal is not something you should take on a regular, long term basis.

• For chronic conditions, you will need to give the treatment a reasonable trial period, about ten or twelve weeks, and I suggest a combination of diet, lifestyle adjustments and perhaps one or two herbs or supplements.

Once you have established a successful treatment, ensure that your diet is varied and reduce herbs or supplements as low as possible to maintain the effect.

CHAPTER 2

EXPLAINING SOME NATURAL THERAPIES

AROMATHERAPY

Aromatherapy, healing through aromas, is divided into two kinds of therapies.
1   The use of essences (essential or aromatic oils) that are obtained from plants. These oils are very concentrated and generally have a strong smell. Most of them are not meant for internal use, except when specifically suggested and in doses of a few drops. There are many books on this form of aromatherapy, giving details of the oils used. Refer to the cautions given on pages 7–8.
2   Osmotherapy, or healing through smell.

ESSENTIAL OILS

Odour molecules can be regarded as a special class of non-toxic, mood-modifying chemicals. Many essential oils also possess demonstrable antiseptic, germicidal, antibiotic and antifungal properties. The Aussie oils – eucalyptus and tea tree in particular – have a deservedly good reputation for these qualities.

Another general feature of essential oils is their use in the gastro-intestinal tract as digestive aids and anti-flatulents. Many of the common culinary herbs are obviously aromatic. They have stood the test of time, not just because they enhance the taste but because the essential oils they contain stimulate salivary flow and digestive juices as well as relaxing internal organs and muscles.

In aromatherapy conditions are treated by using the oils in various ways. Certain oils are clearly anti-inflammatory, such as chamomile, while others such as wintergreen are stimulating. Just rub a few drops on your skin and see the reaction for yourself. The effects of the oils can be via the sense of smell, by absorption through the skin or through the internal dose.

Essential oils applied to the skin can affect underlying tissue, the nervous and circulatory systems. In animal experiments, it took thyme and eucalyptus oils 20–40 minutes to be absorbed into the bloodstream; bergamot, lemon and aniseed oils took 40–60 minutes; citronella, pine, lavender and geranium 60–70 minutes; mint and coriander 100 minutes.

It has been demonstrated experimentally that appropriate volatile oils reduce excitability, restlessness, headaches, palpitations and nerve-related problems. The aromatic substances travel to the brain via the nose, the digestive tract or through the skin and seemingly have a beneficial effect on the way we feel. Some have a demonstrable physical effect.

It is also thought that aromas relate to the part of the brain that accumulates our feelings of things past and how we feel about ourselves, and I am sure we have all had an indication of this when we smell a particular fragrance. This is linked to a particular sensation which we might not be able to match to a past incident, but is probably something in our subconscious memory. Sometimes we can relate these aromas to a known feeling, for example, the smell of cut grass may conjure up conscious memories of a childhood country holiday.

The simplest way of using these oils is to put the whole dried and crushed plants in herbal pillows, or use a little of the extracted volatile oil as perfume, in massage oils or in the bath.

Here are a few examples of disorders for which aromatic oils may be helpful.

Aches and pains	Lavender Wintergreen
Concentration and memory problems	Rosemary Sage
Fainting	Rosemary
Fear and anxiety	Jasmine Lavender Sage
Grief and depression	Hyssop Rose Rose geranium
Headaches	Bergamot Lavender Rosemary Violet
Itching scalp	Rosemary Sage
Nervous cough	Eucalyptus (a few drops in warm water could be gargled or inhaled)
Nervous indigestion	Aniseed Peppermint (use a few drops of either oil in water and take internally)
Nervous tension	Lavender Rose geranium Sandalwood Ylang ylang
Unclean feelings	Lemon Pine Sandalwood

OSMOTHERAPY

For insects, and many other animals, communication by odour is often a major factor in getting a partner, locating food, signalling alarm, avoiding the enemy, establishing boundaries and finding the way home. These odours are often in the form of pheromones.

Every species emits its own particular pheromones. Humans respond to human pheromones, but without consciously noting them. Pheromones can affect other species also. A number of psychologists have reported that male goats and bulls become excited when menstruating women are near them and Charles Darwin noted that apes became obviously aroused in the presence of women in mid-cycle.

Experimentally, when rats that have not been subjected to stress are linked by an air tunnel with deliberately stressed rats, the non-stressed ones not only behave as if they've suffered but actually have high blood cortisone levels, which is the body's reaction to stress.

If rats can communicate stress via pheromones, various forms of human stress may be passed on through airborne stress chemicals. I'm sure you've had the experience of 'feeling the atmosphere' when you visit someone. Perhaps this relates to human pheromones! And, maybe, when you're patting your dog and becoming calm as you do so it is because the animal is releasing anti-stress chemicals? At least some aspects of our relationships to other people and animals may be connected to their 'olfactory envelopes' as well as our conscious thoughts about them.

When Arthur Hasley, an American scientist, was walking in a forest he was struck by the uniqueness of the smell of the river – even when it was not visible. He was intrigued by the fact that it brought back strong feelings of his childhood exploring in that particular area. He related this to the puzzle of how salmon swimming thousands of miles in the ocean could find their way back to a particular mountain stream. It is known from tagging salmon that they do actually return to their own specific birthplace. He wondered if salmon somehow become imprinted with a stream's unique river-bed fragrance before they left for the ocean. Subsequent studies indicated that the fragrance was the cue for salmon identifying their natal stream. This information is not merely nostalgic; it is known that pollutants of various kinds destroy the natural river odours and many fish can no longer find their homes, with the consequence that their numbers are dwindling.

Recent experiments give some examples of humans' responses to odours. British researchers noted that seaside trips were invariably associated with happy memories. In laboratory tests, anxious subjects' forehead muscles relaxed by 17 per cent when they were exposed to relaxation therapy and chemicals that smelt like the sea. There were also sound effects of waves and the odd gull or two! Having associated relaxation with the smell of the sea, subsequently a whiff of sea perfume was enough to stave off attacks of anxiety.

An American researcher asked groups of people to recall events brought to mind by neutral words such as 'house' and 'table'. As they heard the words, they were given a discreet whiff of a fragrance. Pleasant fragrances brought on pleasant memories while the nasty smells evoked unpleasant memories.

The sense of smell has a powerful link to our emotions. When an odour rated as 'very pleasant' is placed under the nostrils, increased bursts of electrical activity occur on the surface of the right hemisphere of the brain. Shortly after the odour is removed, there is a similar burst of activity – as if the brain was confirming that the smell had been pleasant.

Participants in another study were asked a series of questions that would normally increase tension. Some people were simultaneously smelling a perfume called 'Spiced Apple'. The group exposed to the perfume had relatively lower blood pressure, heart rate and muscle tension than the control group. Interestingly, blue chamomile oil, my favourite relaxing oil, has an apple-like fragrance.

Even when we are not conscious of an aroma it can be affecting us. One study showed that when a few waiting-room seats were sprayed with a human male steroid, females invariably chose those particular chairs even though they were not aware of the aroma.

Airborne messengers of various kinds may account for some of our inexplicable behaviour. Conversely, the deliberate use of aromatic substances and perfumes that you find pleasant can relieve stress and improve your wellbeing.

BACH FLOWER REMEDIES

The system of Bach Flowers was discoverd by Dr Bach in the 1930s, who gave up his medical practice and devoted his energies to finding remedies that would help overcome emotional problems. The remedies are prepared from the flowers of wild English plants, and none of them is harmful or habit forming. They are not used for physical complaints but for states of mind and moods, because Dr Bach believed that emotions such as despair, anger and fear hindered the recovery of good health.

The remedies are benign and, with the exception of Rescue Remedy, they are slow-acting. They do not change the personality but act to balance negative emotional states. For example, the remedies for fear give confidence and courage; where there are persistent worrying thoughts the remedy produces the positive side – mental calmness.

There are thirty-eight remedies. Sometimes one remedy only is used but for a particular person it might be appropriate and necessary to prescribe up to six at one time. The usual dose is 5 drops in a little water three times daily.

Some health food stores stock the Bach Flowers and a number of books about the remedies are available. I am sure that Dr Bach did not wish his work to be used for the financial gain of practitioners and I see no reason why people should not self-prescribe with the Bach Flowers; however, there are advantages in discussing your problem with a practitioner.

The following is a very brief summary of the remedies.

Remedy	Emotional characteristics relating to the remedies
1 AGRIMONY	A cheerful mask hides innner torture. Restless at night with thoughts going round and round. Seeks companionship. When stressed can resort to drugs or alcohol.
2 ASPEN	Apprehensive, has fears, bad dreams – all for no known reason.
3 BEECH	A loner: critical, arrogant, trivia annoys, too exacting.
4 CENTAURY	The 'door mat', servile, timid.
5 CERATO	No confidence, talkative, always seeking advice, tends to imitate others.
6 CHERRY PLUM	Fears doing something desperate, has uncontrolled temper.
7 CHESTNUT BUD	Does not learn by experience, repeats the same mistakes.
8 CHICORY	Possessive, self-pitying, a nagger, demands attention, dislikes being alone.
9 CLEMATIS	Dreamy, absentminded, lacks energy, avoids difficulties by withdrawing.
10 CRAB APPLE	Filled with self-disgust, shame, sense of uncleanliness, trival thoughts.
11 ELM	Overwhelmed by responsibilities, subject to attacks of weakness and debility.

12 GENTIAN	Has negative outlook, discouraged by difficulties.
13 GORSE	Feels hopeless, doesn't want to try different treatments.
14 HEATHER	Self-concerned, a poor listener, always wanting to talk about ailments, problems and trivia.
15 HOLLY	Tends to hatred, envy, jealousy, bad temper, suffering – often without a real cause.
16 HONEYSUCKLE	Constantly dwelling in the past, has remorse, homesickness, fear of the future.
17 HORNBEAM	Mentally fatigued, doubts strength to cope although usually does.
18 IMPATIENS	Irritable, impatient, finishes other person's sentences, prefers to work alone.
19 LARCH	Despondent, lacks confidence, expects failure, false modesty.
20 MIMULUS	Fears known things (dark, death, accidents, poverty, other people, etc.), shy, tongue-tied.
21 MUSTARD	Deeply gloomy for no known cause, can lift suddenly without apparent reason.
22 OAK	A plodder, overworks, stubborn, hides fatigue and despondency.
23 OLIVE	Physically and mentally exhausted, doesn't enjoy anything.
24 PINE	Has feelings of self-reproach, over conscientious but never content, often overworks.
25 RED CHESTNUT	Over-concerned and fearful for others.
26 ROCK ROSE	Suffers from terror, extreme fear or panic, bad dreams.
27 ROCK WATER	Uptight, rigid in thought and physique, over-concern with self.
28 SCLERANTHUS	Has varying moods and thoughts, indecisive, unreliable, lack of poise.
29 STAR OF BETHLEHEM	Effects of shock or accidents – can be delayed or immediate reactions.
30 SWEET CHESTNUT	Is exhausted and lonely, feels hopeless and despairing.
31 VERVAIN	Over-anxious, over-conscientious, unable to relax, insomniac.
32 VINE	Dominating, ruthless, inflexible, aggressive pride.
33 WALNUT	Over-sensitive to changes, ideas and atmosphere.
34 WATER VIOLET	Capable, proud, condescending, mental rigidity may be expressed in physical tension.
35 WHITE CHESTNUT	Persistent unwanted thoughts, pre-occupied, lacks concentration.
36 WILD OAT	Uncertain, despondent, talented, feels frustration at not having found a goal in life.
37 WILD ROSE	Apathetic, always tired, resigned to condition.
38 WILLOW	Resentful, self-pitying, irritable, ungrateful.

RESCUE REMEDY

Rescue remedy is a composite of *Cherry plum*, *Clematis*, *Impatiens*, *Rock rose* and *Star of Bethlehem*. It is used where there is shock, sudden bad news, terror, panic, exam stress, fear of speaking in public and other similar situations. This remedy is not meant to be for long-term use. A number of doses of 5 drops may be taken, every five or ten minutes if necessary.

HOMOEOPATHY

The following brief explanation should be considered as a simplified introduction to homoeopathy. There are hundreds of books available on this subject.

Modern homoeopathy began with Dr Samuel Hahnemann (1755–1843), a German physician. It is reported that his work was prompted by his observations when experimenting on himself with various drugs. When he took large amounts of quinine, for example, this brought on the symptoms of malaria; when he took tiny amounts of quinine the symptoms disappeared.

Subsequently he developed the theory and practice of homoeopathy based on the following principles that: what a substance can cause it can also cure; extremely tiny amounts of a remedy are restorative when prepared in a particular way; the patient should be treated, not the disease.

Since Hahnemann's time many hundreds of homoeopathic remedies have been developed using a wide variety of substances.

DISCOVERING HOMOEOPATHIC REMEDIES

Substances are given in high, but not toxic, doses to a number of normal, healthy but sensitive people, and under hospital conditions their responses are noted in great detail. Over a period of time a total picture is built up of reactions to that particular substance. This is called 'proving'. The problems or symptoms caused by these large 'proving' doses are then corrected by using the same substances but in tiny doses.

MANUFACTURING HOMOEOPATHIC REMEDIES

For plant material, the basic procedure is to soak the fresh plant in an alcohol solution. One part of the plant is used to 10 parts of alcohol solution or other substances and there are precise and very detailed instructions of how this has to be done. The result is known as the 'mother tincture' or 1x dilution. Then, one tenth of this is taken out and diluted with 10 parts of alcohol and it is shaken 100 times (this is called succussion). Dilution and succussion can be repeated many times and the more it is repeated, the more potent the remedies become, which is why this procedure is called 'potentising'.

By the time a remedy is 'potentised' twelve times, 12x, readers will appreciate that at a gross chemical level the original substance will not be detectable, as the original substance would represent one trillionth part. Poisonous substances such as snake venom and arsenic can thus be used as the basis of remedies because they may be diluted hundreds, and sometimes thousands, of times.

There are other ways of preparing homoeopathics but whether the end result is a fluid or a pill, the methods require special equipment and the following of strict pharmacopoeial instructions.

HOW DO THESE MINUTE AMOUNTS WORK?

There are many theories as to how homoeopathics work. One relates to the vital force being stimulated; this is similar in principle to the meridians in Chinese medicine. On another tack, Paul Callinan, MSc, has conducted experiments aiming to show that homoeopathic remedies may act at a molecular level by changing 'water bridges'.

However, homoeopaths have always maintained that the remedies work in a subtle and different way from other medications and the system has stood the test of time – and various criticisms.

Whatever the theory, scientific tests do show that homoeopathy works. The results of 70 different trials were published in *Nature*, relating to an antibody solution so dilute that not a single molecule of the original substance was present.[1] However, the diluted solution seemed to alter the chemistry and internal structure of white blood cells. Basically the experiments involved adding one drop of the antibody solution to 99 drops of distilled water and trace minerals, then shaking the mixture. One drop was taken from the new solution, and diluted with 99 drops of water and shaken. After twenty-three dilutions (many thousands of billions water molecules to every molecule of antibody) the diluted water solution attacked white blood cells as if it still contained the antibody. In one experiment, after thirty-seven dilutions the diluted solution was twice as active as a solution that had been diluted only three times! The experiments did not work if there was no shaking after each dilution.

The results were so amazing that the editor of *Nature* wrote an accompanying article, entitled 'When to Believe the Unbelievable', stating:

there was no comfort in the explanation that antibody molecules once embodied in water leave their internal marks, as ghosts of a kind, on its molecular structure for there is no evidence of any other kind to suggest that such behaviour may be within the bounds of possibility ... the results are startling not merely because they point to a novel phenomenon but because they strike at the roots of two centuries of observations and rationalisation of physical phenomena ... when unexpected observation requires that a substantial part of our intellectual heritage should be thrown away, it is prudent to ask more carefully than usual whether the observation may be incorrect.

These experiments are still controversial and some scientists report that they have not been able to duplicate them.

Since hundreds of medical and other practitioners have used homoeopathic remedies successfully for over 150 years, I don't think it is necessary to know precisely how they work. After all, for a number of commonly prescribed pharmaceutical drugs the exact mode of action is not known, in spite of many years and millions of dollars spent on their research.

CLINICAL TRIALS USING HOMOEOPATHIC REMEDIES

Although the individual prescribing system used by professional homoeopaths does not lend itself to standard orthodox clinical trials, there have been a number of tests carried out.

In a randomised, double-blind, placebo-controlled homoeopathic trial of 144 patients with active hayfever 'the homoeopathically treated patients showed a significant reduction in patient and doctor-assessed symptoms scores'.[2] In the early part of this trial, some of the homoeopathically treated patients experienced aggravations, which may have been due to the fact that they were all given the same treatment rather than individually selected remedies. At 30c potency of mixed grass pollens was used.

In the second example, 41 rheumatoid arthritis patients were treated with high doses of salicylate, 54 similar patients were treated with homoeopathics and 100 patients received a placebo.[3] The homoeopathically treated patients, who were given individual remedies, did better than those who received salicylate and did not experience any toxic effects. Thirty-nine per cent of the patients on salicylates dropped out from the study because of toxic effects.

Another successful trial was reported in 1990 (see pages 36–7).

A 1991 review in the *British Medical Journal* indicated that there had been 107 controlled trials using homoeopathy for various problems and eighty-one had given positive results.[4]

CHOOSING A REMEDY

When a patient goes to a homoeopath, a whole series of questions is asked, in addition to all the current symptoms and medical history. Details will be required about likes, dislikes, what aggravates or improves the problems and how times of day and weather affect the patient. The practitioner will place some emphasis on mental and emotional states, and consider any peculiarities as well as the appearance of the patient. The aim of the detailed questioning is to match the patient as closely as possible to one of the many remedies that have been 'proved' (established) in homoeopathic hospitals.

As well as classical homoeopathy, there are now other schools of homoeopathic theory, so treatment may vary somewhat depending on the practitioner's training and philosophy. Consideration is also given to the patient's wishes: for example, someone with flu may wish to be treated only for the acute accompanying symptoms.

When the remedy is found, there is also the problem of selecting the most appropriate potency. As a general rule, the closer the match between the patient and the remedy, the higher the potency. Very high potencies are usually considered to be constitutional treatments, that is, covering hereditary factors and the total picture of the patient.

Dosage

For low potencies (i.e. remedies at relatively low dilutions), the doses are usually around 8 drops three times a day. For really high potencies (extremely high dilutions), only one dose of a few drops may be prescribed. For babies and young children the doses are halved or quartered, fluids being given in a spoon of water and pills crushed or dissolved in a little water.

PRESCRIBING HOMOEOPATHIC REMEDIES

The high potencies, that is above 30x, should be used only by trained and experienced homoeopaths because they are deep acting and incorrect use may cause aggravations. Obviously, no one would use arsenic or other posions in a very low potency.

Many of the plant and mineral remedies up to 12x are used for simple problems and these are safe, non-addictive and therapeutically beneficial. It is preferable to see a qualified professional but you may wish to buy a basic introductory book and use one of the first-aid kits available at health-food stores, which incorporate instructions and some basic remedies. I don't agree with the clichés about a little knowledge being dangerous or that it's better to do nothing than to do your best, because surely you know yourself better than anyone else? My view is that the more knowledgeable and educated you become, the more you are able to help yourself and the better equipped you are to ask relevant questions when you see a health professional. It's very confusing for people to be told to take responsibility for their health and then to be discouraged by warnings of the dangers of self treatment. Self treatment is the oldest, most common and economical form of therapy.

EXAMPLE OF A HOMOEOPATHIC REMEDY

With this example, I have tried to summarise the main points rather than include everything.

Calcarea carbonica
The middle layer of the oyster shell.

TYPICAL APPEARANCE OF THE PATIENT
Fair, fat, flabby, blue eyes, very pale skin; may have thin arms and legs; dry, white tongue; lethargic; clumsy.

GENERAL COMPLAINTS
Night sweats, particularly in children (may be only in one area of the body and be sour-smelling); excessive appetite, often very thirsty; bloating, with gastric pain after eating, plus regurgitation with a sour taste; joint and muscle problems. Children are physically and mentally slow developers, scared of dark, may have nightmares; tendency to travel sickness, trembling or spasms.

TYPES OF ILLNESSES
Respiratory and digestive problems, mainly with excess mucus secretions; constant colds; dry, tickling coughs, worse at night and with the chest sensitive to touch; gallbladder problems; enlarged tonsils and glands; constipation; chilblains.

LIKES
Eggs; salt; sweets; ice cream; oysters.

DISLIKES
Coffee; meat; tobacco; sometimes warm food. Also damp, cold, open air.

PECULIARITIES
Cold hands and feet, but the feet may burn at night. The person is chilly but the slightest exertion makes them hot. Milk may be liked or disliked, but always disagrees and there may be cravings for indigestible articles such as dirt or chalk.

MENTAL AND EMOTIONAL STATES
Anxious, fearful, lacking mental stamina, with a brooding disposition. No initiative. A fear of being laughed at.

USING HOMOEOPATHIC REMEDIES

I recommend taking most natural therapy remedies with food but homoeopathics are quite different. They are taken alone. For most people a convenient time to take them is about half an hour before meals. Pills and drops are dissolved under the tongue. For children and people with sensitive mouths, the liquid homoeopathics need to be taken with a spoon of water. The remedies are held in the mouth as long as possible.

While on homoeopathics avoid spicy foods, garlic, coffee, tobacco, mothballs, perfumes, disinfectants, linaments and other strong-smelling substances. Don't clean your teeth within an hour of taking the remedies.

For serious conditions, and where your own treatments have not cleared up simple problems, you must see a practitioner.

IRIS ANALYSIS

Iris analysis is the art of studying a magnified iris (the coloured part of the eye). Based on practitioners examining the fine detail of thousands of eyes, specific parts of the iris have been linked to specific areas of the body and, in addition, structural irregularities and various types of discolorations in the iris have been related to the health of the individual. The pupil and white of the eye may also be included in this study, which is why some people are now calling it eye analysis.

I have done four courses on iris analysis over the last fifteen years and matched the information with patients' health problems. Here are my conclusions.

• Iris analysis is in its infancy but, in spite of the shortcomings, there is a great deal of empirical evidence to support its use. At this stage it is apparently not a reliable system for diagnosing known, medically defined diseases.

• However, iris analysis may assist our understanding of the underlying causes of illness and may be a guide to appropriate and effective therapies.

• It is especially useful for those who are genuinely sick but have no known medical condition. People in this category have been described as suffering from vertical disease, which means they are walking about but feeling awful and have a range of non-specific symptoms. Often they have had numerous medical

tests, only to be told there is nothing wrong with them. A close study of the eye may give some clues as to why they feel so ghastly and therefore provide a basis for treatment.

• In my experience, the German system of iris analysis correlates more with patients' known conditions than the American or Australian systems that are also taught in natural therapies' colleges here. In Germany, eye analysis is used extensively by medical and naturopathic practitioners and is taught in a more systematic and studious way than the other systems. However, all the systems have some features in common.

• Most natural therapists admit, at least to each other, that with practice they tend to develop their own system and interpretations of iris markings. To an extent, they use intuition. Intuition needs to be supported by training, information, intelligence, observation, discussion, discrimination and physical checks. After all, if we accept that there are good and bad 'fields of influence' inherent in the universe, why would our feelings always be right?

• Every iris, like every human being, is extraordinary and unique. Looking deeply into people's eyes, for any reason, is always incredibly fascinating.

WHAT CAN THE PUPIL OF YOUR EYE TELL YOU?

Iris analysts also study the pupil because experience has shown that the eyes' pupils are especially informative about emotional states.

The pupils of your eyes also react according to your activities. They become larger with pain, excitation, exhaustion, hunger and low light; they become relatively smaller as a result of boredom, eating, mental concentration and bright light. Females' pupils get larger when they see pictures of babies and male pinups. Males' pupils enlarge when they see female pinups and pictures of sharks. Females' pupils get small when they see sharks. In one study, males found large-pupilled women more attractive than small-pupilled – which may explain why Italian women in the old days would dilate their pupils with the drug belladonna (beautiful lady).

A number of eye signs, such as pupil dilation, are used in medical diagnosis.

HOW CAN EYES REFLECT PHYSICAL DISEASE?

• It is not known how or why segments of the iris often reflect parts of the body, and particular health problems or physical and nervous weaknesses can be matched to various changes in the iris. However, in classical acupuncture theory, organ meridians (energy streams) end at the eye.
• There is a connection between how we see things and the brain. Light waves come in through the eye and react with the retina, which triggers nerve impulses to the brain. Without the brain we wouldn't know what our eyes had seen. Signals from the brain gathered from the rest of the body may therefore be transmitted back to the eye. Every body organ is linked, directly or indirectly, to other parts of the body. Other parts of the body may be represented in the blood, the retina, the tongue and so on. For example, in pellagra (vitamin B3 deficiency) the tongue is swollen, bright red and usually sore. So why shouldn't the eye reflect symptoms elsewhere?

• The eye is extremely sensitive. Your pupil size adjusts to the amount of light reaching the retina as well as to physical and mental states. When your pupil size changes, the iris structure adjusts accordingly. Photographic evidence also confirms that when there are changes in your physical and emotional wellbeing there are corresponding alterations in the structure and colour of the iris.
• Josef Deck states that among 72 clinically proven renal patients, 92 per cent showed organ signs in the renal sector of the iris.[5]

Recently I saw a patient who had been under medical specialist care for a serious, long-term kidney condition. She did have a 'kidney–lymphatic iris constitution' but the actual kidney area of the iris was quite good. I told her this but remarked that she had a weakened area about an hour away in the 'iris clock'. She then told me that her kidney X-rays had revealed that one of her kidneys was actually located in the lower part of her back.

As we are all different shapes and sizes, with organs of varying shapes, sizes and placements, why would we expect the iris to conform strictly to someone's chart? We don't expect human structures to be precisely the same as an anatomy chart.

Some cynics may dismiss iris analysis as being completely nonsensical, but even medically there are specific eye signs that reflect a physical problem in the body. There is a relationship between high blood cholesterol and a pale rim around the iris; and in Down's syndrome, one can see grey–white spots in the eye, known as Brushfield's Spots; and patients with Marfan's syndrome and osteogenesis imperfecta have distinct blue sclerae (the sclerae are the 'whites' of the eye). Small, irregular, unequal pupils that do not react to light and do not dilate properly on administration of mydriatic (dilating) drugs are diagnostic of central nervous system syphilis and are called Argyll Robertson pupils.

Arcus senilis is another example of a generally recognised medical problem showing in the iris. This is an opaque, poorly defined line encircling the upper part of the iris, usually in both eyes and commonly showing in persons over fifty years of age – due to lipoid generation and associated with memory loss. When found in younger people it requires further investigation.

TYPES OF IRIS

There are some similarities in all the systems of iris analysis. For example, a perfect eye is considered to be an azure blue or clear brown, with fine, even fibres running radially from the pupil to the edge of the iris; there is no variation in the pattern and no discolorations. In the many thousands of eyes I have looked at, I have never seen a perfect eye, although many people have very strong constitutions. It is interesting that people with a poor iris fibre structure have invariably worked out for themselves that they need to take more care with their diets and lifestyle to avoid getting recurring infections and periods of fatigue. Generally they do not have the same energy levels as people with straight, even fibres. A person with a poor basic constitution usually has spaced, uneven, web-type fibres and a lack of uniformity in colour and structure of the iris.

Of paramount value in the German system is the possibility of distinguishing different constitutional types; this is often helpful in tracing the cause of the problem. For example, with a skin problem, a natural therapist might well find that the patient is clearly a 'kidney constitutional type' and so the treatment would include an appropriate kidney remedy, particularly when this correlates with the patient's family and medical history and presenting symptoms.

Here are two illustrations of constitutional iris types. These examples are very simplified as the full description of each constitutional type would take many pages.

Weak connective tissue type

This is commonly found in a blue eye. The iris fibres show considerable variation, the general appearance is diffuse, honeycombed or web-like. The pupil is often larger than average. People with this type of eye have a tendency to prolapses, varicose veins, haemorrhoids and joint problems because of weakness in the body's structural tissue. Obviously, there are a number of steps people can take to avoid these problems developing.

Hydrogenoid type

A feature of this eye is the clearly defined white flakes resembling small cotton-wool balls that are quite distinct against a blue eye. The white markings are usually concentrically arranged in the outer perimeter of the iris. The main problems relating to this type of iris are rheumatic diseases, dairy allergy and allergic skin problems. The characteristic white markings are thought to indicate a previous but inactive tuberculosis and the patient may also have a 'bronchial' history.

It is important to remember that the constitutional typing relates merely to predispositions (strengths and weaknesses that we have inherited) and we can use this knowledge for preventive measures.

IRIS SIGNS AND DIAGNOSIS OF KNOWN DISEASES

Iris analysis is complex and there are numerous types of signs – lacunae and crypts are common ones. These do have specific meanings but before an analysis is arrived at it is necessary to study the whole iris and relate this to the individual's mental and physical state.

An iris analyst studies the various types of coloured marks overlying the iris. Such marks may appear as heavy felt-like blotches, wispy clouds, long streaks, tiny dots in various configurations, round balls, and some may have other discolorations or markings superimposed over them or there can be underlying discolorations. Sometimes some of these discolorations are significant if found in a particular area and some of them occur anywhere in the iris; many of these are found in a whole range of colours and one needs to distinguish between the shades, because a straw yellow relates to a different problem than, say, ochre yellow.

It doesn't make a lot of sense, though, to look into someone's eyes so that you can tell them their medical history and how they feel. What the patient tells the practitioner is more important. Sometimes a basic physical examination or test will confirm or invalidate suspicions.

If a natural therapist sees someone with an obviously enlarged thyroid it may be of academic interest to look into the iris. However, the wisest course is to refer the patient for medical tests to establish whether the swelling is a tumour, a thyroxine insufficiency or excess, or a euthyroid goitre.

CAN THE EYE FORECAST THE FUTURE?

No, it cannot. Based on your iris constitutional type, your medical history, current health, diet and lifestyle, a competent iris analysist can suggest your potential weak areas. Having done that, the practitioner must be able to make recommendations for preventive action on your part.

THE CRITICS

There have been some medical appraisals of iridology but these have not been what you would term 'studies'. D.J. Stark wrote in 1981 that iridology was 'a drawing-room diversion for the under-educated and under-occupied ... it must be dissected, studied and discredited.'[6] His final shot was that 'Medical practitioners must not dismiss iridology to their patients as utter nonsense without first explaining and denigrating it fully. The people who promote it are super-salesmen.' Russell S. Worrall, OD, is equally scathing in his criticism of iridology.[7] Dr J.W. Piesse, however, considered that the iris is potentially a useful dignostic tool as it could indicate the body's pattern of weaknesses and offered scope for widening our understanding of disease processes.[8]

CONSULTING AN IRIDOLOGIST

Human beings are very complicated. Diagnoses and treatment can be difficult for any practitioner. Whoever you consult should listen to your history and symptoms, examine you and use appropriate diagnostic tests. If you have, say, burning urine, it would make more sense for the practitioner to test your urine rather than look in your eye. If you've got 'vertical disease' and about fifty symptoms, then iris analysis may help select the main area of weakness so that a treatment programme may be recommended.

At this stage of its development, iris analysis is probably more an art than a science but it still requires a degree of training and skill. As a natural therapist, there is no doubt that intuition may play a role in diagnosis. You get a quite different 'feeling' about a patient when you look at a well-lit, magnified eye ... watching the pupil move with each breath, noting the incredible detail and the uniqueness of each iris. You also pick up other things when you're close, such as odours, degree of body tension, skin texture and so on. Of course, intuition is unreliable as the sole means of diagnosis but it is one of many guides to locating possible causes of ill health.

TISSUE SALTS

Dr Schuessler first tested and used these remedies about a hundred and fifty years ago – so they have stood the test of time. They are also known to as Schuessler Biochemical Cell Salts.

The tissue salts are inorganic mineral substances. They are found in human blood, tissues and cells, as well as in the ashes of humans after death and in the earth and soil. These salts are present in extremely minute particles in our bodies and are in a simpler form than the minerals found in foods.

After years of study, Dr Schuessler

found that if the body became deficient in any of these salts, then a disease state followed. His system was not designed to 'cure' a specific problem but to make up for any deficiency so that the body tissues and cells would have the necessary components to function correctly. He considered that the capacity of cells to absorb, to excrete and to use nutrients was hindered if there was a shortage of these basic building materials; correct functioning could be restored by supplying the deficient substances in a molecular form that could be readily taken up by the blood, cells and tissues.

The remedies are prepared by being reduced to extremely fine particles and then used in very small quantities. It is considered that these finely broken-down products are readily absorbed by the body because they are in the same form as the particles of salts normally carried by the bloodstream to the cells and body tissues.

There are twelve tissue salts.

Therapeutic name		Common name
Calc Fluor	Fluoride of Lime	Calcium Fluoride
Calc Phos	Phosphate of Lime	Calcium Phosphate
Calc Sulph	Sulphate of Lime	Calcium Sulphate
Ferr Phos	Phosphate of Iron	Iron Phosphate
Kali Mur	Chloride of Potash	Potassium Chloride
Kali Phos	Phosphate of Potash	Potassium Phosphate
Kali Sulph	Sulphate of Potash	Potassium Sulphate
Mag Phos	Phosphate of Magnesia	Magnesium Phosphate
Nat Mur	Chloride of Soda	Sodium Chloride
Nat Phos	Phosphate of Soda	Sodium Phosphate
Nat Sulph	Sulphate of Soda	Sodium Sulphate
Silicea	Silicic Acid	Silicon Dioxide

These tissue salts (and combinations of them, for they are often used in combination) are stocked by most health-food stores. They are suitable for those who wish to self treat or they may be prescribed by a health practitioner. Some suppliers provide a brochure as a guide to self treatment. There are also a number of books available that give detailed descriptions of the salts. The products are sold either under the common name or the therapeutic name.

DESCRIPTION OF THE TISSUE SALTS

Calc Fluor

This is for general tissue weakness and flabbiness. It is taken for conditions such as varicose veins, weak muscles, fragile blood vessels, haemorrhoids, weak ligaments and cracked skin. Another use is where there is deficient enamel of teeth and for babies' teething problems. It is also recommended where there is hardening of the arteries and hard swellings generally. A further indication for its use is when conditions are aggravated by cold and moisture and improved by warmth.

Calc Phos

Generally used to promote growth and strength in the young and for convalescence, especially when there is poor absorption and when the person is pale and weak. It is recommended to help broken bones heal and for blood and circulation problems that cause cramps or numbness, or for people with constant cold hands and feet. It is also used in cases of constant colds, indigestion, chilblains, a tonic for childbearing women and

when the problems are aggravated by weather changes.

It is considered to be the main remedy for the transition periods of life.

Calc Sulph

This salt is indicated where skin eruptions, such as pimples, continue to discharge or where there is thick, yellow mucus anywhere in the body. It can also be helpful where there are frontal headaches with nausea; as a liver tonic and cleanser; and where there is sensitivity and touchiness of the nerves. Some specific uses include pimples during adolescence, skin slow to heal, chronic respiratory infections, weakened memory and sore lips.

Ferr Phos

Used for a range of inflammatory conditions, particularly those that cause discharges. It can help bedwetting, listless children with poor appetites, and also insomnia caused by concentrated study. A common use is to increase resistance in the early stages of any illness. Another indication is for people with pale yellow faces that are easily flushed from excitement. Some specific conditions include coughs, colds, chills, flu and other feverish states.

Ferr Phos is often combined with Kali Mur (potassium chloride) to reduce the severity of viral and bacterial infections. When used for this purpose and at the beginning of an infection, you can take quite high doses for a short period. For example, a tablet every 10–15 minutes for 1 hour, then continuing with one every hour for the rest of the day, after which you would take the dose on the label until the problem abated.

Kali Mur

This salt is for secondary stages of inflammatory problems, particularly with greyish-white mucus. It has been used successfully for some cases of eczema and a range of blistery skin problems such as shingles. Another use is in swollen and congested conditions such as blocked eustachian tubes, jaundice, fluid retention, sluggish liver with constipation and light greyish stools. Where the menstrual blood is dark and clotted, and also in cases of leucorrhoea, this remedy may help. A general indication is where there are dull, aching pains in any part of the body and where starchy and fatty foods are badly tolerated. Pain is aggravated by movement and improved by warmth. The tongue may be coated white or grey. Some other uses include swollen and inflamed joints, asthma and chronic inflammations generally.

It is used in combination with Ferr Phos for coughs, colds, chills and feverish conditions such as flu.

Kali Phos

The most common use of this tissue salt is where there are nervous conditions, including moodiness, poor memory, anxiety, fears, weak muscles and for cramps from over-exertion. It can also be used for insomnia, headaches, hair problems, nervous skin rashes and palpitations; also asthma relating to nervous agitation. In addition, it can help ulcers or indigestion related to anxiety or excitement.

It may relieve nerve pain, usually in conjunction with Ferr Phos.

Kali Sulph

This tissue salt is for discharges that are yellowish and slimy, whether they are from the skin or the respiratory passages. It is indicated when there is a feeling of heaviness in the body, vague feelings of anxiety or sadness, pains of rheumatism or neuralgia that move to different parts of the body. Also, it is used in many catarrhal conditions including bronchitis and jaundice. Cool, fresh air is generally preferred while closed-in warmth aggravates. The patient is worse towards the evening. This remedy can also help scaly skin, brittle nails and depression.

Mag Phos

The indications for this remedy are sharp, shooting or constrictive pains resulting in problems such as headaches, earache, toothache, cramps, flatulence or rheumatism. It is suggested for continued hiccups, squinting, menstrual and other colicky pains. Commonly the type of person who needs this remedy is highly sensitive, restless, nervous, often thin with little stamina and frequently with profuse sweating. Relief is usually felt from warmth and pressure.

Nat Mur

With conditions showing watery, transparent discharges this is the principal remedy; these include hayfever, watery eyes, blisters, skin conditions, flu and also loss of taste or smell. It is generally indicated where there is an imbalance of fluid, such as in chronic constipation with very dry stools, or where there is fluid retention and diarrhoea.

People needing this remedy often have cold hands and feet, a sensitive and cold spine, pasty face, numbness and pins and needles in toes, fingers, lips and tongue. Aggravation comes from moist, cool weather.

Nat Phos

One of the remedies used for gout and acute arthritic problems. It may also help nausea, sour breath and sour sweat, and offensive odour in front of the nose. Other indications include all acidic conditions such as heartburn; and also frequent urination or diarrhoea.

Nat Sulph

Generally this salt has a stimulating effect on the liver, gallbladder, pancreas, intestines and the urinary system; it also helps all natural secretions, so it could be used in cases such as rheumatoid arthritis where there is swelling in the joints. A number of other conditions may be helped with this remedy, for example, gastric upsets, vomiting in pregnancy, earache with noises in the ears, excessive sleepiness and soft swellings. Problems are worse in the morning and with moisture, and helped by dry warmth.

Silicea

Basically for those who are easily fatigued, with little body heat. Also headaches that are brought on readily from study, nervous exhaustion or digestion problems. Other conditions include mouth and tongue ulcers, irritating coughs, brittle nails, pimples and generally for blockages and weakness, as well as a remedy for elderly people. A feature of this remedy is that it is indicated for 'old-looking children' who have thin arms and legs, largish heads and abdomens. Warmth helps the patient; movement and cold, moist conditions aggravate.

SIDE EFFECTS

There is a caution in the use of these tissue salts. The small particles of the salts are bound together in tablet form with lactose (milk sugar) so people with lactose intolerance cannot tolerate this form of therapy. Apart from this, there have been no noted adverse side effects.

DOSE

There are varying strengths of tissue salts on the market so generally be guided by the instructions given on the labels. Tissue salts are not swallowed with water but dissolved under the tongue. The dosage is typically one tablet three times daily. However, for problems such as headaches, I suggest you take one tablet every 10 minutes for an hour or more and then one every hour for the rest of the day.

If you have recurring headaches, pain or infections you can use the salts at the standard dose but get health practitioner advice to establish the cause of the problem. Long-standing problems usually need many months of treatment.

CELLOIDS

These are a variation on the tissue salts and the indications for their use are similar except that the tablets are generally swallowed with water. You could think of tissue salts being akin to homoeopathic minerals and celloids being low-dose, assimilable minerals.

CHAPTER 3

ARTHRITIS AND OTHER JOINT AND MUSCLE PROBLEMS

No one has a 'cure' for arthritis but thousands of people find that their symptoms are reduced or even disappear through dietary changes and natural therapies.

The causes of most forms of arthritis are unknown. Experts may put it down to ageing, allergies, infectious organisms and so on. However, not every old person has osteoarthritis, most of us can consume common foods without them causing an inflammatory reaction and if you're inflicted with pneumonia, klebsiella-induced (infectious) arthritis is not the inevitable outcome.

Inherited characteristics are important but we also 'inherit' dietary and lifestyle habits. If you suffer from arthritis you should admit that you're sick and need to make changes, but getting people to change their habits is a naturopath's nightmare. People on quite dreadful diets invariably say things like, 'I eat a balanced diet', 'I've eaten like this all my life' or 'My mother ate a packet of chocolate biscuits a day and lived till she was ninety'. It's quite possible that the way you eat may suit your taste buds but not your body.

A Swedish medical study on vegan diets and arthritis concluded that although the joint condition did not always improve, patients making dietary changes invariably reported that they 'felt better'. Perhaps just doing something to help yourself is therapeutic, so the sooner you start the better.

Lolling around is a popular pastime,

but arthritic joints need movement. Of course during acute, inflamed phases, more rest is required. Resigning yourself to semi-invalidism and taking drugs is easier than changing habits, but a day doesn't go by without my hearing 'If only I'd known this would happen ... '

We do know that personality doesn't cause arthritis. It's bad enough getting old or being in pain without blaming yourself. However, feeling helpless doesn't make you stronger. Also, you know from experience and observation that when you're upset your neck and back muscles can get really tight. When these muscles are tight, your joints and body usually feel uncomfortable. Constant muscle tension can also restrict blood and nerve flow.

Learning relaxation and meditation techniques is a good, but usually slow way of reducing muscular and mental tension. Most people need a lot of practice before they feel the benefits and you will probably have to try various techniques to find what suits you. The Bach Flower remedies (see pages 13–14) also help re-balance your emotions and nervous functioning.

Regular therapeutic massage can be beneficial to the circulation, nervous system, muscles and joints of arthritis sufferers. Don't have a massage while your joints are in an acute, swollen, inflamed phase, though – at least, not on the affected joint itself. When a joint is going through a severe flare-up, rest is usually the first stage of treatment; cool or warm compresses of water, herbs or apple cider vinegar may be helpful. Spa baths, massage mattresses and chairs are other soothing luxuries that may make your life more enjoyable if you can afford them.

Massage sandals may help feet, legs and lower back problems as they stimulate circulation. Initially they should be worn for only about ten minutes a day, gradually increasing the time. They are not comfortable for heavy work, walking long distances or over rough surfaces, but they are useful when travelling. An alternative is a small massage mat that can be used while sitting or standing. Both the sandals and the mats may be too hard for your feet initially without socks, and remember that they need regular cleaning and drying in the sun. You can also buy vibrating massage pillows to soothe aching muscles and joints.

Exercise can help, and you're never too old to start swimming lessons, to set up your own cooking or walking group, take up dancing, music or painting. If nothing else, learning new things is diverting. Buddha likened the body to a fragile and unreliable vessel and recommended making a citadel of your mind. Discover your inner self.

Your outer self also needs all the help you can give it. Warming volatile oils, such as wintergreen, act as rubefacients – which means they make the skin red and somewhat irritated. This dilates the blood vessels underneath, causing an increased blood flow, so the oils can be beneficial if applied to the joint area. Some skins may be too sensitive to handle this. In such cases lavender oil is more sedating than wintergreen oil and it also helps relieve pain.

Infra-red lamps provide warmth which is usually soothing for joint and muscle pain; they can be used once or twice daily for 5–10 minutes. Ensure that you have the correct type of lamp and do not use it if you are likely to fall asleep, because the heat builds up. It is obviously more restful if someone can supervise you but always set an alarm or timer to be on the safe side. Don't have the glare of the lamp in your eyes.

Cigarette smoking generally restricts circulation, and tends to aggravate arthritic conditions, so it should be eliminated. Dry skin brushing stimulates the circulation. You can buy skin brushes or loofahs at health food stores; use them daily before showering. This also helps to remove dead cells from the surface of the skin and thereby improves elimination of waste products via the skin.

Steam baths also help with elimination via the skin. You can do this yourself by putting an electric frying pan filled with water under an old kitchen chair and using some large blankets to keep the steam in.

One cup of Epsom salts in a deep, hot bath is another old remedy that promotes sweating and often eases muscle and skeletal pain. When using these types of heat treatments, I suggest you use a little crushed ice in a small towel to keep the forehead or back of the neck cool.

It is very important to ignore those who tell you that there's nothing you can do. If you're not sure how to start, see a qualified natural therapist (members of the Australian Natural Therapists' Association have done the equivalent of a three-year, full-time course) or take a holiday at a health farm. Some are more therapeutic than others so make enquiries about the staff, food, exercise programme and facilities before you book in. Alternatively, what about a 'water cure' to Rotorua in New Zealand or Europe? It has been reported that sulphur baths and mud packs gave significant improvement to some sufferers for up to three months. The benefits may be due to the chemicals in the water, moist heat, muscle relaxation, rest, reducing stress or simply doing something that makes you feel better generally. A travel agent can give you details of special trips to spa areas. Assuming you can afford such a holiday, it would possibly be just as enjoyable and more useful than doing the rounds of the tourist attractions. Holidays are some of the easier – but more expensive – ways of learning about different foods and treatments.

A natural therapist always endeavours to match the treatment to the individual. As a guide, a particular patient might be put on the following regime.

• A gluten-free diet. For everything eliminated from the diet, substitutes would be given.

• At least three fish meals (not shellfish) per week.

• Instructions to avoid all processed oils and margarine, and keep fatty foods to a minimum.

• 1 dessertspoon virgin olive oil to be used per day in salads or in cooking.

• Evening primrose oil (3000 mg per day in divided doses afer meals).

• Celery seed extract (30 drops twice daily).

• A combined vitamin and mineral supplement.

• An external remedy.

This programme, together with gradual dietary improvements and exercise, would be followed for three months. Depending on the patient's progress, the programme might be continued with lower doses of celery and evening primrose or a new regimen could be tried. If you're doing your own programme, consider using professional help if you don't improve rather than lurch from one scheme to another.

It would be impossible to cover all the

complexities of joint problems in a few pages. I will give a very brief description only of the more common forms of arthritis together with a selection of remedies suitable for self-treatment. Medical books, the Arthritis Foundation pamphlets and your health practitioner will provide you with the intricate details of what is happening to your joints – if you want to know about this. Always get a professional diagnosis before beginning treatments because not all joint pain is arthritis.

Basic categories of arthritis

	Examples
1 Degenerative	Osteoarthritis
2 Inflammatory	Ankylosing spondylitis, psoriatic, reactive and rheumatoid
3 Crystal	Gout
4 Soft tissue	Fibrositis

OSTEOARTHRITIS

Description
This is the most common form of arthritis and is now being called osteoarthrosis. It is basically wearing of the joint structures. Cartilage, which covers bony ends of joints and functions as a joint cushion, starts to erode, placing a strain on the surrounding muscles and ligaments. The skin covering bones is very sensitive and loss of cartilage usually causes pain.

In response to this erosion, the body tends to produce additional bone in the weak area. These additional growths are commonly called nodes or spurs. If fragments of them chip off, they can cause extreme pain. These bony growths can also press on a nerve fibre. If, for example, this happens on the spine, you

could experience tingling sensations, numbness, weakness or excruciating and variable pain in limbs, muscles and bones.

Causes
Ageing, genes, over use, injuries, obesity, poor blood supply. Inappropriate diet and aggravating exercise are also implicated. As part of the ageing process we must expect a certain degree of joint and muscle change but many elderly people are fit and flexible. One of my aunts taught yoga until she was seventy-nine! Long-distance road running causes joint wearing, although former athletes commonly assess themselves as being healthier and fitter than other people.

Treatment
HERBS
Taken internally
• *Aloe gel* • *Celery seed* • *Devil's claw* • *Feverfew* • *Gotu cola* • *Horsetail* • *Meadowsweet* • *Willow* • *Yucca*

NOTE *Celery seed is a concentrated substance and much stronger than the rest of the plant.*

Applied externally
Volatile oils: • *Lavender* • *Rosemary* • *Wintergreen*
FROM THE KITCHEN
• *Alfalfa* – tea or sprouts • *Apple juice* • *Celery juice* • *Chamomile tea* • *Dandelion coffee* • *Ginger* • *Globe artichoke* • *Green bean broth* • *Lemon balm tea* • *Wheatgrass juice* • A handful of *parsley* or *watercress* can be juiced as well.
DIET
Vegetarian or semi-vegetarian recommended as large-scale surveys (based on

self-reporting) show that vegetarians have a lower incidence of arthritis than meat-eaters.

Boron

A trial showed that 70 per cent of osteo-arthritis patients improved from taking boron supplements.[1] Arthritic bone contains less boron than healthy bone. Boron will also reduce the loss of calcium from osteoporotic women. A loss of 117 mg calcium daily in the urine was reduced to 64 mg by taking 3 mg of boron per day.

Boron supplementation in New Zealand and Australia has been more successful than in some other countries in treating arthritis. This may be due to our high fluoridation, as boron is antagonistic to fluoride. A too high fluoride intake leads to a condition similar to arthritis in its early stages.

In Australia at present, boron is available only on prescription from a medical practitioner. It is usually combined with calcium.

You can increase the boron in your diet yourself, by filtering the fluoride out of your tap water. Boron is an essential nutrient for plants and is taken up by them from the soil. Soluble chemical fertilisers inhibit the uptake of boron from the soil; processing reduces the boron content of food and so does boiling vegetables in water – unless you use the water. The best food sources of boron are prunes, almonds, raisins, linseed meal, parsley, dates, apples, peaches, hazelnuts and organically grown vegetables.

Supplements
• *Green-lipped mussel* • *Organic mineral formula* • *Vitamin C with bioflavonoids* • *Niacinamide*

TISSUE SALTS OR CELLOIDS
• *Calc Fluor* • *Silicea*

EXERCISE

Swimming, walking, gentle yoga and tai chi are usually the most helpful exercises. You're never too old to learn. If you don't move your joints they not only get stiffer but the muscles around them become weaker and smaller.

At the end of this chapter I have given specific information on posture as well as detailed instructions for some basic exercises.

FIBROSITIS

Description

Muscle or joint pain in one particular spot or in several different places, usually with specific 'trigger points'. There are no actual joint changes that can be detected by a standard X-ray, which explains why it has been described as psychogenic (produced by the mind) rheumatism. It is also called muscular rheumatism.

Causes

Unfit muscles, allergies, diseases, viruses or other infections, hormonal imbalances, drug reactions, poor posture, injuries and repetitive use. Stress, fatigue, anxiety, insomnia and various emotional problems are also linked to fibrositis.

Treatment

Once a diagnosis has been confirmed, aerobic exercise is one of the best therapies – starting gradually of course. Improve your posture, avoid working in the same position for long periods of time and, if needed, invest in a quality mattress and pillow. Sometimes particular chores, such as vacuuming, seem to make people worse so if possible get someone else to do these jobs. Driving may be another aggravating factor; if so, try to use public transport.

Learn relaxation and meditation techniques to relieve physical and mental stresses and to help you get better quality sleep.

Remedies depend on the individual and the possible cause.

HERBS
Taken internally

To relax muscles: • *Chamomile* • *Lemon balm* • *Valerian* • *Wild yam*

Anti-inflammatory and antiviral herbs: • *Echinacea* • *St John's wort*

Applied externally

Aromatic oils: • *Bergamot* • *Marjoram* • *Rose* • *Rosemary*

OTHER

Some of the remedies given under Osteoarthritis (pages 30–1) can also be tried. Massage should be gentle at first to avoid aggravation.

The *British Medical Journal* reported that homoeopathic Rhus tox 6x (one part of the plant to a million parts of the solvent) gave symptomatic improvement to a distinct subgroup of fibrositis sufferers.[2]

GOUT

Description

A metabolic condition where there is a fault in the chemical mechanism by which the body deals with uric acid, that is, too much is produced or too little excreted in the urine. Uric acid may be converted by your body from purines (which occur in high quantities in those foods listed to avoid on page 33). Your body can also manufacture uric acid from other substances. When there is too much uric acid circulating in the body, the blood desposits it in the form of crystals called 'tophi' in various parts of the body,

commonly in the ears, but also in organ tissue such as the kidneys.

There is usually a sudden onset of gout, frequently involving the base of the big toe but feet, knees and elbows are often affected. The particular area becomes red, swollen and extremely painful. Usually only one joint is involved and sometimes there is accompanying fever, headache and a fast heartbeat. During recovery, the area is often scaly and itchy.

Gout requires a medical diagnosis because it can be confused with some more serious infections, or even a bunion or chilblain.

After several years of attacks, the chronic form of the disease may set in, where joints are permanently damaged and deformed, and kidney cells may be destroyed.

Following the initial attack, there may be months or years with no symptoms.

Causes

Hereditary. Ninety per cent of gout sufferers are men, usually over thirty years of age. Traditionally considered to be the result of excess rich food and alcohol. It may be due to a particular enzyme defect or various disorders, including kidney malfunction, cancer, and sometimes psoriasis. Certain other diseases cause a decrease in the excretion of uric acid, for example, diabetes. Some pharmaceutical drugs, such as Moduretic, cause high blood levels of uric acid and give gouty symptoms. Lead toxicity can also give similar symptoms.

Treatment

Acute attacks require professional treatment, as do severe recurring cases because of the potential damage to joints and kidneys. However, as the pharmaceutical drugs may have unpleasant or serious side effects, it would be worth consulting a qualified natural therapist to attempt to offset further attacks and the recommendations given below are more in the nature of support therapies.

In my opinion, as gout is not fully understood, there does not seem to be justification for strong life-long pharmaceutical intervention following one attack, particularly in young people.

HERBS
Taken internally
• *Celery seed* • *Barberry bark* • *Burdock* • *Devil's claw* • *Globe artichoke* • *Nettle*

Applied externally
Oils: • *Basil* • *Benzoin* • *Chamomile* • *Juniper* • *Lavender* • *Rosemary* • *St John's wort* – for itching

FROM THE KITCHEN
Taken internally
• *Corn silk tea* • *Dandelion greens* • *Dandelion root coffee* • *Fennel seed tea*

Applied externally
• *Chamomile tea* • *Fenugreek tea* • *Marshmallow tea* – as warm or cold compresses
• *Chilled apple cider vinegar* – as a cold compress often gives relief to swollen, hot or itchy conditions; dilution about 1 tablespoon to ½ cup of water.

DIET
It is important to have a very high fluid intake – at least 2–5 litres per day – to help flush out the uric acid via the kidneys. I would suggest at least one litre of water, the balance being a selection of *herbal teas* and recommended *juices*, including carrot, all vegetables, unsweetened pear or apple. If available, unsweetened cherry and cranberry juice is highly recommended.

Try to include in your diet: *alfalfa, fenugreek* and other sprouts; a high *vegetable* intake (vegetarians rarely suffer from gout); 250 g *cherries* per day, preferably the black variety; 2–4 pieces of *fruit* daily (not citrus, plums or obviously acidic fruit); *blueberries, loganberries* and other blue–red berries; *carob, almonds, buckwheat, coconut, corn, buttermilk, millet, sweet potatoes, yams.*

If the attacks are intermittent, it may be worthwhile writing down everything you had to eat or drink for the previous 24 hours, because some gout sufferers are sensitive to certain foods.

The worst feature of any restricted diet is that one runs the risk of deficiencies or a build-up of a particular toxin (natural or otherwise) so a wide variety of foods must be eaten. There are hundreds of foods which people never try, so I suggest you introduce at least one new food each week. Some new foods you may like to include are tofu, hijiki, wakame, nori. You will find ways of using them in a macrobiotic or Asian cookbook. These products are often stocked in health-food stores or Asian stores.

Foods to avoid
Some experiments have shown that foods high in purine do not necessarily increase the levels of uric acid; however, it would be prudent to avoid the following:
• *Liver* • *Kidneys* • *Anchovies* • *Sardines* • *Sweetbreads* • *Brains* • *Meat extracts and gravies* • *Fish roe* • *Mussels* • *Herring* • *Yeast supplements*

Naturopaths also recommend that you avoid alcohol, coffee and all sugary foods. Supplemental bran should be used cautiously.

Apple cider vinegar can cause a problem, especially if taken generously. A friend of mine was big on supplements to help with her digestion. I suggested that she have apple cider vinegar in water before meals instead because it is a weak acetic acid and therefore increases stomach acidity. Instead of taking the customary *teaspoon* of apple cider vinegar before meals my friend swallowed about half a cup. I'm not sure how she managed this! A few weeks later, she rang me to say that her big toe had become swollen and painful. A doctor had diagnosed gout and prescribed a pharmaceutical drug without doing a blood test. Now what my friend had was an unusual condition which I called excessivitis or vinegaritis. I told her to stop both the drug and the vinegar. Her symptoms completely disappeared within a week and never returned.

Supplements

• *Bromelain* • *Vitamin B complex* plus additonal *B9* (folic acid) • *EPA oil* • *Magnesium* • *Vitamin E*

TISSUE SALTS OR CELLOIDS

• *Ferr Phos* • *Nat Phos* • *Nat Sulph*

OTHER

Homoeopathic remedies can be helpful. I have had good results with diet plus Urtica 1x and other remedies.

You've probably heard of desperate people using bee or ant stings to relieve arthritic pain. Beatings with fine birch stems and nettle are other heroic treatments I wouldn't be game to try. James A. Duke, PhD, reported in an American herbal magazine that he could not get full relief from gout pain in his elbow – even from prescribed drugs – so he decided to sting the area with nettle. He wrote: 'The sting caused a momentary forgetfulness of the gout, and be it cause and effect or coincidence, my gout subsided by nightfall. As a matter of fact, I walked and ran several miles in the afternoon with no pain at all.'

It is thought that the external stinging agent may stimulate natural cortisone activity in the area. The problem is that insect and nettle stings may cause severe allergic reactions in some people.

RHEUMATOID ARTHRITIS

Description

The most common of the inflammatory joint diseases. It may start at any age and be mild or severe. Diagnosis is confirmed by signs, symptoms and biochemical tests.

Causes

There are a number of different possibilities. First, it may be triggered by various infections, including bacteria or unknown viruses. Live bacteria and debris from microorganisms have been found in arthritic joints. A British survey of 500 patients with acute rheumatoid arthritis showed that *all* of them had raised levels of antibodies to *Proteus* – a bacteria commonly involved in urinary tract infections. The rubella vaccination is another suspect. The state of the bowel wall and intestinal bacterial balance have also been linked to joint inflammation.

Second, allergies, vitamin and mineral deficiencies or imbalances are also implicated. Sufferers often have low selenium levels, while some have excess iron deposits. Male sufferers tend to have below average testosterone levels.

Contributing or precipitating factors include poor diet, inability to cope with stress, trauma, overuse of joints, obesity and dampness.

The immune system may malfunction in a similar way to that described under ankylosing spondylitis.

Over-riding all these possibilities is genetic bad luck.

Treatment

HERBS

Taken internally

For inflammation and fluid retention:
• *Burdock* • *Devil's claw* • *Meadowsweet*
• *Nettle* • *Reishi* • *Wild yam* • *Willow*
• *Yucca*

For strengthening the gastro-intestinal system: • *Aloe gel* • *Dandelion* • *Gentian*

There aren't any herbs that specifically treat a disordered, over-reactive immune system. If you use natural remedies as far as possible to treat infections there is less likelihood of disturbing your immune system and bacterial balance compared to doing nothing or taking antibiotics.

Applied externally

Mustard and hot chilli powder as a poultice or plaster, mixed with warmed castor oil and linseed meal, as described in Chapter 1. Alternatively, mix a little *chilli powder* into Sorbolene or other base and use it as a rub. Aromatic oils can be included as well, selecting from *chamomile, eucalyptus, hyssop, juniper, lavender, rosemary, St John's wort* and *wintergreen*. Make additions one at a time in case you have an allergic reaction.

FROM THE KITCHEN

• *Chamomile tea* • *Horsetail tea* – these can be flavoured with ginger

DIET

Water fasting and vegetable juice diets reduce joint stiffness, pain, swelling and biochemical indications of rheumatoid arthritis. You also lose weight. However, you can't do this for more than about a week, it needs practitioner supervision and is not appropriate for the very young, the elderly or thin people.

A successful treatment programme was reported in the *Lancet*[3]: 7–10 days on herbal teas, garlic, vegetable broth (no spinach or silverbeet), decoction of potatoes and parsley (the patient has the juice only), carrot, beetroot (not the tops) and celery juice. Then other foods were introduced one at a time – if a reaction occurred, that particular item was omitted for a week. If on re-introduction it caused the same effect, it was eliminated from the diet. During the first 3–5 months, the patients were asked not to eat food that contained gluten, meat, fish, eggs, dairy products, refined sugar or citrus fruits. Salt, strong spices and preservatives were not allowed, nor alcohol, ordinary tea and coffee. After five months, patients were allowed to test the re-introduction of dairy and gluten-containing food (wheat, oats, barley and rye).

Compared to a control group, after one year on the programme the dieters showed a significant decrease in swelling and stiffness, with improvement in strength and biochemical markers.

This study was done in Norway and, for the first three months, patients who did not use a daily cod liver oil capsule supplemented their diet with vitamin D. In warm climates, patients receiving even small periods of exposure to the sun should not need this. A daily cod liver oil capsule would not be harmful. Patients were told not to take Omega-3 oils because this might invalidate the testing of the diet.

The doctors concluded that this type of diet seemed to be a useful supplement to conventional medical treatment.

I recommend that rheumatoid arthritis sufferers dramatically change their diet and lifestyle, in addition to using specific oils and natural remedies. As you will see in Chapter 16, 'Recommended Herbs', some spices, such as turmeric and ginger, have therapeutic properties and should not be automatically excluded from your diet on a long-term basis – unless you react badly to them.

Food allergies and intolerances

As well as the foods avoided and tested in the Norwegian study, there are other known irritants to rheumatoid patients, including the nightshade family (common potatoes, tomatoes, capsicum, chilli, egg-plant and tobacco). Occasionally, arthritics get dramatic improvement if they completely avoid these substances. You need to stay off them for three months to test the effect. Sweet potatoes are not part of the nightshade family and are okay. Other reported allergens are beef, all pre-served and processed meats, chicken, corn and black walnut.

You might ask, 'What can I eat?'. It's highly unlikely that you will be allergic to or intolerant of all the foods men-tioned. I bet there are lots of foods you've never tried. Some options are given in Chapters 13 and 15.

Oils

Some trials show that fish oil (marine lipids) therapy gives a modest improve-ment to rheumatoid arthritics. However, when quality oils are used over a long period the results are more impressive. A trial conducted by the University of Glasgow gave patients Efamol evening primrose oil and Efamol Marine. After three months, the patients were told to withdraw their aspirin-like medications as far as possible, while continuing with the oil therapy for a further nine months. Eighty-nine per cent of the people taking Efamol and 95 per cent of those taking Efamol Marine were able to reduce their drugs by half or completely come off them. Interestingly, 32 per cent of those

taking a placebo were also able to come off their drugs.

Other trials have shown good results with olive oil. I would recommend an oil supplement long term plus the daily use of a dessertspoon of virgin oil or cold-pressed corn oil in salads or cooked dishes. Don't brown oils when cooking them. Avoid margarine and processed polyunsaturated oils and keep the rest of the fat intake very low. Fish oils generally have benefits to the heart, circulation and skin. A high fish diet has been related to a low incidence of heart disease and rheu-matoid arthritis.

Supplements

• *Manganese* • *Zinc* • *Vitamin C with bio-flavonoids* • *Vitamin B5* • *Royal jelly* • Possibly *calcium*

NOTE **Do not take iron unless you have a test showing a deficiency. Excess iron interferes with the metabolism of other minerals; ferrous sulphate in particular may lead to constipation and unwanted storage in body tissues.**

TISSUE SALTS OR CELLOIDS

• *Ferr Phos* • *Nat Sulph* • *Nat Phos* • *Silicea*

OTHER

Homoeopathy

In a double-blind clinical study, two homoeopathic physicians were involved in prescribing for patients. The patients had either ceased to improve on anti-inflammatory drugs or were deteriorating when they were admitted to the trial. The remedies were individually pre-scribed, the ones most frequently used being Arnica, Arsenicum album, Bryonia alba, Calcarea carbonica, Causticum, Ignatia, Lachesis, Lycopodium, Natrum muriaticum, Nux vomica, Opium, Pulsatilla, Rhododendron, Rhus tox, Ruta, Sepia, Sulphur, Sycotic co. and Thuja.

There was a significant improvement in subjective pain, articular index, stiffness and grip strength in those patients receiving homoeopathic remedies whereas there was no significant change in the patients who received placebos.[4]

ANKYLOSING SPONDYLITIS

Description
This problem has similarities to rheumatoid arthritis. It commonly starts in the lower spine and young male adults are the most frequently affected. Characteristically, there is increasing stiffness and in severe cases the back can become rigid. Other joints may be damaged, particularly the larger ones. Sometimes the patient has unusual accompanying symptoms such as abdominal and chest pain.

Causes
Research has shown a connection to an over-abundant population of undesirable intestinal bacteria, such as *Klebsiella*. Journals are now referring to ankylosing spondylitis as Klebsiella-reactive arthritis, enteropathic arthritis and infectious arthritis. A wide range of microorganisms, together with genetic susceptibility, are linked to various forms of inflammatory arthritis.

It is likely that the immune system becomes weakened and the microorganisms persist, probably in the intestines. Even in the absence of symptoms, a high percentage of patients have inflamed intestines, thereby increasing gut permeability. In other words, live microorganisms, bits of them or other substances (antigens), leak through the intestinal wall

instead of being excreted. These substances get into the circulatory system, are carried to the joint tissue and trigger an inflammatory or autoimmune reaction. Part of the *Klebsiella* bacterium resembles a tiny portion of human joint tissue (a sort of molecular mimicry) and the theory is that the body's defence system becomes confused; in its attempt to get rid of the harmful agent it also starts attacking the joint tissue.

Our bodies produce stress hormones, so do bacteria. Another theory is that the body can't discriminate between the two hormones and this may account for reported cases of joint reactions following accidents or other major stresses.

Treatment
HERBS
• *Celery seed* • *Echinacea* • *Garlic* • *Reishi* • *St John's wort*

DIET
The *Klebsiella* bacterium loves starch and the strategy being adopted by Dr Ebringer of King's College Hospital, England, is that patients cut out bread, pasta, cereals of all sorts, rice, potatoes and all sugary foods. Vegetables, fruit, eggs, cheese, fish and meat are all allowed.

This is not a quick cure – or a very naturopathic one – but the majority of ankylosing spondylitis patients have had their disease process halted from following this diet. Anyone considering doing this would need detailed dietary advice and monitoring.

At the time of the writing this book, I haven't used this programme but suggest it would be enhanced by supplementation with quality lactobacillus and bifidobacteria products, in addition to a herbal formula. After six months, some starchy foods could be cautiously re-introduced, starting with small quantities of corn, then dried beans, lentils and whole grains.

PSORIATIC ARTHRITIS

Description

Sometimes the associated joint problem is similar to rheumatoid arthritis but frequently there is a particular pattern. Typically skin lesions come first, and psoriasis of the nails is common. However, the skin and joint problems can occur together and relapse simultaneously. The end joints of the fingers and toes are often affected, although any joint may be involved. Fewer joints are involved than in rheumatoid arthritis, there may be high uric acid levels (see gout) and there may be new bone formation near to joint capsules and tendons, often in the heel bone, which may cause severe pain. The spinal column may become involved, particularly at a later stage.

Treatment

Basically the same as for rheumatoid arthritis. I suggest *Efamol Marine* as the most effective supplement. The best dietary oil is linseed but it must not be over-heated in cooking. The rest of the diet is low-fat, with no margarine or processed polyunsaturated oils.

Refer also to Chapter 12, 'Skin and Related Diseases', *sarsaparilla* being one of the most recommended herbs for psoriasis.

DRUG-INDUCED ARTHRALGIAS

This is another category of muscle and joint pain. Some of the drugs that have been implicated in producing pain were listed in the *Australian Adverse Reactions Bulletin*, November 1989.

Sole suspected drug	Number of reports
Trimethoprim-sulphamethoxazole	54
Hydralazine hydrochloride	30
Mianserin hydrochloride	29
Carbimazole	27
Methyldopa	20
Nitrofurantoin	20
Hepatitis B vaccines	18
Quinidine	16
Iron dextran	16
Amoxycillin trihydrate	14
Metoprolol	11
Carbamazepine	9
Cimetidine	9
Nifedipine	9

ANTI-ARTHRITIC PHARMACEUTICAL DRUGS

If people wish to have a reasonably complete assessment of any pharmaceutical drug, I suggest they read the Australian *MIMS Annual* which is available in most libraries. The current edition lists nineteen contraindications and precautions for Naprosyn, as well as over thirty possible adverse reactions, many of which are severe – including ulcers and fatal hepatitis. Voltaren, advertised as 'the world's most popular anti-inflammatory' has an even longer list of side effects.

Dr R. S. Mendelsohn wrote in *Confessions of a Medical Heretic*:

... a torrent of advertisements in medical journals has heralded the coming of such anti-arthritis drugs as Butazolidin, Indocid, Naprosyn, Tolectin and others ... Millions of prescriptions have been written. And in just these few years, this new class of drugs has a record of side effects that promises to rival antibiotics and hormones as genuine public health menaces. Just reading the information supplied by the manufacturer of Butazolidin and thinking that your doctor actually is prescribing the stuff to you is enough to make you ill. This is a potent drug; its misuse can lead to serious results. Cases of leukemia have been reported in patients with a history of short and long term therapy. If you read further you find that your doctor is setting you up for a possible 92 adverse reactions. Use the lowest effective dosage. Weigh initially unpredictable benefits against risk of severe, even fatal reactions. The disease condition itself is unaltered by the drug.

After reading that, you have to wonder why the drug company would bother marketing the stuff ... In the case of at least one anti-arthritis drug, Naprosyn, the sacrifice has graduated into a farce. Though the FDA has discovered that Syntex, the drug's manufacturer, falsified records of tumors and animal death during the safety tests for its drug, the government is uanble to remove the drug from the market without long and tedious proceedings.

For over a decade medical researchers have known that patients with both rheumatoid and osteoarthritis who have taken nonsteroidal anti-inflammatory drugs (NSAIDs) show a striking increase in intestinal permeability – even from suppositories.[5] When the bowel wall loses its selectivity there is increased absorption of carcinogens and other harmful substances.

The *British Medical Journal* has reported that people taking corticosteroids or NSAIDs were more likely to have the most serious complications of diverticular disease.[6] The extension of contamination outside the colon was strongly associated with all of these drugs. Such pharmaceutical drugs – and aspirin – cause changes in the intestinal wall, leading to a reduced level of villi (microscopic hairs) and lactase (the enzyme required to digest milk sugar) as well as high levels of wheat intolerance.

The gastrointestinal side effects of modern arthritic drugs may partially explain why some of the old natural therapy remedies and diets are not as effective as they once were. For example, Scandinavian people have a long history of high tolerance to dairy products. In the past, practitioners such as Dr Waerland successfully used soured milk products and whole grains as part of the clinical treatment of arthritis. But the results of the trial of a restricted diet regimen on rheumatoid arthritis sufferers (see page 35) showed that these two foods are now apparently poorly tolerated by many arthritic Scandinavians. Rheumatoid arthritics may have a higher incidence of intestinal malfunction that can be related to food sensitivities. Current anti-arthritic medication is aggravating or causing this problem.

May & Baker Pharmaceuticals have published a free booklet entitled *Diet and Arthritis* (being circulated by the Arthritis Foundation of Australia at the time of revising this book). It advises you to eat at least four servings of bread or cereals a day and 1 tablespoon of butter or margarine, plus 300–600 ml of milk to drink and, predictably, includes a warning 'It is important that you remain on prescribed medication unless directed otherwise by your doctor'. A cynic might think it was a regimen specifically designed to aggravate your digestive system and your joints!

In 1989 the *Journal of Rheumatology* printed a review which concluded that there was no firm evidence that commonly used drugs halted the progression of severe arthritis.[7] Dr McDougall, an American doctor, wrote in his *Newsletter* in 1989:

... the powerful drugs prescribed, often in a less-than-honest manner by many doctors, can be the cause of death and disability of the very patients they're supposed to save. One study found more than half of patients undergoing the best drug treatment science had to offer were dead or severely disabled at the end of 20 years.

Recent reports in the Australian media have also sounded the alarm about the long-term dangerous effects of these drugs in elderly people. A quote from the *Australian Prescriber*:

Although the risk of a catastrophic reaction for an individual is low, the sheer prevalence of usage of NSAIDs in Australia means that 30 per cent or more of all cases of massive gastrointestinal bleeding in the over-60 age group can be attributed to NSAIDs. In this age group, the mortality of major gastrointestinal bleeding is approximately 10 per cent.[8]

Seventy-four known cases of colitis caused by NSAIDs were reported in *Archives of Internal Medicine* in 1992[9], while an 1992 article in *General Practitioner* warned that NSAIDs are unlikely to relieve muscle or tendon injury pain and may in fact delay the healing process.[10]

Is there any justification for the use of these anti-arthritic drugs? Yes – for pain relief. Be warned, though: you can't come off these drugs suddenly. Generally, you would need to follow a total alternative programme for about three months before attempting to reduce long-standing anti-arthritic medication.

ARTHRITIC PAIN

Unfortunately, natural therapies have few effective painkillers. Here are some that help over a period of time.
• *Feverfew* • *Meadowsweet* • *Willow*
• *Wood betony* • *Calcium Phosphate* and *Magnesium Phosphate* – taken together in celloid or tissue salt form • *DL-Phenylalanine* • External use of *chilli*.

Some people are allergic to hot chillies so always use a chilli remedy weak the first time and test it on a small area of your body. You can cut a fresh chilli in half and simply rub it on the painful joint, or mix a little chilli powder into Sorbolene or a similar base and rub it in. Another option is to make a chilli infusion (tea) and apply a warm compress of it over the area. The burning heat is quite diverting. Wash your hands thoroughly after handling chilli because if you touch your eyes with 'chilli fingers' it causes stinging pain.

Acupuncture, biofeedback, homoeopathy and hypnotherapy are all used for pain relief.

Massaging with aromatic oils and linaments often gives relief.

A NATUROPATHIC VIEW OF ARTHRITIS

Natural therapists have always considered factors such as a wholefood diet, elimination, digestion and organ function when treating joint problems. Nowadays we use words like 'dysbiosis' rather than 'toxic bowel', but the principles remain the same. Scientists have now confirmed the connection between malfunctioning intestines and an inflamed joint – as explained in the previous sections on rheumatoid arthritis and ankylosing spondylitis.

Endotoxins (bacteria, viruses and metabolic wastes) enter the body from the intestines and lungs in both health and disease. These toxins may be destroyed in the liver or pass into body tissues via lymphatic or blood circulation, so when naturopaths treat the bowel and liver for complaints in other parts of the body it is not without reason. Habitual constipation also encourages the reabsorption of toxins.

Apart from circulating toxins, joints may also be affected by poor digestion. At a simple level, if you have low stomach acid you cannot break down foods properly, so the nutrients cannot be absorbed effectively in the small intestines, with the result that your joint tissue and other cells may not get all the nutrients they need.

In naturopathic practice, it is quite common for people to say that they had a particular infection some time ago and have never been well since. It is no longer weird to consider that they may have a low-grade residual infection. Herbalists have commonly prescribed and still use what are classed as 'blood cleansers', such as garlic, echinacea and sarsaparilla, to help rid the body of residual infection.

Why a wholefood diet? Chapter 15 gives some specific and compelling reasons why you should eat food that has a close relationship to something that has grown. We can't choose the air we breathe but we can choose what our hands put in our mouths.

Promoting circulation is another naturopathic approach. You can see the connection because blood carries needed nutrients to joints and organs as well as carrying unwanted waste products to the liver, spleen and kidneys for recycling or elimination.

Elimination via the skin is another concern. Traditionally, for a wide range of joint problems, people have used hot baths and herbs that promote sweating, and elimination of waste products with the sweat. Hein Zeylstra, writing in the *British Journal of Phytotherapy*, suggests adding a large quantity of Epsom salts (1–2 kg) to a bath that should be as hot as possible.[11] Affected joints should be rubbed with a brush (or loofah, not a scrubbing brush!) for 5–10 minutes and you should stay in the bath for a further 10–25 minutes. Don't dry off with a towel but wrap yourself immediately in a large, clean, cotton sheet and go straight to bed, covering yourself with several blankets. The Epsom salt solution absorbed by the sheet will draw off heavy perspiration and for this reason the mattress should be protected with plastic or a thick blanket. The following morning the sheet is often tainted with products excreted through the skin, sometimes the colour is yellow-orange. (When I did it there were obvious yellow stains on my sheet!) He warns that people with weak hearts or hypertension may not be able to tolerate such a treatment, but for healthier people the suggestion is that it be done once a fortnight until the sheet does not get stained.

Don't try this during heat-wave conditions. If you don't like hot baths, use a little crushed ice wrapped in a small towel to keep your head cool during and after the bath.

A theme running through this book is that most of us need to make changes in the way we think and behave if we want to improve our health by making our bodies stronger. Giving up things you like isn't easy. At first it may seem that everything you like is either fattening or unhealthy but there are lots of pleasant, healthy foods and activities. You can still have a few treats. As James Thurber said: 'You might as well fall flat on your face as lean over too far backward'. You can possibly make it easier for yourself: in a large-scale study of American patients recovering from heart attacks, the group learning yoga and meditation had more success at sticking to dietary and lifestyle changes.

WHY AREN'T NATURAL THERAPIES 'PROVED'?

• It costs millions of dollars to prove a health remedy, through scientific tests and human trials, before it is approved by governments. Drug companies can recoup this money through selling their drug, but since no one can 'own' a plant or nutrient there is no economic reward for proving a natural remedy.

• Pharmaceutical drugs are tested by themselves and are expected to work in a specific way in a specific area of the body irrespective of whatever else is happening in the body. In fact the scientific testing procedure is not as rigorous as one might expect. Even after drugs are licensed scientists may not know specifically how the drugs are working (their 'mode of operation'), and not all the scientists involved in a study necessarily agree with the published conclusions.

• Herbal remedies cannot be restricted to one particular constituent for testing, as they contain hundreds of different substances. They cannot be standardised either, as the remedies vary according to climate, soil and season.

• The idea of testing one plant component at very high concentrations for possible toxic effects makes no sense to naturopaths, as no one ever takes a remedy at these concentrations. If this was the yardstick for safety in the real world, potatoes, peanuts and many common foods would be classified as poisons, for potatoes contain tiny amounts of alkaloids that are more acutely toxic than strychnine, and the aflatoxins in peanuts are potent carcinogens and liver toxins.

• Naturopaths aim to treat the whole person, that is, by using various means to get the body strong enough to heal itself. Patients are encouraged to change their lifestyle, and to participate positively in their treatment. These elements of naturopathic treatment are not possible to assess under scientific drug 'proving' regimens.

• Many scientific trials use laboratory animals in testing, which naturopaths find difficult to accept philosophically and ethically. Rats and humans are completely different, in any case.

Naturopaths can argue that the safety of our products has been proved by the many millions of humans who have used them; surely such long-term human trials at least show that the remedies are not hazardous? Can we not conclude that the use of natural therapy remedies would not have continued had there been no benefits? As Dr J. A. Duke said: 'We give all those ancient cultures credit for knowing what in their environment is edible and what is toxic. Why in the world don't we give them credit for knowing what is medicinal?'

I can't believe that all the thousands of people who have successfully used natural therapies, special diets or some other forms of non-drug therapy, are all lying, suffering from delusions or had spontaneous remissions. Indeed, many doctors have written about their patients' frequent improvement from 'unofficial cures'. Dr Bieler wrote in *Food is Your Best Medicine* that 96 per cent of his patients who were suffering constant pain and were badly crippled by arthritis were left with only minimal pain and stiffness or had completely recovered after following his dietary programme.

Dr R. Bingham stated in the *Journal of Applied Nutrition* that if every available mode of therapy was used arthritis could be successfully treated, arrested and sometimes cured.[12] He employed a combination of diet, exercises, hydrotherapy, herbs and drug therapy.

Dr Jean Monro reported on a case of severe rheumatoid arthritis where the patient was only able to walk with a Zimmer frame.[13] The patient tested positive for many food and inhaled allergens. She was put on a diet which excluded all the suspected allergens. When foods were re-introduced it was found that eating eggs caused her severe joint pain. Her treatment involved avoiding chicken and eggs for two years, a homoeopathic de-sensitising programme, a rotation diet, a multi-vitamin supplement, an organic food diet, filtered water, plenty of fresh air and exercise and the avoidance of man-made chemicals. Three years later she no longer needed the homoeopathics, could walk twenty kilometres, sail a small yacht singlehanded and was running an outward-bound school.

Naturopathic journals and patient files are full of cases that have responded favourably to a holistic approach to arthritis.

WEIGHT

In my practice, nearly every arthritis patient I see is overweight. If you had to carry a 5 kg bag of potatoes all day, you'd be aware of the load. With bodyweight you're not so aware of the additional pressure of even a few kilograms – expecially to the legs and feet.

The weight may be due to lack of exercise – which is understandable if you're in pain. Swimming may be the only non-aggravating exercise for some people. It's possible that your current diet, lifestyle and medication simply don't agree with you. If you're overweight and aching, some major changes should be made. I can assure you from personal experience that in time you'll see most of your old habits as pathetic – even shocking.

My arthritis was first diagnosed over twenty years ago. I didn't know a thing about natural therapies or good health. After a week on prescribed medication my stomach was already upset. Over the next three years I did a full-time naturopathic course, became vegetarian, cut out the alcohol, chocolate and processed foods, lost about 10 kg without dieting and took up yoga. Although I still have some morning stiffness, I've only had to resort to painkillers for about two weeks. Given my family medical history, I'm glad I didn't listen to the experts who told me that 'Diet doesn't make any difference, you'll just get steadily worse, so keep taking the medication as the benefits outweigh the risks and when you're older we can give you a hip and knee replacement'!

BUNIONS

Description
Painful swelling at the base of the big toe.

Causes
Inappropriate shoes or shoes that are too tight. Flat or weak feet.

CAUTION **Needs to be distinguished from gout, arthritis and injuries.**

Treatment

Severe cases are best treated by a podiatrist.

HERBS

Hot poultices or foot baths: choose from
• *Calendula* • *Chamomile* • *Lavender*
• *Mustard* • *Rosemary* – these can be followed by an ice pack, or a packet of frozen peas applied for several minutes over a small towel • *Comfrey ointment*
• *Pennyroyal oil*

DIET

• *Buckwheat* • *Ginger* • *Chilli*

Supplements

• *Calcium* • *Vitamin E* (the oil from a capsule can also be used externally)

OTHER

Massage sandals help stimulate the circulation in the feet, but you need to ensure that the straps do not aggravate the bunion.

Walking barefoot on the seashore is another suggestion.

An old-fashioned remedy is to paint over the affected area with a combination of iodine and castor oil.

Of course, you might need to throw away some of your shoes.

CARPAL TUNNEL SYNDROME

Description

Periodic or constant pain in the inside wrist area, often accompanied by burning or tingling, with pins and needles in the fingers. The pain may radiate up the arm to the shoulder and neck and is worsened by physical activity, including unscrewing lids, lifting objects and so on. In some cases the pain only comes on at night. In severe cases the muscles may become weak and small.

A professional diagnosis is required for Carpal Tunnel Syndrome because there are other causes of wrist pain and workers' compensation may be involved.

Causes

Pressure on the median nerve, usually resulting from: strenuous repetitive use of the hands; injuries; fluid retention. It is also a feature of a number of diseases, including rheumatoid arthritis, hyperparathyroidism and diabetes, to name a few. Nutrient deficiencies have also been implicated.

Treatment

HERBS

Taken internally
• *Nettle* • *Scullcap* • *Valerian* • *Yarrow*

Applied externally
Hot hand baths with chamomile flowers, followed by a gentle massage with • *St John's wort oil* • *Mustard* and hot *chilli powder* plaster

FROM THE KITCHEN

• *Chilli* • *Cinnamon* • *Ginger* • *Celery and parsley juice*

The aim is to stimulate the circulation because you want to drain the breakdown products and bring nutrients and oxygen to the area; and to relax the tension and reduce fluid build-up.

DIET

High *fruit* and *vegetables* (except citrus, spinach, rhubarb).

Supplements

Vitamins B2 and *B6* in addition to a combined *vitamin and mineral* supplement taken at a different time of the day. You may need to take these for up to fifteen weeks.

OTHER

• *Acupuncture*   • *Chiropractic/osteopathic*
• *Massage* – including back and neck
• *Posture improvement* • *Stress management*

CRAMPS – SKELETAL MUSCLE

Description

Painful, spasmodic contractions that may occur in any part of the body. There are also smooth muscles in the walls of the 'tubes' within the body, such as the intestines and blood vessels, but in this context the recommendations specifically relate to cramps in the external muscles.

Causes

There are a number of possibilities, including poor circulation, excessive or irregular exercising, arterial spasms, insufficient sodium in relation to water loss through sweating or diuretics, repetitive work without appropriate breaks and calcium, magnesium or other mineral deficiencies. Intermittent claudication, peripheral vascular disease, thrombosis and other conditions such as diabetes, hypoparathyroidism and hyperaldosteronism may also be related to cramps but such conditions need practitioner consultation. Blood pressure problems and anxiety attacks with hyperventilation may also cause cramps.

Treatment

HERBS
• *Ginkgo* • *Scullcap* • *Valerian* • *Wild yam*

FROM THE KITCHEN
• *Chilli, hot* – internally or in a bath
• *Ginger* • *Turmeric*

DIET

Check for *sodium deficiency*. This is rare but may occur when taking diuretic drugs, with diarrhoea, vomiting or on some diets. Professional advice should be sought in such cases.

A friend of mine used to visist her elderly father once a fortnight and they always went out to dinner to a Chinese restaurant. He used to say it was the only night his leg cramps eased enough to let him get a reasonable night's sleep. She at first thought it was 'all in his mind', but eventually suspected it might be dietary as he cooked for himself. They tried a number of strategies without success. When he added a pinch of salt to his evening meal, the cramping was markedly reduced.

If you're one of those no-salt fanatics and you suffer from cramps, you might try adding a tiny quantity of sea salt or salt-reduced Shoyu (a type of soy sauce) to one of your meals.

Supplements
• *Vitamin B2* • *Calcium and magnesium* – either as a mineral supplement or as tissue salts • *Vitamin C* • *Vitamin E* • Athletes might try *carnitine* or coenzyme Q

OTHER

Calf muscle cramps are often relieved by hyperextension of the foot, that is, pulling the toe back towards you.

An old-fashioned remedy for nocturnal leg cramps is to put a piece of camphor in the bed.

Wear warm socks in winter. Hot foot baths are also helpful.

Daily walking is one of the best things you can do, although in most cases this will need to be built up gradually. Exercising increases collateral circulation, that is, the blood vessels develop extra branches and increase their flexibility.

Use a footstool whenever you are sitting, practise deep abdominal breathing (it acts as a pump for the venous circulation), avoid tight clothing, do ankle circling exercises and avoid sitting or standing still for long periods of time.

Further suggestions for improving circulation are given on pages 126–7.

REPETITIVE STRAIN INJURY (RSI) AND TENOSYNOVITIS

Description

A painful, crippling problem, affecting the fingers, hands, arms, neck and back. The condition may affect one small part of the body or be more generalised. The pain may be constant or intermittent, and is usually worsened by movement. The affected area may feel 'boggy' and there may be associated headaches and other problems.

Causes

It is generally considered to be work-related, that is, in association with repetitive movement and stress. There are many theories as to the exact cause including postural faults, excess fluoride, stress, lead toxicity, nutrient deficiencies such as calcium, magnesium and vitamin B12, as well as psychosomatic causes.

Treatment

The use of filtered water and dietary improvements are a good start. Light yoga and tai chi together with relaxation techniques will reduce general muscular and mental tension.

Many people work all day in discomfort and most employers are now more aware of the importance of appropriate furniture, allowing breaks from repetitive work, providing footstools for office workers and so on. A rigid posture with only a small group of muscles constantly working is bound to create muscle and joint tension. The obvious example is keyboard work where the arms, back and neck are fixed into a position with only the fingers moving.

One advantage of having a massage or physiotherapy is that you become aware of how much tension you have in some groups of muscles; when you do yoga or tai chi, you realise that one side of your body is invariably stiffer than the other. Such new awareness should help you to adjust your working and postural bad habits to prevent further problems developing.

HERBS

Taken internally
• *Chamomile* • *Ginseng* • *Lemon balm* • *Scullcap* • *Valerian*

Applied externally
Oils: • *Lavender* • *Marjoram* • *Wintergreen*
• An overnight *poultice* of any of the arthritic remedies

CAUTION **Always do a small test area first in case of allergic reactions.**

DIET

Supplements
• *Bromelain* • *Vitamin C with bioflavonoids* • *Calcium* • *Magnesium* • A *multi-vitamin* that includes *B12*

TISSUE SALTS OR CELLOIDS
• *Ferr Phos* • *Kali Phos* • *Silicea*

OTHER
Complete rest and splints are a last resort.

SPRAINS, STRAINS

Treatment

As for Bruises (see page 189).

Additional herbs internally
• *Horsetail*

Additional supplements
• *Multi-mineral*

CAUTION **Before starting treatment, make sure there are no broken bones.**

BASIC EXERCISES AND POSTURE

• Immediately following injuries and in flare-up, inflamed stages of arthritis, rest and elevation are indicated. Generally cool or moist warm compresses are best. If you use a compress of ice or a bag of frozen peas, make sure the area is covered with a towel otherwise you can cause a nasty 'ice burn'.

• Swimming is generally recommended but not always convenient. Rebounders (bouncers) are good for most people as well as exercise bikes and dancing. I have patients in their seventies who are having swimming and dancing lessons.

• Learn yoga or tai chi. Some forms of yoga are strenuous, so check with the teacher before enrolling. You could tape some of the classes so you do some of the exercises every day.

• New exercises should be introduced gradually. At first some soreness and a little pain may be experienced, but severe or prolonged pain is an indication that you are doing too much too soon, or that the particular exercise is inappropriate for you.

• For arthritis, a number of short exercise programmes are better than one long one. Never exhaust yourself.

• As a general rule, do more exercises on the side or areas that are the least flexible.

• Walking is also good but do not walk for long periods if the lower part of the body is painful. Two short walks are better than one long one.

• If you are bedridden for any reason, remember to exercise as much as you can; particularly the ankles and abdominal breathing.

• Avoid long periods of the same activity, particularly knitting and similar repetitive movements.

• Find interesting activities, mental and physical. Don't sit around feeling sorry for yourself. Look in your local newspaper, there will be many activities listed you could try.

• Have planned rest periods.

• Early correction of posture faults, including feet problems, may prevent joint and muscle problems later.

SOME BASIC EXERCISES

The following is a small selection of the type of exercises you can do; a physiotherapist or a natural therapist with qualifications in exercise therapy could give you more.

The exercises given are relatively easy, and rely on regular repetition for improvement. If you don't exercise a joint, it becomes less flexible and this is worsened if the muscles around it start to waste away, so it helps to exercise even when the problem has set in. As stated under the general guidelines, you need to start gradually and within your own limits.

All the exercises should be done evenly and slowly. I like to incorporate the breathing into the exercises because it helps relax the muscles. I also prefer to exercise on a sheepskin rug.

These exercises are intended as a guide because what you do depends on your individual mobility.

You can record the instructions on cassette as it's hard to do exercises while you're reading! Make sure the pace is extra slow and allow plenty of time between each exercise.

Neck
COMBINATION STRETCHING AND RELAXING

Check in a mirror first, so that you know your head is straight and your chin is level.

• Sit on a firm chair with your back straight, shoulders relaxed, head straight, chin level.

• Close your eyes and slowly turn your head to the right as far as you can without strain. Hold in that position and each time you breathe out imagine that your neck is more flexible and turns just a little more. Breathe gently and evenly and do not force or strain. Stay in that position for six breaths.

• Slowly take the head back to the centre, keeping the eyes closed.

• Take a few deep breaths, then repeat on the left side.

• Then turn the head slowly back to the centre. Take a few deep breaths.

• Now do the same procedure with the head gently dropping forward.

• Bring the head up slowly.

• Next raise the shoulders up toward the ears, open your mouth and ease the head back. Then slowly return the head and drop the shoulders down.

Each time you return the head to the centre take deep breaths, but otherwise you should be breathing gently and evenly.

MOBILISING

From the same sitting postion, gently and slowly rock your head from side to side.

MOBILISING AND STRENGTHENING

• Kneel on all fours.

• Drop chin towards the breast bone.

• From that position, slowly turn your head to the right, looking up to the ceiling.

• Take your head back to the breast bone.

• Now slowly turn your head to the left, looking up to the ceiling, and return to centre.

NECK AND BACK MOBILISING

• Kneel on all fours.

• Bring your right knee up towards your face at the same time as you take your left ear towards the right knee.

• Slowly take your head and leg back to their original positions.

• Now look up to the ceiling and take your chin up slowly, as you lift the right leg up behind you as high as you can, keeping the knee slightly bent.

• Slowly return to the starting position.

• Repeat with the left knee.

Back
GENTLE STRETCHING

• Lie on your back, knees bent, feet flat on the floor. Place your hands behind your head with the elbows flat on the floor.

• Cross your bent right leg over your left leg, just above the left knee.

• Use the weight of your right leg to gently push your left knee to the right side. Hold for a slow count of five. Feel that you are melting down with each breath out.

• Return, uncross your legs, and repeat with your left leg over the right.

Knee-to-chest raise

• Lie on your back, legs straight.

• Bring your left knee up to the chest as far as comfortable, then slowly straighten the left leg upwards; bend your knee again and clasp your hands around the knee.

• Slowly return the left leg to the floor and then repeat the exercise with the right leg.

MOBILISING

Cat hump
• Kneel on your hands and knees.
• Breathing out, drop your head forward and pull your abdomen in as far as you can, humping your back upwards.
• Breathing in, lift the head up and look at the ceiling as you fill the abdomen with air, arching your abdomen downwards.

Tail wagging
• Kneel on your hands and knees.
• Turn your head sideways to the left as far as possible, at the same time gently swing the left buttock sideways to the left.
• Then gently swing sideways to the right with your head also turning to the right.

Spinal twist
• Sit on the floor with legs stretched out in front.
• Place your hands on the floor to the side of the right thigh.
• Keeping your left hand firmly on the floor, raise your right hand to shoulder level with the elbow straight and take the arm slowly backwards turning as far as possible. Keep your eyes on your right hand.
• Return slowly to the starting position and repeat on the other side.

Spinal twist – sitting on a straight-backed chair
• Back straight, shoulders relaxed.
• Raise both hands in front to shoulder level.
• Turn slowly to the right side, keeping your arms parallel.
• Slowly return to the starting position, lower the arms, then repeat on the other side.

Spinal twist – on floor
In this exercise, the head turns with the body.
• Lie on your back, legs straight.

• Stretch both arms out sideways, level with the shoulders.
• Breathe in, and as you breathe out raise the right leg about 30 centimetres. Hold for a few breaths.
• Breathing out, take the right leg over to the left side, keeping the knee as straight as possible and put the right foot on the floor. Relax in that position for a few breaths.
• Breathe in, slowly bring the right leg up and back to the starting position.
• Repeat on the other side.

Back arch
• Lie on your back, knees bent, feet flat on the floor and slightly apart. Hands by your sides, palms down.
• Keeping your shoulders on the floor, lift the buttocks off the floor as high as comfortable. Hold for a few seconds.
• Slowly lower yourself down, relax.
• Repeat two or three times.

Standing back stretch
• Stand with the feet slightly apart.
• Stretch the hands above your head, keep the arms parallel and feet flat on the floor.
• Bend forward without hunching over, until your arms are parallel to the floor.
• Slowly return, stretch up and slightly backwards, then back to the centre.
• Keeping the arms close to the ears, bend slowly to the right, then back to the centre, then to the left side. Return to the centre.

Shoulders
LOOSENING
• Stand, back straight, shoulders relaxed, arms at the sides.
• Raise the right shoulder up towards the right ear, then let it flop down.
• Repeat with the left shoulder, then both shoulders together.

MOBILISING
• Sit, back straight, shoulders relaxed, fingers on the shoulders and elbows by the side.
• Breathing in, take the elbows up and slowly back as you bring your shoulder blades together.
• Breathing out, take the elbows down and forward till they meet in front.
• Repeat.

STRENGTHENING
• Stand with feet slightly apart, back straight, chin level.
• Breathing in, slowly take the arms out and up above the head.
• Breathing out, slowly lower the arms back to the sides.
• Repeat this with each arm, from the front, side and back.
• As a strengthening exercise, place a small book in the hand, gradually increasing the weight.

Hips
STRETCHING
• Kneel on all fours.
• Stretch your right leg backwards in line with your body.
• Keeping the leg relaxed but straight, take it sideways as far as comfortable.
• Return to the centre and starting position.
• Repeat with the other leg.

MOBILITY
• Lie on the right side, right arm extended, head resting on the right arm.
• Bend the left knee, bringing it towards the chest.
• Straighten the leg and slowly take it forwards, stretch the leg, relax, then slowly take it backwards.
• Return to the centre and repeat on the other side.

Knees and ankles
• Sit upright on the floor, knees bent, feet on the ground, both hands under your right knee.
• Raise the right leg, point the toes, then bring the toes back towards you. Repeat this six times while the leg is raised.
• Return to the starting position and repeat with the left leg.

The same procedure can be used for toe stretching and curling; and ankle circling.

Standing on your toes and doing half squats will strengthen your knees and ankles as well as keep your feet flexible.

POSTURE

• When you are sitting, standing and walking, straighten your back, keep your chin level and imagine that the top of your head is rising. Then consciously relax the shoulders because holding yourself rigidly upright is just as bad as slumping. Look in the mirror to check that you are not lop-sided. Don't attempt to be perfectly still.
• Avoid sitting or standing for long periods. When you are standing you can move from side to side or gently rock backwards and forwards. Don't paint or do craft work without a break for movement every half-hour. When carrying a shopping bag, change arms regularly.
• Choose your furniture with care. While you are working, a chair that supports the lower back is usually preferable. For armchairs, it is generally better to have a high-backed chair for neck support, with a firm seat and a fairly straight back. Use a footstool while sitting.
• A good mattress is important. The worst type is the 'saggy-in-the-middle'

variety. Ripple mattresses are probably the best but very expensive. At least have a firm mattress with a firm support under it. Cheap cotton mattresses have no 'give' and are not suitable for people with back problems and they have the added disadvantage of holding moisture. If you change your mattress, be prepared to have a backache for a few days, while your body is adjusting.

• A small, soft, non-rubber pillow is best for the head, neck and shoulders. If you use a pillow under the knees while doing a relaxation session, always do stretching exercises before standing up.

• If you have been sitting or lying down for some time, always move the joints before standing up.

• Analyse some of the movements you do; for example, when you write don't forcefully grip the pen because that can cause tension up your arm to your neck.

A technique for relaxation and visualisation is given in Chapter 10, 'Nervous and Immune Systems'.

CHAPTER 4

COMMON CHILDHOOD AILMENTS

PARENTAL PRESCRIBING

This chapter is not intended to be a guide to treating serious childhood diseases but to help the process of recovery in common, mild and long-term conditions. A number of the suggestions could be adjunct treatments in more serious cases, such as using echinacea or homoeopathics to strengthen the immune system.

You should be aware that many childhood ailments are self-limiting, that is, given a reasonable diet, environment and time, the conditions apparently clear by themselves. However, from your own experience you know that a mild head cold can travel to the throat and then to the chest; and a cough can develop into a more serious chronic problem. If you treat common ailments with non-harmful remedies and energise the body, you may prevent a worsening of the condition or low-grade health over a protracted period.

The simplest and most natural remedy is a good diet and rest, but it's not always possible to get children to accept either. You can, however, ensure that they are sufficiently warm (or cool), taking in adequate fluids and having regular bowel motions.

I recommend that you do a first-aid course so that you can recognise serious signs and know what to do in an emergency. Also, have a basic medical guide in your house to help you understand more serious illnesses and complications.

Natural therapies are useful therapeutically, have minimal side effects and function as preventives, but if your home treatments do not bring results within a reasonable time or the condition worsens, then seek the advice of a qualified health practitioner.

An article in the *British Medical Journal* investigated mothers' perceptions of their children's illnesses and how they routinely coped with their minor ailments.[1] The conclusion was that 'generally mothers should be treated as competent in caring for a child whose health and behaviour are causing concern, and in these cases the skills of the general practitioner should be viewed as complementing those of the mother. Mothers do not invariably expect a prescription from the doctor. Many doctors seem not to appreciate that the bulk of illness in the community is negotiated without professional intervention.'

Parents should be at the head of the team caring for their children's health. This doesn't imply that you should initiate a health debate while your baby is struggling for breath or bleeding heavily. But there are times when all you need from a consultation is reassurance, basic advice about making your child more comfortable or perhaps a few tips on improving nutritional intake.

Good nutrition is obviously a major factor in ensuring good health, but often it is easier to talk about than to enforce. If children won't eat reasonably – and particularly if they get more than their share of ailments – then at the very least give them a broad spectrum combined multi-vitamin and mineral supplement.

NOTE **Nutritional supplements should not be given to children under six months without practitioner advice.**

There are some 'grown-up' therapies that are useful for young people. For example, a number of yoga breathing techniques and stretching exercises would be strengthening for those with chronic respiratory problems. Yoga might also be considered as an alternative for children who don't like team sports or athletics, although some form of aerobic activity should be encouraged. Most yoga exercises are excellent for posture, balance, co-ordination and concentration. Relaxation techniques have been shown to reduce stress problems such as headaches as well as improving learning ability and self-discipline in children.

Of course, some natural remedies are not suitable for young children, such as hot chilli, garlic oil, horse chestnut, the internal use of essential oils, fasting and very hot external treatments. Additionally, try every natural therapy on yourself before attempting to give it to a child. Then you will get a reasonable idea of how much you will need to disguise the taste or dilute the remedy.

DOSES FOR CHILDREN

For natural therapies, it is neither practicable nor necessary to measure specific percentages based on your child's weight. The following is a guide.

Age of child	Fraction of adult dose
Babies	⅛
2–5 years	¼
6–9 years	⅓
10–13 years	½
14–16 years	¾

With delicate, sensitive or small-built children, go down to the category below. When giving liquids, I suggest you use drops. As droppers differ quite markedly, you need to use a small medicinal measurer and count how many of *your* drops equal 1 ml. With the droppers I use, there are about 20 drops to the ml, therefore if an adult dose is say, 5 ml, this equals 100 drops, making a dosage of 25 drops for a three-year-old. Most bought remedies will have the children's dosage specified on them.

Generally, herbal extracts and other supplements are best taken with or after meals, either in a little water or juice. Tablets may be crushed into rice or barley malt – or jam.

Some children will drink weak herbal teas. Chamomile and mint combine quite well to make iced tea which can be served with slices of lemon and orange; rosehip, lemongrass and most others are quite pleasant cooled and mixed into apple or pear juice. Dried herbs can be mixed into food: aniseed powder can be included in biscuits, fenugreek in rissoles, slippery elm powder in cooked or mashed fruit.

FEVER AND TAKING TEMPERATURE

I suggest you have a little practice taking temperatures while your children are well. You will discover that they will have natural fluctuations, rather than steady, 'normal' temperatures. Temperatures may be raised or lowered for a number of reasons.

• Usually temperatures are lower in the morning and in cold weather, even as low as 35.5°C.

• After exercise, temperatures are higher, sometimes up to 40°C.

• You may not be taking the temperature correctly, i.e. not shaking the mercury down enough, or the thermometer may be faulty.

• The patient may be 'normally' somewhat higher or lower than average. The

average is 37°C but the normal range for people is 36–37.2°C.

• If you are taking a child's temperature under the arm the reading will be 0.5°C lower than from a thermometer under the tongue, and you should add on this amount to get a true temperature. Conversely, a thermometer in the rectum will register 0.5°C higher than normal, and this should be subtracted.

Although a fever is the body's mechanism for fighting infection, febrile convulsions can occur in an infant whose temperature is above 39°C. Although a few febrile convulsions leave no apparent side effects, I would suggest that if a child's temperature is 39°C or higher you should put the child to bed and seek the advice of your practitioner.

EMERGENCIES

If someone in your family needs emergency treatment it's very hard to think clearly. When you're panicky, the telephone book seems more confusing than usual! I suggest you make a simple list of appropriate emergency numbers near the phone.

AMBULANCE
FIRE
NEAREST HOSPITAL
POISONS INFORMATION
POLICE

In life-threatening situations, always dial 000.

NATURAL THERAPIES ESPECIALLY SUITABLE FOR CHILDREN

Four systems are especially suitable for children: aromatherapy, Bach Flowers, homoeopathy and tissue salts. They have almost no side effects and are relatively easy to give to small children. Herbal remedies and supplements also give excellent results but children often resist taking them unless their taste is disguised.

These four systems are discussed in more detail in Chapter 2, 'Explaining Some Natural Therapies' and the following is a brief description specifically relating to children.

Aromatherapy

Babies and young children have somewhat different smell and taste perceptions to adults, which is why you need to be especially careful about potentially harmful cleaning agents, chemicals and medication.

It is thought that the primitive sense of smell is quite developed in young babies and it has been suggested that this may affect their behaviour. One reported experiment showed that six out of ten babies could distinguish the odour of breast pads worn by their mothers compared to those worn by another nursing mother.[2]

Another study in a French hospital indicated that babies seem to be able to recognise the perfume their mothers wore when pregnant. Doctors asked mothers-to-be to use just one perfume they liked during the last three months of pregnancy. After the birth, their babies became calm when anyone wearing that particular perfume approached their cots. Whether the unborn baby 'smells' in the same way as it does after birth is not known, but some kind of memory does seem to exist.

It has been suggested that an extremely upset mother might unwittingly convey airborne stress chemicals to her child.

Since aromas such as lavender are demonstrably sedating to the nervous system, I suggest that mothers wear a few drops of lavender oil as a perfume to offset stress in both the mother and child. For a gentle sedating effect, another option is to place about three drops of the oil on a tissue under the baby's pillow. For colicky infants, give baby a gentle, abdominal massage with a few drops of chamomile oil.

Aromatic plant oils are extremely strong. They are not given internally to children and a few drops externally is all you apply at one time. Otherwise, they are used as outlined in Chapter 2.

Bach Flowers

This is a gentle, slow-acting support therapy for a wide range of nervous and emotional problems. There are thirty-eight remedies in the system and people are matched to one or a number of them. Here are a few examples of particular Bach Flowers remedies as they relate to children.

ASPEN	For thin, delicate quivery, over-sensitive children with vague fears. May have night terrors or frightening dreams.
CHESTNUT BUD	A remedy for children who keep making the same sort of mistakes, often with self-pity. Slow learners often benefit from this remedy.
CHICORY	A remedy for damaging, tantrum-prone, over-clinging children, who won't let parents out of sight.
CLEMATIS	Recommended for children who are constantly bored, dreamy, inattentive, with slow reflexes, slow to answer and often rambling conversationalists.

| LARCH | Usually good for children who lack confidence, cling to parents, hate being alone, won't try new things, have fears of failing at school or games. |
| WALNUT | Especially for those who are physically and emotionally over-sensitive. A good remedy for helping transitions, such as going to school or having a new baby in the house. |

These remedies are usually taken for a least a month. The children's dose is 5 drops, three times daily in a little water. The exception to this is Rescue Remedy. It is a combination of the five fear/shock Bach Flowers and is used in emergency situations, such as visits to the dentist, tantrums, over-excitement, major upsets, injuries and so on. It is not taken all the time. The dosage of Rescue Remedy is 5 drops in a little water. If necessary, repeat dose every 10–15 minutes until the 'drama' subsides. It may be dropped around the mouth or on the wrist if the little patient won't swallow it. Mother might want to take some too!

Homoeopathy

Homoeopathic medicines are prepared from minerals, plants and other substances and used in extremely minute doses. Due to the process of potentisation (which involves shaking the remedies), the inherent value or energy of the material is released and the body's natural healing ability is enhanced.

Generally, the remedies are best prescribed by a qualified practitioner but there are home remedy kits available through health-food stores. These kits contain around twenty different remedies which are safe for children and adults. They are easy to use, low in dosage, not habit-forming and virtually tasteless.

Here are two examples of homoeopathic remedies commonly prescribed for children.

CHAMOMILLA (a symptomatic remedy)	General complaints: irritability, constant dissatisfaction, restlessness, impatience, won't tolerate opposition, anger over trifles, tendency to whims, wants constant attention, moans piteously if can't have own way, nightmares, sluggish bowels, thirsty, hot, teething – especially where one cheek is red and hot, the other cold and pale. Problems are worse from heat, anger, open air, wind and at night and improve with being carried and petted, warmth, wet weather.
	Chamomilla is also indicated for diarrhoea, especially if the stools are greenish, vomiting bile and coughs with rattling mucus.
	This remedy is derived from German chamomile.
NATRUM SULPHURI-CUM	Produced from sulphate of sodium and is one of the remedies used in treating asthma in children.
	Used when wet weather, humidity and damp houses worsen complaints. There's a tendency to jaundice, warts, thick yellow nasal mucus, flatulence, colic, yellow and watery bowel motions.

The best results usually follow from looking at the total constitution of the child and treating accordingly, not just an immediate ailment.

Tissue salts

These may be likened to homoeopathic minerals. They are produced in a finely broken down, energised form so that they may be more readily taken up by the cells. I generally use them as adjunct remedies. There are twelve remedies, most of which are appropriate for babies and young children. Like homoeopathics, they are matched to the individual.

Taking Calcium Phosphate as an example, this would be used when the child matches some of the following: poor growth and defective development, bone and tooth disorders, slow comprehension, anxiety over trivia, poor appetite and pain after eating, bedwetting, cold hands and feet, chronic enlargement of tonsils, nervous irritability, frequent colds, cramps or twitching. Aggravated by cold weather and exertion. Salt cravings.

ASTHMA

Description

A disease of the bronchi (airways to the lungs) because of oversensitivity to a variety of things. Some asthmatics react to only a few irritants, others to many. Once the irritant or allergen hits the smooth muscles in the bronchi linings, the airways tighten and less air can get through. The reaction also causes the linings to swell and there is an increase in mucus secretion which may be stringy or thick, thereby adding to the breathing difficulties. This secretion is given the rather horrible name 'sputum' to distinguish it from the normal and necessary mucus secretion. The result is asthma: a tight feeling in the chest, wheezing, coughing and shortness of breath.

Your doctor can give you information about the equipment currently available for home use to measure breathing capacity. The Asthma Foundation has many pamphlets, including one called 'Asthma in the Very Young—what parents of children under 5 should know about asthma attacks'.

Generally, the advice is that wheezing itself is not a serious problem in an infant that is happy, eating and sleeping well. An emergency exists when there is rapid panting, unusual chest movements, inability to rest or eat and obvious shortness of breath. Lips and mouth turning bluish is an indication of oxygen deprivation and emergency treatment is required.

Causes

The main cause is not lung weakness but hereditary allergies or sensitivities. For instance, when an asthmatic inhales dust mite particles, the linings of the body's respiratory system react as if the dust mite material was dangerous organisms. This alarm reaction leads to swelling, mucus build up and breathing difficulties.

Asthmatics are sometimes put into two broad categories.

ALLERGIC (most young children)	Often seasonal – worse with summer grasses and spring pollens, moulds, feathers, animal fur, various foods, some drugs (such as aspirin). Other contributing factors are hypochlorhydria (low stomach acid) and permeable bowel (the intestinal lining lets certain particles be absorbed instead of being excreted).
NON-ALLERGIC	Triggers include exercise, cold weather or weather changes, smoke, fatigue, emotional upsets, excitement, petrol fumes, viral or bacterial infections and virtually anything dusty or perfumed.

Quite often it is hard to make a distinction between the two types. Primarily there is a genetic predisposition that is aggravated by external factors: mothers smoking during pregnancy, passive smoking, modern lifestyles and naturally occurring allergens.

Evidence from New Guinea and Australian Aboriginal groups shows that when country people move to cities there is a dramatic increase in asthma attacks among them, possibly due to dust mites in household furniture, smoking or other pollutants.

Treatment

Taking natural therapies does not necessarily mean coming off pharmaceutical drugs: this may never be possible with severe asthmatics. Basically the natural treatments aim to:
• strengthen mucous membranes
• prevent and treat infections
• reduce allergic reactions
• relax smooth (internal) muscles, skeletal muscles and the nervous system
• dissolve sticky mucus
• reduce the need for drugs
• prevent the necessity for starting drug therapy in mild cases.

Physiotherapy and osteopathy are helpful for releasing structural tensions.

ALLERGIES

Skin tests are fairly reliable indicators of exactly what inhaled allergens the child is reacting to. Many allergens are extremely difficult to avoid completely. However, if you know, for example, that your child has an allergy to grasses and pollens you should not organise the family's summer holidays on a farm.

Food tests are not reliable, but may provide a guide as to which foods should be avoided and tested. Some information is given in Chapter 13, 'Food Allergies', or you can consult an allergy specialist.

Inhaled allergens

Firstly, smoking should not be allowed in the house.

Dust-mite populations may be lowered by using cotton or synthetic blankets instead of wool, cotton curtains or holland blinds rather than venetians. Don't give an asthmatic child fabric toys, avoid leaving clothes lying about because the shed human skin on them feeds the mite, don't have carpet and, if possible, have furinture that can be wiped rather than covered with thick fabrics. An uncluttered house is easier to clean than one filled with decorative furniture and ornamentation, and an efficient vacuum cleaner collects particles rather than spreading them.

Moulds are another common allergen. Unfortunately, combating them also requires regular and thorough cleaning, especially in bathrooms and kitchens; there are anti-mould products on the market which are helpful. Yeast and mould foods are covered in Chapter 13, 'Food Allergies'.

If pollens are one of the asthma triggers, you can keep windows closed when the particular irritants are about. Sensitive people may also react to fallen leaves and garden debris.

Pets may have to be banned.

There's a limit to what you can do financially and physically. I know people who have almost pulled their houses apart to eliminate dust, moulds, formaldehydes and chemicals, without dramatically improving their children's health.

Negative ionisers remove particles from the air and are worth trying.

Food allergies

Sulphur dioxide and metabisulphite are comon offenders, triggering asthma attacks. Other additives and colouring agents are known triggers. This includes monosodium glutamate, benzoate, nitrites, tartrazine, amaranth, coccine and binders in tablets and medications. Some drugs, including aspirin and penicillin, may also cause adverse reactions.

Immediate food sensitivities causing asthma include eggs, fish, shellfish and nuts (especially peanuts). Delayed reactions may be caused by meat, chocolate, wheat, citrus fruit and food colourings.

At least some children with chronic respiratory problems improve if they avoid or markedly restrict their intake of dairy foods. I suggest parents should enforce complete avoidance for at least one month as a trial. The drawback with casual trials is that children can be sensitive to a number of foods and other substances, not just one, so food allergens can be difficult to pinpoint.

HERBS

Taken internally

• *Echinacea* • *Elder* • *Fenugreek* • *Garlic* – there are now special products available for children • *Hyssop* • *Liquorice* – powdered root, not the confectionery

Qualified herbalists and homoeopaths have other remedies that are individually prescribed.

NOTE *There is always a possibility of sensitivity reactions to herbs. Make sure you read Chapters 1 and 16.*

FROM THE KITCHEN

• *Chamomile* – a weak tea flavoured with lemon and honey • *Thyme* can be used regularly in small quantities in salads, sandwiches and cooked meals

DIET

You can see that a wholefood diet automatically excludes a number of potential irritants, as well as providing maximum nutrients. Flavonoids and carotenoids are especially beneficial to asthmatics; these are found in vegetables and fruit. Excess dietary salt should be avoided.

Supplements

For poor eaters: • *Vitamin A* • *Vitamin C and bioflavonoids* • *Vitamin B12* injections have been used successfully in the USA. A study showed that vitamin B12 in the form of intramuscular injections, together with hydrochloride supplementation (if the stomach acid was low), plus magnesium and vitamin B6, gave good results. Patients were tested and taken off dairy products and other allegens *only* if they reacted to them.

TISSUE SALTS OR CELLOIDS

• *Kali Phos* • *Mag Phos*

NOTE *All new foods and supplements need to be introduced cautiously. There has been one case of a fatal reaction to royal jelly.*

OTHER

People with sensitivities and allergies can react to mock irritants, for example, artificial flowers. If this can be demonstrated, relaxation techniques can be taught to young children (and adults) to help with anxiety and known irritants. Yogic breathing techniques and exercises will assist but many young children can't or don't want to do them on a regular basis. Most adults don't like exercising either.

However, once they overcome the initial shyness, most young children love a massage. Aside from postural drainage with pounding, there are many techniques that parents can learn. Get a physiotherapist or a trained massage therapist to show you some of them, because they need to be rhythmical, with the wrists relaxed. If you're tense or in a hurry it might be more beneficial to use a vibrator. An asthmatic attack can be brought on by inappropriate or heavy massage.

Activities like swimming and singing should be encouraged.

For older children, inhalations can be used to clear the nasal passages. Weak, tepid, salt water nasal drops may help clear mucus in younger children. Breathing in through the nose is important because this regulates the air temperature before it gets to the bronchi and filters out some of the irritants.

In the old days, warm poultices or compresses were used on the back or chest to relieve chest tightness.

Homoeopathics can help overcome allergies, treat symptoms and strengthen the physical and emotional characteristics of the individual.

PHARMACEUTICAL DRUGS AND SOME OF THEIR PROBLEMS

Why go to all this bother when you can use a drug? Pharmaceuticals may save lives but mild asthma is not a death-threatening condition. The head of a large pharmaceutical company once boasted: 'Show me a drug without side effects and I'll show you a drug that doesn't work.'

Asthma is on the increase or is being more frequently diagnosed; deaths from asthma are increasing; the use of pharmaceutical drugs is also increasing. At the time of writing this chapter, a number of warnings had been issued regarding asthmatic drugs such as Ventolin and Berotec. The *New England Journal of Medicine* reported that the risk of death from asthma is associated with the regular use of these inhaled bronchodilators.[4] The company that makes Berotec warned that

an asthmatic's likelihood of having a fatal attack more than doubles for every can of the drug used per month over the previous year.[5] Of course, people who use the most of these types of drugs presumably have the most severe asthma. Until recently, these drugs have been used regularly to prevent attacks. Now most experts are suggesting that they be used only to relieve attacks and that other drugs be used as preventives.

The *British Medical Journal* reported that 46 per cent of seven-year-olds in Melbourne had some degree of asthma in 1991, compared to 19 per cent in 1964.[6] Eighty-three per cent of children with a history of wheeze during the previous 12 months had used a bronchodilator such as Ventolin.

The over-use or incorrect use of such drugs may account for the increased death rate and severity of asthma because:
• continuous use of this category of inhalants can cause problems such as mouth and throat irritations and infections indicating weakening or damage to the mucous membranes; these membranes are the first line of defence against harmful microorganisms and any damage would tend to expose the airways to an increased reaction to inhaled allergens
• the drugs not only reduce the inflammatory reaction but also reduce heparin – one of the body's own healing agents
• bronchodilators tend to increase mucus secretion; this may be sticky and form plugs.

The *British Medical Journal* concluded that 'continuous bronchodilator treatment without anti-inflammatory treatment accelerates decline in ventilatory function.'[7] In other words, an asthmatic tendency may be reinforced by using drugs. I recommend that parents get complete information on drugs from a source such as *MIMS Annual* so they can at least read the full picture of cautions, contraindications and adverse reactions – based on the manufacturer's research and trials. At least you will then be able to recognise adverse reactions. Don't be put off by the opening technical segments on each drug. Ventolin carries a warning of cardionecrotic effects and the possibility of myocardial lesions (heart muscle damage). Large doses of fluorocarbon propellants can produce heart irregularities in animals. It's not very encouraging to read that 'Data in humans are meagre'.

Asthma medication in propellant form is not used for young children. However, if they take the same types of medication as tablets or syrups it means that the chemicals are absorbed into the whole body, not just the air passages, so that higher doses have to be used. Side effects include tremors, insomnia and behaviour problems.

Mothers often tell me they have been reassured that corticosteroid inhalers are without side effects. Common reactions include local infections and sore throats – which is not a good sign if someone is expected to be on a drug for life. Animal studies show an increase in foetal damage where the mother is given the drugs but damage to humans is uncertain.

I suggest using a tepid salt-water gargle with one drop of tea tree oil added after using corticosteroid inhalers. Children who can't gargle could use it as a mouth rinse.

Safety during pregnancy (the possibility that the drug may affect the foetus) has not been demonstrated for a number of asthmatic drugs. Theophylline, a commonly prescribed drug, carries a warning 'Should only be used in pregnancy if the expected benefits outweigh the potential risks'.

I think you should do as much as reasonable to keep your family's drug use minimal.

BEDWETTING
(nocturnal enuresis)

Control at night is usually reached at four or five years of age. Up to seven years, one in five children occasionally wets the bed; at ten years this ratio is one in fourteen children and at fifteen years about one in thirty-three.

Causes
The bladder strengthens variably as children age and the problem usually corrects itself. Bedwetting may relate to allergies, emotional problems, kidney or bladder disorders, intestinal worms, hormonal imbalances, infections and drinking too much before going to bed. Constantly wanting drinks may be a ploy to find out what is going on, that is, an anxiety signal, or it may indicate diabetes. Some congenital handicaps such as spina bifida and certain diseases cause bladder control deficiencies. Antibiotics and other drugs may upset the normal bacterial balance and chronic constipation may cause pressure on the bladder.

Basically, when the bladder gets irritated or there is pressure on it, it behaves as it were full.

Treatment
A medical check may establish the cause.

Depending on the age of the child, discuss things that are affecting the family rather than excluding them completely or talking about problems in hushed tones. What a child may be imagining is possibly worse than reality. Many children (and adults) are scared of the dark, so try leaving a dim light on in the hallway or the bedroom.

HERBS

Taken internally

• *Bilberry* • *Clivers* • *Corn silk* • *Horsetail*
• *Marshmallow* • *Shepherd's purse*
• *Valerian* – 1 tablet crushed in honey before bed

Applied externally

• Lower back massage with *cypress* or *pine oil*

DIET AND FLUIDS

No drinking after dinner. During the day you must ensure that the child has a sufficient fluid intake as this flushes out toxins, irritants and unwanted substances. If children won't drink water, try diluted fruit juices.

Check for allergies. Orange juice is a common bladder irritant; also soft drinks and food colourings.

Red- and blue-coloured *berries* are recommended as bladder cleansers and strengtheners. Of course, young children can't safely eat cherries or similar fruits because of the stones, but you might be able to obtain cherry or cranberry juice.

TISSUE SALTS OR CELLOIDS

• *Ferr Phos* • *Kali Phos* • *Silicea*

BEHAVIOUR PROBLEMS

Description

Just about everybody is an expert on what *you* should do with *your* child. 0.1–10 per cent of children are said to be hyperactive, depending on the expert and your patience and energy quotients. Attention deficit disorder is said to affect about three per cent of children and is characterised by extremely disruptive or constant activity, severe lack of concentration, emotional changeability, co-ordination problems, impulsiveness, specific learning difficulties, speech and hearing disorders and neurological irregularities.

Causes

The causes include brain chemical and hormonal imbalances, allergies of various kinds, food chemical sensitivities, drug reactions, junk food, lead toxicity, nutrient deficiencies, fluctuating blood sugar levels, refined sugar and family problems.

Occasionally I see children who are having difficulties at school and their mothers have not noticed that they can't see or hear properly. A few children are just bored or undisciplined. Toddlers often make little sense and there's no logical explanation for their unreasonable behaviour.

Treatment

Extreme cases need professional diagnosis and support.

HERBS

Taken internally • *Chamomile* • *Evening primrose oil* • *Valerian* – for settling down at night-time

DIET

Some children may need to eat six small meals a day to regulate their blood sugar levels and brain function. A few of the meals can be in liquid form if they don't want to stop and eat. Fruit smoothies can be blended with many different foods.

Make sure your children eat something for breakfast. If they won't eat first thing, then give them a largish morning tea. The brain uses 25 per cent of the body's energy and in the USA junk foods and missing breakfast were shown to lower academic results. Another survey of 276 delinquent teenagers (who had committed serious crimes) showed that those who were subsequently given healthy foods had a 50 per cent reduction in their antisocial acts. For problem eaters, a child combined multi-vitamin and mineral supplement may help.

Some strategies for picky eaters are given in Chapter 15, 'Nutrition'.

Allergies

Treating a hyperactive child when you suspect food allergies is controversial and difficult because there are so many possibilities. Foods implicated include apples, cheese, chocolate, dairy products, corn, eggs, fish, grapes (also sultanas and raisins), melon, oats, oranges, peanuts, salicylate-containing foods, soft drinks, soya products, tomatoes, tea, wheat and many food additives.

Supplements
• *Vitamin B complex* • *Zinc* (neither if taking a combined multi-vitamin and mineral supplement)

TISSUE SALTS OR CELLOIDS
• *Kali Phos*

OTHER

Consider *Bach Flowers* and *Homoeopathy*.

Look for some unusual or stimulating activities. I recently visited a Police Citizens Youth Club and was surprised at the discipline and attentiveness of the children in the martial arts class.

COLD SORES
(herpes simplex)

Description

These are usually preceded by a stinging or shooting, itchy pain; then a red patch and small blisters appear, sometimes accompanied by swollen glands and a fever. The lesions are commonly located on the lips but can be on the gums, tongue and other parts of the body. In severe cases, the child may not want to eat or drink but it is essential to give him or her fluids. Outbreaks last 3–21 days. Unfortunately, they are quite infectious.

Causes

A virus that is usually persistent and recurring. Attacks may be associated with: respiratory tract infections; exposure to sun and wind; dietary factors; environmental or emotional stresses.

Treatment

HERBS

Taken internally

To help build up the immune system:
• *Echinacea* • *Garlic* • *Reishi* • *Thyme*

Applied externally
• *Tea tree oil* – to prevent spreading to other parts of the body • *St John's wort oil* – for itching and anti-viral activity • *Thuja* or *lemon balm ointment* – anti-viral • *Aloe jelly* – healing • *Calendula ointment* mixed to a paste with liquorice powder and calcium ascorbate powder – combines healing, soothing and anti-viral activity

FROM THE KITCHEN

A little *crushed ice* in a washer often gives relief.

DIET

Aim for a diet high in *lysine* (fish, chicken, dairy products, beans, yeast, sprouts) and low in arginine-rich foods (chocolate, carob, nuts, wheat, lentils, peanuts, peanut butter, oats). Avoid known allergens.

Supplements
• *Vitamin C* • *Zinc sulphate*

OTHER

Externally
• Finely crushed *aspirin* mixed into a little Sorbolene or an ointment

COLIC

Description

Some of the symptoms include irritability, drawing up the legs, wind, belching, redness in the face, crying and distress. The problems occur after feeding. Of course, there can be other causes of abdominal pain and if in doubt consult a health practitioner.

Causes

Feeding too fast or overeating, anxiety, excitement, taking in air, allergies, unsuitable food for a small child and toxic substances.

During breastfeeding, some foods the mother eats or drinks can occasionally irritate the baby, particularly onions, garlic, legumes, chickpeas, lentils, cabbage, broccoli, cauliflower and coffee.

Treatment

No remedies are a substitute for burping, cuddling and rocking. Walks outside always seem to help – at least the screaming doesn't sound as loud. Going for car rides is another old treatment but it's not very convenient. One American magazine suggested putting the baby on the washing machine but if your machine is like mine, the baby would be terrified and you'd have to hold the baby very firmly! You'd think some inventive person could produce a safe, alternative rocking system for busy and exhausted mums.

HERBS

Taken internally

• *Aniseed* • *Basil* • *Caraway* • *Chamomile*
• *Dill* • *Fennel* • *Lemon balm* • *Peppermint*

During breastfeeding you may use these liberally for yourself in cooking and as herbal teas. The herbs can be used in combinations, but generally at a total strength of around 1 teaspoon per cup of water. Teas will keep for a few days in the fridge. For an infant you would further dilute them and give in dessert-spoon doses, perhaps with some diluted pear juice. A pinch of the herbs can be mixed into food for children who are on solids.

Applied externally

A gentle abdominal massage using a few drops of aromatic oil often helps. *Bergamot chamomile, peppermint* or *rosemary* oils are suitable.

DIET

If the problem occurs periodically, note down all the foods taken in the two previous meals and eventually you may be able to trace the cause.

Supplements

• *Lactobacillus acidophilus* and *bifidobacteria* – there are special formulations for babies

TISSUE SALTS OR CELLOIDS

• *Mag Phos*

THE COMMON COLD

Description

All colds are not identical because there are at least twenty different viruses involved and individuals react differently to them. Colds usually start with a runny nose, sneezing, stuffy head, mild headache, watery eyes, general malaise, aching and a slight fever. The nasal passages become blocked and often the throat becomes sore and infected; there may be loss of taste and smell. Most people feel tired.

The symptoms usually subside in a few days and the majority of children are 'back to normal' in about one or two weeks.

Cause

A virus that apparently attacks randomly. Those who don't 'fight it off' may have lowered resistance due to physical or emotional stresses, that is, following chills, during teething or at times of change such as starting play school. It's also part of building up the immune system.

Treatment

The aim of treatment is to reduce the severity and duration of symptoms as well as preventing secondary bacterial infections. Select a few remedies and give them with food, otherwise the little patient will get an upset tummy.

HERBS

- Catnip • Chamomile • Echinacea • Elder
- Garlic • Hyssop • Peppermint • Rosehip

Some of these can be powdered or crushed and combined in equal proportions, simmered in fresh lemon juice, water and a little honey or barley malt; the tea can be sipped warm or cooled and added to vegetable or fruit juice. For a young child, use about ½ teaspoon herbs to 1 cup water.

DIET

Mainly fruit, vegetables and fluids for the first few days, to get a 'flushing' effect.

Supplements

- *Vitamins A and C* – if the patient won't eat fruit and vegetables.

TISSUE SALTS OR CELLOIDS

- *Ferr Phos* • *Kali Mur*

OTHER

Rest and 'tincture of time'.

Older children can have an *inhalation*, using a few drops of an aromatic oil such as lemon. For babies and toddlers put about 4 drops on a handkerchief under a pillow.

For blocked nasal passages, with thick congestion, you can drop in a weak, tepid *saline solution*, sucking it out with a dropper. Of course, the dropper should not be inserted more than 8 mm (¼ inch) into the nose.

Older children might be willing to sniff up some *sodium ascorbate* powder – as described in Chapter 11, 'Respiratory System'.

Influenza (Flu)

The basic treatment is the same as for a cold, but you might want to add in an additional supplement, such as *propolis* (a natural antibiotic substance produced by bees) or *reishi* (a medicinal mushroom), and continue this for some weeks after the symptoms have abated.

CONSTIPATION

Description

Infrequency or difficulty in passing hard, dry faeces.

Cause

Functional or structural abnormalities – which would be medically diagnosed. In infants it may be that the intestines are still relatively immature.

In older children, the causes and treatment are similar to those of adults – see pages 81–6.

Treatment

Babies are best treated by a practitioner-prescribed remedy, such as homoeopathic dandelion 1x or a matched constitutional remedy.

Gentle abdominal and lower back massage is helpful. When you massage the abdomen use small circular and stroking movements. Remember that the colon runs up the lower right abdomen, across the body below the waist-line and down the lower left abdomen. For massage purposes, add a few drops of marjoram to almond oil if the baby is agitated; for placid infants use rosemary oil.

HERBS THAT CAN BE GIVEN TO TODDLERS AND OLDER CHILDREN

• *Dandelion* • *Psyllium* • *Slippery elm*

DIET

The fluid intake may need to be increased.

For older children reduce meat and increase dietary whole grains, cereals, fruits, vegetables, legumes, and nuts and seeds (crushed for pre-schoolers). These foods speed up transit time and help develop healthy intestinal mucus production. Increasing dietary fibre also reduces the chance of developing appendicitis by about 50 per cent.

Don't use wheat bran because it tastes like sawdust, sometimes it blocks the intestines and causes gas. Try adding a little rice bran to dishes, or perhaps barley and oat bran.

If children refuse to eat fibre-rich foods, you might be able to disguise them in rissoles, muffins and smoothies. Fruit juices contain very little or no fibre.

Supplements

Bifidobacterium infantis is a pure strain of bacteria isolated from the gastrointestinal tract of a healthy baby. It helps introduce healthy microorganisms into the digestive tract.

Sodium ascorbate powder can be used as a laxative but you need to start with a pinch once a day with food and work out the dosage individually so that you avoid a gastric upset or colic. The aim is to have a normal bowel motion. When using largish doses of vitamin C, you need to build up slowly to the therapeutic quantity and taper off rather than stopping suddenly. Your body gets used to large quantities and then has to adapt to lesser amounts.

OTHER

Exercise is important to stimulate the digestive systems of people of all ages. Sadly, some children get very little. Not everyone likes standard athletics and sports so, within reason, encourage dancing or the types of physical things young people enjoy.

COUGH

Causes

Viral or bacterial infections. Getting a reasonable number of coughs, colds and minor infections is normal as it helps activate the immune system. Occasionally, a persistent cough is caused by a foreign body such as a peanut or seed lodged in the airways or lungs. Inhaled irritants, allergies and asthma may be responsible. Coughs may also be secondary to certain diseases such as cystic fibrosis.

NOTE **Coughs lasting for more than three weeks or getting worse require practitioner advice.**

Treatment

HERBS

Taken internally

• *Aniseed* • *Fenugreek* • *Garlic* • *Liquorice* – not the confectionery • *Marshmallow* • *Peppermint* • *Sweet violet leaves* • *Thyme* • *White horehound*

Too many remedies upset the stomach. Some of these are available in tablet form or they can be taken in the same way as suggested under The Common Cold (page 64–6).

Applied externally

Poultices are especially helpful for harsh or irritating coughs because of the reflexly soothing action. Also, the little patient appreciates something being done to help, rather than only a pill to swallow. Poultices are best applied at night for 15–20 minutes. Linseed meal, fenugreek or slippery elm powder are some suggested poultices. Before applying the poultice, use eucalyptus or a similar oil as a chest rub (see page 5).

For a dry cough, a *humidifier* is often helpful.

DIET

If possible, avoid dairy products, sweets and greasy foods – especially when the cough is very congested.

Supplements

• *Vitamin A* or a *cod liver oil* capsule

A number of studies show that respiratory illnesses in children are reduced by *vitamin A* supplementation. Massive doses are not recommended. I suggest a trial of at least three months of around 450 micrograms per day (retinol equivalent is the modern way of describing this vitamin).

• *Vitamin C* • *Zinc* (not long-term)

TISSUE SALTS OR CELLOIDS

• *Ferr Phos* • *Kali Mur* • *Calc Sulph*
• *Silicea* – after the cough has cleared

OTHER

If the coughs are recurring, some of the suggestions under Asthma (pages 57–61) may be used.

Playing wheelbarrows is a form of *postural drainage* – if the coughing child is the barrow! Handstands against a wall is another good exercise, but you will need to give a little support initially, i.e. by standing to one side and holding the child's thighs or waist. Start with a few seconds and gradually build up to a few minutes at a time. Of course, these types of exercises are not appropriate for babies or performing while children are acutely sick and weak.

CRADLE CAP

Description

Scaly, crusty, somewhat yellowish covering that commonly appears on the scalp of babies and young children. It usually has a thick, oily look and is best treated early because it can spread to the face, ears and neck.

Cause

Excessive secretion of the sebaceous glands.

Treatment

OILS

Every night you should gently massage the scalp with one or a combination of the following oils: • *Almond* • *Apricot kernel* • *Evening primrose* • *Olive*

Shampoo daily adding a few drops of *tea tree oil*, using a rough washer and gentle circular movements.

NOTE **Make sure you don't use too much oil or shampoo as they are extremely unpleasant in the eyes.**

DIET

It usually helps to eliminate all greasy foods, chocolates, sweets, soft drinks and cakes from your affected child's diet.

Supplements

For children not being breastfed:
• *Vitamin B6* or *B complex* • *Magnesium* (a low dose for a month)

DIARRHOEA

Description

Watery stools. This is a common infants' symptom and an occasional, mild bout needs only home treatment and watching. Persistent or violent diarrhoea needs urgent medical attention because a child can quickly dehydrate.

Causes

Teething, infections, food and heavy metal poisoning, allergic reactions (to dairy products and citrus in particular), microorganisms in drinking water, malabsorption diseases, antibiotics and some other drugs, including those which contain magnesium and aluminium, and emotional stress. Some serious disorders, such as coeliac disease, also cause diarrhoea if gluten-containing foods are not avoided completely.

One study of children with long-term diarrhoea showed that fruit juices were the cause, including apple, pear, grape and orange. The diarrhoea was worse if the juice contained sorbitol (additive 420).

Treatment

Fluid replacement is the primary aim but this does not mean excessive quantities. Sugggested fluids:
• 500 ml boiled, cooled water with 1 dessertspoon table sugar or glucose powder and a pinch of salt dissolved in it
• rice or barley water, with a teaspoon of rice or barley malt and a pinch of salt added to 500 ml fluid. To make the rice or barley water, add about ¼ cup white rice or pearl barley to 500 ml water and simmer for 20 minutes, then cool and strain.

For babies give at least a few tablespoons every few hours, aiming to give sufficient to prevent dehydration but not so much that it goes straight through the digestive tract. In a day you should not give more than 150 ml for each kg of bodyweight. For children over two, let them sip half a glass of the fluid every 2–3 hours during the day and a small quantity if they wake during the night. Increase the quantities according to the child's weight and tolerance.

HERBS

Sage, raspberry leaf and *thyme* can be used as tablets, weak tea or added to a broth. *Rosehip* is rich in tannins and vitamin C but it may be too acidic for some.

DIET

Prolonged diarrhoea can lead to malnutrition but this doesn't happen in a few days. Ensure the child avoids all fatty foods, such as meat, fat, eggs, dairy products, ice cream, chocolate, custard, bacon, preservatives and colourings. Initially, don't serve raw vegetables and fruit.

First foods can be plain chicken broth (with the fat skimmed off), white rice, steamed potatoes, cracker biscuits or other plain low-fibre cooked food. Vegetable soups and plain pasta are usually well tolerated. Try cooked apple or pear as the first fruit, then raw, ripe banana and raw grated apple (without the peel). Fruit juices, soft drinks and acidic fruits usually aggravate.

Supplements

A little *slippery elm powder* can be mixed into cooked apple.

Gastric upsets may be caused by even a mild vitamin A deficiency.

Lactobacillus acidophilus and *bifidobacteria* supplements are recommended as long-term correctives for diarrhoea.

Children aged 1–44 months with acute diarrhoea were reported to recover more quickly when given 5 mg *folic acid* every eight hours.[8]

Wherever there is a problem with nutrient absorption I would suggest a combined multi-vitamin and mineral supplement.

NOTE *Children with gastric upsets may not be able to tolerate many supplements because they are concentrated substances. There is no need to give supplements unless the problems become chronic (long-term).*

ECZEMA
(atopic dermatitis)

Description
Often begins as a rash on the cheeks and head, then in the creases of the elbows and legs. It reddens, becomes raised and is often oozy. There is accompanying itching, discomfort and pain. The lesions can be widespread and often they form sores that can get infected, leaving behind very dry patches.

Causes
Like asthma and hayfever, it is usually hereditary, with a history of allergies in the family. Dairy foods may aggravate but almost any food or pollutant can be the trigger.

Treatment
Breastfeeding solely for at least six months will reduce the incidence. Breastfeeding mothers should try to avoid cow's milk, eggs, fish and peanuts in their diet if there is a family history of allergic tendencies.

NOTE *These herbs and supplements should not be given to infants under the age of six months.*

HERBS
Taken internally
• *Fenugreek* and *golden seal* – these have to be given in tablet form crushed in honey because of the taste! • *Heartsease*
Applied externally
As a cool compress or wash: • *Calendula petals* or *chickweed leaves, flowers and stems* or *sweet violet leaves and flowers* • *Liquorice powder* mixed into Sorbolene or other base – to soften and soothe • *St John's wort oil* – to prevent itching • *Evening primrose* and *fish oils*

FROM THE KITCHEN
• *Chamomile tea* – strained and poured into the bath water • *Cabbage poultice* • *Bran* or *oatmeal baths*

To make a cabbage poultice use the whole outside leaves, with the main stems removed and the leaves rolled soft. Place directly over the lesions in a few layers and bandage firmly onto the area. Do a test patch first because cabbage sometimes causes inflammation after a few hours and the leaves need changing. It's better to use organically grown cabbage.

To make a bran or oatmeal bath, put about a cup of bran or oatmeal in a stocking (with the top tied in a knot); let hot water run over it and add a dessertspoon of bicarbonate of soda to the bath. When the water cools to tepid, the bath is ready and the stocking is removed.

DIET
Consider allergy tests and a 1-month avoidance trial of dairy products.
Supplements
• 1 tablet per day of *cod liver oil* and

evening primrose oil – for young children you will have to cut the capsules and disguise the taste of the oil in something like barley malt or a little jam • *Zinc* (short-term) • *Vitamin C*

OTHER

Homoeopathy is appropriate for babies and small children.

Avoid soap and friction. Soap tends to be alkalinising – use Sorbolene or a similar base instead (some people have skin reactions to Sorbolene) or try a special neutral soap, and ensure it is unscented and uncoloured. Don't allow children to have bubble baths, either.

Wool next to the skin can be very irritating.

Don't use talcum powders.

Sweat tends to aggravate the dermatitis so nylon clothing should not be worn in hot weather. Showering after activity is a good idea but not always feasible, especially for schoolchildren. During exercising or sweating, it sometimes helps to rub a slice of lemon over the skin to keep it slightly acidic.

Smoking and pets may need to be banned from inside the house. Controlling house dust mite is another suggestion.

Generally, it's better for the skin not to be covered excessively so have rooms reasonably heated in winter rather than letting the child 'stew' inside layers of heavy clothing.

Constant scratching further aggravates the skin, and is difficult to prevent, which is why external soothing remedies are suggested – even though they may not cure the eczema. A simple procedure for making up herbal and essential oil ointments is given in Chapter 1, 'Using Natural Remedies'.

NOTE **Ointments with heavy, tacky bases tend to suppress normal skin functioning. Commerical ointments also invariably contain many different substances, any one of which can cause an adverse reaction. Always test a small area first before applying anything new.**

GLUE EAR
(otitis media)

Description

Inflammation of the middle ear that causes pressure on the eardrum. A common indication is that the child pulls at the ear or puts a hand over it. There may be itchiness, throbbing pain, discharge and associated diarrhoea or respiratory infection. Medical attention is obviously required if there is a discharge and pain.

Causes

Ear problems often follow recurring respiratory infections. It is also possible that the discomfort may be referred pain from teeth or the throat. Foreign bodies, insects or impacted wax may be the cause. Allergies or food sensitivities may contribute to the blocking of the eustachian tube, which connects the eardrum to the upper respiratory system. In some cases it may be simply that the eustachian tube is relatively immature or smaller than normal.

When there is tobacco smoke in the home, children are more likely to have ear problems. There is also a higher incidence in bottlefed babies than breastfed.

COMMON CHILDHOOD AILMENTS ❖ 71

Treatment

Within reason, treat coughs, colds and other minor infections promptly. The remedies I have suggested help improve immune system functioning and, together with wholesome food, should prevent long-term low-grade infections and secondary complications.

HERBS

Taken internally

• *Echinacea* • *Fenugreek* • *Garlic* • *Golden seal* • *Reishi*

Applied externally

• *Calendula* or *mullein oil* – a few drops in each ear for chronic problems • *Lavender oil* – a few drops in the ear may help ease the pain • *Tea tree* or *garlic oil* ear drops – for infection

FROM THE KITCHEN

• Fresh *lemon juice*, diluted 50:50 with tepid water and dropped into the ears • *Olive* or *almond oil* may be used externally, in drops, to soften impacted wax

DIET

It is worth ensuring the child avoids dairy products for a month to see if they contribute to the problem. Other associated allergens are eggs, wheat, corn, oranges and peanut butter.

TISSUE SALTS OR CELLOIDS

• *Ferr Phos* • *Kali Mur*

OTHER

A *foot bath* or *foot massage* is diverting and may help ease the pain. Try applying finger pressure in the area below and between the third and fifth toes.

In the old days, they used to put a clothes peg on the tip of the ring finger or on the tip of the fourth toe!

CAUTION **Never insert anything down towards the eardrum.**

A warm, partially filled hot-water bottle over the ear is another reliever.

Deep breathing and deliberate yawning may help to open ear blockages.

GROMMETS

Since the early 1970s, controlled medical studies have shown no benefit from the placement of tubes in the ear drum to treat middle ear infections. Little patients with the problem in both ears had a grommet placed in one ear only and – you've guessed it – the outcome was the same in both ears! Grommets may cause scarring and permanent perforation. At least some medical practitioners are now recommending pain relievers and tincture of time. I've found homoeopathy, plus herbs and dietary improvements, to be very successful.

ANTIBIOTICS

A Dutch medical study concluded: 'We find no difference between co-amoxiclav [an antibiotic] and placebo with regard to the resolution of acute otitis media'.[9] The report cited other studies showing that the symptoms and fever resolve within the same time in placebo- and antibiotic-treated groups.

Antibiotics have many possible side effects. A basic problem is that they upset the body's natural bacterial balance with the result that another infection is likely to follow or an upset digestive system.

If antibiotics are really necessary, follow with a course of *lactobacillus acidophilus* and *bifidobacteria*, plus *garlic* or *echinacea*. There is probably no benefit in taking these at the same time as the antibiotics because the drugs will largely offset the supplements. In cases of long-term antibiotic therapy, the supplements can be used but need to be taken at a different time of day from the drugs.

HIVES (urticaria)

Description

A skin reaction to something eaten, touched or in the air. The skin becomes red, lumpy, itchy; the reaction may be sudden or delayed.

In very sensitive people, the reaction can be dramatic. If there is extreme swelling or difficulty breathing seek emergency treatment.

Causes

Particular foods, additives, chemicals, certain drugs, insect stings and garden plants. It can be brought on during exercise, by temperature extremes and emotional stress.

Treatment

Tracing the offending item or items is sometimes difficult because the reaction is not always immediate. If you suspect a particular plant, get it identified by a horticulturist or the Department of Agriculture. There might also be a sensitivity to other plants in the same family.

HERBS

Taken internally

• *Alfalfa* – tea or tablets • *Aloe* – in tablet form • *Nettle* – in homoeopathic form

Applied externally

• *Chickweed ointment* – may alleviate the itching • *Liquorice powder* mixed into Sorbolene – for skin redness • *Chamomile tea* – as a cold wash

FROM THE KITCHEN

Cold water with about 20 per cent *apple cider vinegar* is usually helpful as an external wash.

Give plenty of water to drink, with a little bicarbonate of soda added or Andrews Liver Salts as this will help flush out the disturbing substances.

According to folklore, if the rash is actually caused by nettle, then crush some yellow dock leaves and lightly rub over the affected area.

Supplements

If the problem is recurring: • *Vitamin C with bioflavonoids* • *Vitamin B12*

TISSUE SALTS OR CELLOIDS

• *Ferr Phos* • *Nat Phos*

INSECT STINGS

Extreme reactions to stings are quite rare. However, if you are not sure of the type of sting, ring your nearest Poisons Advisory Service. Dramatic reactions with shortness of breath need emergency care, otherwise keep calm because the child's screaming is usually disproportionate to the injury.

Treatment

Once you have established that there is no danger and removed the sting – if any – a small ice pack can be applied to the affected area and the little patient can rest with the limb elevated. A little 'treat' usually helps.

NOTE **Never put ice directly on the skin as this causes a burn.**

HERBS

Applied externally

• *Chickweed* or *golden seal* ointment
• *Lavender* or *St John's wort oil* to prevent itching • *Tea tree oil* – to prevent infection

FROM THE KITCHEN

• Malt vinegar dabbed, undiluted, on the affected area
• *Turmeric powder* – mixed to a paste with water and plastered over the sting

TISSUE SALTS OR CELLOIDS
• *Nat Mur*
OTHER
• *Homoeopathic Apis 6x*
External insect repellants
• *Citronella oil* • *Lavender oil* • *Pennyroyal oil*

CAUTION **These oils cannot be used around the eyes.**

It is said that insects prefer to land on people who are low in vitamin B1!

NAPPY RASH

Description
Most babies experience at least some degree of this problem. The skin around the anus, genitals and between the legs becomes red and if not treated this can spread, becoming even more inflamed and tender. Blisters can form and a secondary fungal or bacterial infection can set in, which makes the whole condition much harder to treat.

Causes
Faeces and urine in contact with the skin can lead to various types of skin complaints.

Treatment
Take action at the very first sign. Change nappies frequently, let baby go without napkins for short periods, in the fresh air if possible.

Some soaking solutions, washing powders and detergents are irritating to young skins so make sure nappies are thoroughly rinsed, or try different brands. Don't use talcum powder or scented soaps. For a trial period, use Sorbolene or a neutral soap. Don't use plastic pants while the rash is present.

HERBS
Applied externally
• *Evening primrose* or *almond oil* – applied after bathing • *Aloe jelly* – not if it stings

A number of herbal ointments may be helpful. I think they are better in a non-greasy base, such as Sorbolene, with one or more of the following:
• *Calendula* • *Comfrey* • *Liquorice* • *St John's wort*

CAUTION **Avoid strong-smelling aromatic oils and test everything on a small area before applying all over.**

To prevent infection, a few drops of *tea tree oil* can be added to the bath water after the baby's face has been washed. *Oatmeal baths*, as described under Eczema, pages 69–70, are usually soothing. Zinc cream is commonly used as it forms a barrier; however, this is suppressive and I would not suggest it as a long-term treatment or preventive.

SLEEP PROBLEMS

Like adults, babies and children have individual sleep requirements. They can have difficulty getting to sleep, wake up through the night or wake up very early.

Causes
They need a 'winding down' period before sleep as it's unlikely they'll settle quickly if they are excited. Dreams and darkness often scare children so a low light in the room and a little soft music may help. Respiratory complaints, teething, colic or any pain and discomfort will disturb sleep patterns.

Treatment

For babies, there's no substitute for rocking, walking and singing. Telling or reading stories is good for older children. If you're too drowsy, you could make or buy some talking books but parents' voices usually work better. You can also buy relaxation tapes with dolphin and other sounds that appeal to children, and lullabies on cassette work for some.

The theory that crying is good for the lungs is not highly regarded these days. One study has shown that babies whose mothers responded to their cries within two minutes during the first few weeks of life were crying for their mothers least by the end of the first year. The general consensus is that you can't spoil babies but toddlers need 'taming'.

Don't let a little insomniac wear you down – you can get help from early childhood centres.

HERBS

Herbal pillows or toys stuffed with dried aromatic herbs – see Chapters 1 and 2 for suggestions. • *Scullcap* or *valerian* – one tablet crushed in a little barley malt before bed

DIET

Supplements

• *Vitamin B complex*

TISSUE SALTS OR CELLOIDS

• *Kali Phos* – does not have an immediate effect

OTHER

Massage with a pleasant-smelling sedative oil such as chamomile, lavender, marjoram, melissa or clary-sage. Volatile oils are strong: dilute these in almond or apricot kernel oil.

Also arrange fresh air and exercise during the day – appropriate to the age of the child.

SORE THROAT

This is very common in infants and is often accompanied by a blocked nose, fever, headache and swollen glands in the neck. The tonsils are invariably very swollen but this is not a cause for alarm unless there is difficulty breathing or the tonsils are badly infected.

Causes

Viral or bacterial infection. Unfortunately, these may be contracted from impure drinking water, swimming pools – even some beaches. The incidence is usually higher if the diet is poor. Other aggravations include emotional stress, allergies, exposure to cigarette smoke and teething. Excess crying or screaming also makes the throat sore.

The cause may also be mumps or other serious diseases.

Treatment

Try to find and remove any aggravating factors.

HERBS

The remedies given under coughs and colds generally help strengthen the immune system.

Older children may agree to use some of the remedies listed in Chapter 11, 'Respiratory System'.

Inhalations or vaporisers are quite effective for throat conditions. A few drops of *lemon oil* is one of the best additives to the hot water.

FROM THE KITCHEN

Cut up an onion, cover with 2 teaspoons honey, let it stand for a few hours. You will be surprised how much liquid is formed. Encourage the patient to sip a little of the *juice* throughout the day.

A cold *apple cider vinegar compress* on the throat may ease the swelling.

DIET

Supplements

• *Vitamin C* • *Propolis* – as liquid or tablets dissolved in water and sipped slowly.

TISSUE SALTS OR CELLOIDS

• *Calc Sulph*

SUNBURN

Prevention is the most important factor, using sun block and a hat. However, you can't supervise children all the time. PABA, one of the B vitamins, may help prevent sunburn if taken regularly as a supplement through warm weather.

Treatment

HERBS

Applied externally

• *Aloe* – the pure jelly straight from your garden is an effective treatment. Scrape the inside part from the leaves and apply 2–3 times daily. This is not a preventive or blocking agent • *Tea tree oil* – diluted in water

OTHER

Plenty of *water* to drink.

Bathing in cool water with *apple cider vinegar* added.

Don't prick or burst any blisters.

At a later stage, use a *moisturiser* such as vitamin E, avocado or almond oil.

NOTE **Severe sunburn needs medical attention.**

TEETHING

The first set of teeth appear over a period from about six months of age to thirty months. During this time, many babies become cranky, have bouts of diarrhoea, skin rashes or coughs and colds. Sleeping patterns can be disrupted.

Treatment

Taken internally

• *Catnip* • *Chamomile* – small quantities of weak tea help with irritability. (Many children won't take herbal teas but in these cases appropriate homoeopathics are usually well tolerated. The homoeopathic form of chamomile gives good results but unless you have a home remedy kit you will need a homoeopathic consultation to obtain this.)

Applied externally

• *Clove* or *sage tea* – let cool and gently massage into the gums

---

NOTE **Clove and sage oils are too strong for use on babies and young children.**

DIET

Fruit juices should be kept minimal and extremely diluted. They are quite high in natural sugars and low in fibre. All sugary foods should be avoided: even some baby rusks have added sugar. A piece of apple or carrot, tied inside a handkerchief so baby can't choke on chewed fragments, is healthier than most commercial biscuits. More dietary information is given in Chapter 15, 'Nutrition'.

Do not bottle feed longer than absolutely necessary as this can affect the structure of the teeth and jaw.

To strengthen gums

• *Vitamin C and bioflavonoids* • *Calc Fluor* – Tissue salt or Celloid

To strengthen teeth

• *Calc Phos* – Tissue salt or Celloid

VOMITING AND NAUSEA

The general recommendations are basically the same as for Diarrhoea (see pages 68–9).

Treatment

HERBS
Ginger is now available in tablet form and is quite effective for treating all mild cases of nausea, travel sickness and vomiting. Tablets may be crushed in barley malt, honey, jam or juice.

NOTE *Fluid replacement is important. If the problem persists longer than a day and the child can't keep any food in the stomach, then get medical advice. This applies to sudden, violent vomiting also.*

OTHER
Some common anti-emetic pharmaceuticals (and anti-diarrhoeals) contain aluminium and other chemicals that are poorly tolerated by young people.

CHAPTER 5

DIGESTIVE PROBLEMS

In the system of herbal medicine practised by the early USA herbalists, it was considered that the stomach was the 'throne of the vital powers' which means that this organ governed the important functions of circulation, respiration, digestion, assimilation and the activity of the various secretions. According to Dr Swinburne Clymer (1895) 'the stomach is in almost every instance the seat of disease. When this organ is diminished, the power of generating heat and nervous energy is diminished, and consequently the actions and functions of other organs become weakened.'

Aside from the mixed metaphors, this is not as strange as it may sound because unless your stomach breaks down your food, you will not absorb the nutrients effectively. Therefore, at least some of the cells in your body will be deprived; in time they will not function optimally, and health problems will follow.

Many of the suggestions in this chapter could be considered preventive and certainly should be used at the early stages of digestive problems. When you consider the delicate and unique structure of the whole of the gastro-intestinal tract, you will appreciate that a constant minor irritation can lead to more serious complications. In certain circumstances, the best treatment may be simply to give the stomach a brief rest. Fasting is complicated and requires expert supervision, but you could try a day or two on fluids and blended soups.

Problems in the gastro-intestinal tract may be very difficult to diagnose. Sometimes a successful 'cure' is effected because a particular irritant or allergy is removed from the diet or environment. Often, the problem requires a medical diagnosis.

The possibility of heavy metal toxicity, such as aluminium or lead, should also be considered.

When you are nervous, angry or emotionally upset the autonomic nervous system functions in such a way that the energy is directed to areas other than the digestive tract, which is why it is better not to eat during acute stress. This also happens during times of physical activity so it is sensible not to exercise vigorously directly after a meal or to eat while working.

Digestion starts in the mouth, with the partial breaking down of starches. The food stays in the stomach for a few hours while it is subjected to the acidity in the stomach, the gastric juices and the peristaltic action.

By the time the food has entered the small intestines it should be mushy (chyme). It is then broken down to molecular size by pancreatic enzymes and bile, allowing the nutrients to be absorbed through the wall of the small intestines into the bloodstream. In the large intestines, water, some minerals, and other substances are reabsorbed.

If the food is not broken down and the digestive enzymes are not adequately secreted, then the nutrients are not only poorly absorbed but there may be consequent irritant effects.

When the passage of food through the digestive tract is too rapid, then the stools are watery and the person may become dehydrated and lose some essential minerals; fluid replacement is therefore very important.

If the transit time is too slow, there is a build up of faecal matter and metabolic waste products, as well as the possibility of developing bowel pockets, infections and other intestinal problems.

Many commonsense rules should apply.
• Do not over-eat. Small, regular meals are less stressful for the digestive system.
• Chew properly; have teeth and jaw problems checked by a dentist.

• Avoid drinking with meals. Although fresh fruit and vegetables contain a high percentage of water, it does not seem sensible to dilute the gastric juices more than necessary, especially where there is a digestive problem.
• If you suffer from an intermittent gastric problem, note everything you have had to eat or drink that day. You may trace an allergen or toxin.
• A number of commonly ingested substances and drugs may cause or aggravate digestive problems: for example, coffee, cigarettes, alcohol, excess orange juice and certain pharmaceutical drugs.
• When introducing new remedies or foods, try one at a time. With dried beans and legumes, always pre-soak, cook well and have very small quantities to start with, as otherwise they will give you wind.
• Changes in bowel patterns and rectal bleeding must always be medically checked.
• Beware of faddish and restrictive dietary recommendations, such as those giving lists of food combinations to avoid; remember that you absorb nutrients at a molecular level so that the body does not distinguish between, say, the glucose from a carrot and the glucose from an apple.

If you enjoy fruit after a meal without ill effects, there is no reason why you should stop simply because someone writes mythological biochemistry about the human gastrointestinal system not being able to absorb carbohydrate with protein. Any food composition table will show that the majority of foods have a wide range of nutrients in them, plus hundreds of other constituents, and a normal digestive system can sort these out perfectly.

Antacids

In addition to laxative and drug abuse causing or aggravating gastric problems, there are also problems with the over-use of antacids. Bearing in mind that the stomach must be very acidic in order to break down the food particles, it follows that antacids reduce this acidity. There is also the possibility that more acid will be secreted to compensate; eventually, this can deplete the secretory function. In other words, if you take antacids, you should be certain that your digestion problem is one of excess acidity.

The other difficulty with antacids is that some of them contain aluminium. Aluminium toxicity can be a problem for certain individuals, and it is aggravated by the fact that a number of everyday products such as table salt, toothpaste and deodorants contain it. Some individuals excrete aluminium less efficiently than others and they are more likely to suffer from excess.

If you read antacid labels you will see that some contain calcium and magnesium in sufficient quantities to be toxic, or at least cause imbalances if the medications are taken liberally. Excess of one mineral can interfere with the absorption and metabolism of other essential minerals such as iron or zinc.

Digestive tonics

Some digestive tonics are bitter-tasting and it is considered that these work by reflexly stimulating the gastro-intestinal tract and surrounding organs such as the liver and pancreas. Although I recommend that herbal extracts and tablets are taken in a little water after meals, in the case of digestive tonics they are usually more effective sipped slowly half an hour before meals. Because the reflex action starts in the mouth, these bitter herbs are probably not as effective if sweetened with honey. They can be taken as a long, cold, pre-meal drink, with the addition of chopped lemon, including the rind, peppermint leaves and mineral water.

APPETITE – LACK OF

Description

Except in the elderly, this is not common, but I do see people in my clinic who have lost interest in food and do not have adequate kilojoule and nutrient intake. One suggestion is that they complete a diet diary for one week, so that they can see for themselves what they are eating; I suggest this is taken to a practitioner for evaluation.

Some individuals have small stomachs and it is difficult for them to eat large, or even normal, quantities at one time; it would suit them better to have small, regular meals, with a snack in between.

Causes

Chronic conditions such as anorexia nervosa and serious diseases such as cancer require practitioner advice. Early warning signs of more serious tendencies are noticeable weight loss and fatigue.

A general lack of appetite may have many causes such as prior over-eating, recovery from an illness, emotional upsets (others may eat excessively), allergy to a commonly eaten food, teeth or sinus infections, excess alcohol, cigarette smoking and over-concern with weight.

Treatment
HERBS
• *Bergamot* • *Burdock* • *Centaury* • *Dandelion* • *Fenugreek* • *Gentian* • *Golden seal* • *Rosehip*

FROM THE KITCHEN
• *Basil* • *Cardamon* • *Chicory* • *Endive*
• *Ginger* • *Paw paw juice* or *papain tablets*
• *Pineapple juice* or *bromelain tablets*
• *Radiccio*

All the *culinary herbs* are digestive tonics, especially those that are somewhat bitter-tasting, including coriander, fenugreek, marjoram, oregano, sage, tarragon and turmeric.

DIET
Having meals served attractively and in harmonious surroundings may help. More time in food preparation may be required. Blended soups and juices provide concentrated nutrients.

Hearty eaters love to see a plate piled high but for those with tiny appetites large servings are a turn-off. In Chapter 15, 'Nutrition', I have given some tips for picky eaters.

Supplements
• *A combined multi-vitamin and mineral –* after breakfast • *Vitamin B1* • *Zinc –* after dinner • *Digestive enzymes –* taken with meals

TISSUE SALTS OR CELLOIDS
• *Calc Phos* • *Nat Phos*

BAD BREATH
(halitosis)

Causes
Dental cavities, gum infections, inadequate dental hygiene, over-eating, excess alcohol, cigarette smoking, stress, hayfever, sinusitis, allergies or enzyme deficiencies. A problem in any part of the digestive system may cause breath odour. As well as garlic, certain other foods may cause or aggravate this problem, for example, fish, raw onions and cabbage.

Treatment
HERBS
• *Aniseed* • *Caraway* • *Dill* • *Fennel*
• *Ginger* • *Meadowsweet* • *Peppermint*
• *Spearmint*

FROM THE KITCHEN
• *Cinnamon* • *Cloves* • *Parsley* • *Paw paw*
Chlorophyll is the pigment that makes plants green, and it has a mild deodorising effect internally. In cases of bad breath, chlorophyll capsules, tablets or juice may be used, but generally speaking I suggest it is sufficient to add basil, parsley, watercress, sprouts and green leafy vegetables to your normal diet, either in salads or lightly steamed.

DIET
Have fruit and vegetables only for 1–3 days. Some juices may be helpful, such as: • *Beetroot* • *Carrot* • *Celery* • *Cucumber* • *Paw paw* • *Pear* • *Wheatgrass*

Supplements
• *Charcoal tablets –* charcoal is an absorber of toxins and 1-2 tablets with each meal may be useful as a short-term, symptomatic treatment of bad breath and flatulence • *Lactobacillus acidophilus and bifidobacteria* • *Digestive enzymes*

BURPING AND BELCHING

Causes
A number of factors may cause this, such as: over-eating, excess alcohol, inadequate chewing, underactive gastric functioning, nervous indigestion, allergies, excess acidity, hiatus hernia.

Treatment
HERBS
• *Agrimony* • *Alfalfa* • *Aloe* • *Centaury*
• *Chamomile* • *Fennel* • *Marshmallow*
• *Meadowsweet* • *Slippery elm*

FROM THE KITCHEN
Use all these in cooking and salads:
• *Alfalfa* and other *sprouts* • *Basil* • *Bay*
• *Lovage* • *Oregano* • *Savory* • *Tarragon*
TISSUE SALTS OR CELLOIDS
• *Nat Phos*

COLIC – INTESTINAL

Description
Colic usually refers to abdominal pain caused by spasmodic contractions of the intestines. This is more common during the first three months of life and is covered in the previous chapter.

Causes
Several factors may contribute, such as eating too quickly, swallowing air, anxiety, allergies, infections, malfunctioning digestive organs and some drugs.

CAUTION **Occasionally the cause may be related to toxicity, for example, arsenic, aluminium, lead – this would require a professional diagnosis. Abdominal pain can also be caused by a number of serious diseases and severe or persistent pain requires prompt medical checking. In some cases, people are frightened of the possible diagnosis but it is more stressful not knowing what the problem is.**

Treatment
HERBS
For symptoms: • *Aniseed* • *Catnip* • *Chamomile* • *Cinnamon* • *Cloves* • *Dandelion* • *Dill* • *Ginger* • *Peppermint*
   Other remedies depend on the cause of the problem.

FROM THE KITCHEN
• *Caraway* • *Cardamon* • *Cumin*
DIET
Check for allergies by making a note of everything eaten or drunk during the two meals prior to the attack.
Supplements
• *Vitamin B3* • *Calcium* • *Vitamins A and D combined* • *Lactobacillus acidophilus* • *Bifidobacteria* • *Pectin*
TISSUE SALTS OR CELLOIDS
• *Mag Phos*

CONSTIPATION

Description
Hard or inadequate bowel movements. Inadequate, infrequent or incomplete bowel motions may result in discomfort, headaches, nausea or anxiety. Ideally, people should have one bowel movement a day but this can vary individually depending on nerve signals to the intestines, eating habits, physical activity and stress.

Causes
Numerous. Could be something simple such as stress, insufficient food or liquid intake, inadequate dietary fibre, excess protein – especially meat and cheese – refined foods or poor bile flow. It could also be related to liver or thyroid underfunctioning.

   Other causes include inadequate fluids, pregnancy, antacids, metabolic disorders, structural abnormalities, psychogenic disorders, tumours, strokes, old age – particularly when related to physical inactivity – spinal cord trauma, constant use of enemas and laxatives. Constipation is also a side effect of some pharmaceutical drugs.

NOTE **Sudden blockages, bleeding or changes in bowel habits must be checked by a medical practitioner.**

Treatment

Generally, a well balanced, varied, high-fibre diet with adequate fluid and exercise, together with a reasonable lifestyle, should ensure appropriate excretion.

HERBS

• *Aloe gel* • *Chamomile* – to relax intestinal muscles • *Dandelion* • *Psyllium* • *Senna* • *Yellow dock*

DIET

Some people find that a glass of hot water with the juice of half a lemon is helpful when taken first thing in the morning, especially if followed by a brisk walk.

The fluid intake should be adequate – depending on temperature and level of activity, about 6–8 glasses being the minimum daily requirement.

Breakfasts

Fruit such as prunes or figs with cereal and 1–2 tablespoons of rice bran make an ideal breakfast for someone with constipation. Dried fruits should be pre-soaked in water; also it is better to use sun-dried products because the types commonly sold contain a sulphur compound.

One of my favourite winter breakfasts is freshly ground whole rye and whole wheat, cooked with dried apricots, and topped with a little dried coconut and almond meal. If you're not worried about your weight serve with some sour cream. There are many variations of this recipe. You can use any whole grains and grind them before cooking, or soak overnight.

Another breakfast suggestion is buckwheat seeds cooked with raisins, apple and cinnamon.

This type of breakfast does not need added sweeteners or milk although some people prefer it with a little yoghurt or buttermilk. I have never known anyone to put on weight through the reasonable use of whole grains.

Bran

Wheat bran, especially in large quantities, may cause problems because it can be difficult to digest; it may also cause bad breath, anal irritation and itchy skin. For most people, bran acts as a bulk fibre laxative but for sensitive people it can cause bloating and even constipation, especially if there is insufficient fluid intake. Wheat may cause allergic-type reactions, so try rice bran, linseed meal, oat or barley bran or slippery elm powder.

Bran contains phytic acid, which may prevent the absorption of certain minerals, and although some researchers doubt that the phytic acid is a problem it would be wise not to eat more than 1–2 tablespoons per day.

In any event, it doesn't make sense to mill the bran out of grains so that you can eat refined flour, and then have to eat bran separately in order to get sufficient fibre for the bowels to function adequately. Why not eat the whole grain in the first place, because as well as the fibre, it also contains vitamin E, other vitamins and minerals, about 50 per cent of which are lost in the processing to white flour?

If you look in health food stores, you will see that it is possible to have a different cereal every day of the week. As a bonus, many of these have no added sugar, salt or additives, but you need to read the labels. I am not suggesting that you have a wide variety in the one meal. Have two or three grain-type foods daily, selecting from barley, brown rice, buckwheat, millet, oats, polenta (corn), rye, soya grits, wholemeal pasta and other relatively unprocessed starches.

Some commercial whole-grain breads consist of a large proportion of refined flour (sometimes called baker's flour) with a few whole grains thrown in. In the old days we used to mix white flour with water to make paste, so it is not surprising that it can block up the human intestinal tract, just as it can stick paper together. White flour does have the advantage of a long shelf life and it does make breads and similar foods lighter.

Other dietary suggestions

Raw grated vegetables, such as beetroot, sliced zucchini, as well as the common salad foods all help relieve constipation. Foods such as broccoli, cauliflower and green beans may cause flatulence when eaten raw, so you may need to steam them for a few minutes. You could try, for example, blended beetroot, apple and yoghurt with a little water and bran. Eating beetroot is also one way of finding out your 'transit time', that is, the length of time your digestive tract takes to digest, absorb and eliminate. Ideally, you should see the beetroot colour in your stools within 24 hours. Three or four charcoal tablets after breakfast is another way of testing the transit time.

In some cases, up to 30 ml olive or linseed oil, taken internally, may help constipation by providing stimulus to the gallbladder as well as lubrication. Most people tolerate this amount of oil quite well, especially if taken with some pure lemon juice as a salad dressing, but it is high in calories so all other dietary fats must be eliminated.

TISSUE SALTS OR CELLOIDS

• *Nat Mur* – for regulating fluid • *Nat Sulph* – for 'toxic' bowel • *Kali Mur* – for mucous membranes

OTHER

Constipation may be related, also, to repeatedly ignoring the urge to defecate because of worry about not getting to work on time, embarrassment about using other people's toilets or unwillingness to interrupt activities. This type of constipation may have its onset in childhood.

Lack of exercise is a problem for bedridden or handicapped people but deep abdominal breathing helps in such cases. A yoga teacher can give you some special exercises. Brisk walking, gentle skipping and bouncers are also recommended.

ENEMAS

CAUTION *Generally, I do not recommend enemas, however, for constipation and intestinal cramps an occasional use should not be harmful if there are no structural defects in the bowel. One or two enemas a year may be helpful, especially if used in conjunction with a short elimination diet.*

In the case of irritable bowel I would suggest one every second day a week, then once weekly for 4–6 weeks.

Don't use when there is diarrhoea, inflammation or bowel diseases.

A catnip enema

Use a *gravity feed enema* (obtainable from pharmacies). Make a catnip infusion: add 2 tablespoons dried catnip leaves to 600 ml water. Bring to boil and let stand for 10 minutes. Strain.

The bathroom is the best place to administer an enema. Make sure the rest of the household knows you will be in there for about 20 minutes so you will be undisturbed.

Prepare everything you need. Cover the floor with a plastic sheet, old towelling or newspapers. Arrange a pillow and have a book or radio to pass the time. Have a rug handy in case you feel cold. Fit up the enema kit and hang the container about 65 cm (2½ feet) above where you are going to lie.

• Pour the *strained* catnip infusion into the enema container, having first remembered to secure the tap at the end of the tube.

NOTE **The infusion should be bloodheat (tepid).**

• Set an empty jug on the floor, release the tap on the catheter and allow some of the infusion to flow into the jug *to make sure all the air is out of the tube*.
• Turn off the tap. Empty fluid in the jug back into the enema container.
• Return the jug to floor and put the end of catheter into it.
• Lie on your left side with your knees up, making yourself comfortable.
• Grease the nozzle of the catheter with a little K-Y jelly.
• Relax.
• When you feel ready, gently push the catheter into the rectum, bearing down gently as you do so to open the ring of the muscle.
• When the catheter is properly in place, turn on the tap until you feel the catnip infusion flowing in. Don't let it flow too fast. Give yourself plenty of time. Hold up the tube to ease in the last of the catnip.
• Turn off the tap and remove the catheter, which is placed in the jug.
• Massage your lower abdomen to spread the enema.

• Try to relax – read or listen to the radio for 15 minutes; later you will be able to hold for much longer.

NOTE **The first time you have an enema you may be able to hold for a few minutes only.**

Catnip is not the only herb suitable for an enema – chamomile, lemon balm and peppermint are also suggested and are used in the same way.

One of the edible oils may also be used as a retention enema, that is, using about 150–200 ml of oil and, hopefully, retaining it in the bowel overnight. This may not be possible on your first attempt.

Freshly ground coffee beans, simmered in water for 20 minutes, strained and then used in the same way as catnip, are also stimulating for the liver and gallbladder and, as well, they have the added advantage of acting as a painkiller. This may have a role in the treatment of chronic headaches, especially migraines, where there is a relationship with allergies or digestive problems. I must confess that most of my migraine patients are unwilling to try this mode of therapy so I have not been able to test it adequately.

To sum up, enemas should be used after giving consideration to the possible benefits and the fact that they interfere with the normal bowel reflexes.

LAXATIVES

The abuse and over-use of laxatives is widely known but some people are helped by them as long as the remedy is not irritating and is being used appropriately.

In *Current Medical Diagnosis and Treatment* it is said that normal movements may range in frequency between 3–12

CAUTION Laxatives should never be used as a means of losing weight.

To have frequent watery stools means that one is losing essential body fluids and electrolytes (minerals). The food you eat cannot be properly absorbed if it passes too quickly through the intestinal tract; also, undigested food may cause irritation and inflammation.

Seek practitioner advice where there is intestinal obstruction, undiagnosed abdominal pain and vomiting. Professional advice is also required for constipation during pregnancy and lactation.

stools per week. My own belief is that it is probably ideal to have at least one bowel motion daily but there is no need to be concerned about missing an occasional day.

From the thousands of patients I have seen, I have noticed it is extremely rare for a vegetarian to be irregular, although occasionally this happens where there is excessive cheese in the diet.

Long-term constipation and constant straining may contribute to haemorrhoids, bowel pockets and general malaise. There is some reabsorption through the colon wall and although I do not think we should think of ourselves as carriers of 'bowel toxins', there are metabolic breakdown products that can cause problems if they build up excessively.

A special test (urinary Indican) will show whether or not excessive toxins are being reabsorbed through the bowel wall. If you are concerned ask your health practitioner or doctor about this.

Some laxatives are habit forming and it is preferable to use them only as a last resort.

Laxative herbs can be divided into different categories.

1 Aperients
Such as dandelion. These have a very mild effect.

2 Laxatives
For example, psyllium. The stools are normal, but there is an improvement in regularity.

3 Cathartics
For example senna and cascara. At a low dose the stool is not watery. At a higher dose the user may experience griping, which is why it is recommended that these be combined with an anti-spasmodic herb such as chamomile, fennel or ginger. Aloe might also be classed as a cathartic depending on the product and the quantity used.

4 Purgatives
Such as castor oil. These have a more powerful action and are accompanied by watery stools and abdominal discomfort. Some of the herbs and plants in this category are not used even by herbal practitioners and are therefore clearly not part of home remedies.

Another way of classifying laxatives is to group them according to their action.

1 Providing bulk
These are usually classed as hydrophyllic colloids which means that they absorb water and swell, thereby helping to promote a normal bowel function. Examples are bran, linseed meal, slippery elm powder.

2 Stimulants to the nerves controlling the muscles in the bowel wall
Viewed in comparison with pharmaceutical drugs, one report states that the

standard preparations of aloe, cascara and senna are 'undoubtedly safe even if they are consumed in enormous quantities'. The theory behind this is that when the laxative starts to work by stimulating the colon wall, you will then have a bowel motion, taking the rest of the laxative out of the system. My advice is that, apart from occasional use, seek professional advice because these laxatives, especially in large quantities, can irritate the bowel wall to the extent that the linings are damaged and the mucus secretory function is impaired.

Senna tea is relatively mild; the pods are somewhat stronger. To use the pods, soak 6–12 of them in freshly made tea or ginger root decoction, stand covered for about 6 hours and drink the fluid before bed.

3 Promoting bile flow
Dandelion and chicory are mild examples of such laxatives.

Olive oil combined with lemon juice may also be considered but you would need to watch the total fat intake.

Herbal practitioners have access to a range of herbs in this category and olive oil and lemon juice may be used in conjunction with these herbs.

4 Relaxing spasms and tension
Chamomile and valerian are two herbs in this category.

5 Normalising secretions of the gastro-intestinal tract
Depending on the patient's condition, it may be helpful to firstly soothe the intestinal walls with something like slippery elm powder. For constipation you need to use 1–2 tablespoons, either with a cereal or mashed into fruit or yoghurt. Some of the bitter herbs stimulate the flow of gastric and intestinal secretions, as indicated under Appetite – Lack of (see pages 79–80)

CROHN'S DISEASE

Description
An inflammatory intestinal disease related to immune malfunction and abnormal intestinal permeability. Sections of the intestines become non-functional, inflamed or ulcerated. There are recurring episodes of pain (especially in the lower right abdomen), diarrhoea, fever, weight loss and fatigue. There may be mucus and blood in the faeces.

NOTE **All these sorts of symptoms require a medical diagnosis.**

Causes
Probably genetic. Aggravated by food intolerances, alcohol, infections and some drugs, especially arthritic medication (NSAIDs). [1]

ALLERGIES AND INTOLERANCES
The following table lists the foods Crohn's sufferers are most likely to react badly to.

Food	Crohn's sufferers – percentage intolerant [2]
Wheat	69
Dairy	48
Yeast	31
Corn	24
Potato	17
Tap water	17
Banana, tomato, wine, eggs	all 14

Other foods poorly tolerated by Crohn's patients include baker's yeast, nuts, carbonated drinks, shellfish, pickles, most dried beans, broccoli, Brussels sprouts, chocolate, cocoa, lamb, onions, peas, peppercorns, radish, tomato, turnip, refined sugar, red meat, carrageenan-containing foods (additive 407), garlic, strong seasonings and raw fruit.

Following a period off all suspected food irritants, patients are re-introduced to single foods one day at a time, while they keep a detailed diet diary. Once they avoid their particular food irritants, patients usually remain symptom free. Most people require expert help and supervision to establish and keep off troublesome foods. Foods least likely to aggravate are lean chicken, rice and some vegetables.

An elemental diet reduces intestinal inflammation and permeability but this is an extremely difficult regimen to follow for both the doctor and patient. This is a programme of no normal foods but specific types of carbohydrate, protein and fatty acids.

Another possible irritant is toothpaste.[3] Toothpaste contains magnesium aluminium silicate and other abrasive compounds, some of which are absorbed and are known to irritate mucous membranes. Crohn's patients should buy toothpastes that are aluminium free, and avoid swallowing any.

Treatment
HERBS
To soothe, in powder or tablets: • *Liquorice* • *Marshmallow* • *Slippery elm*
To strengthen and heal (these may not be tolerated during periods of diarrhoea): • *Aloe* (with caution) • *Barberry* • *Echinacea* • *Golden seal* • *Psyllium* • *Raspberry leaf* • *Turmeric*

NOTE **All herbs and supplements should be introduced singly in case any of them cause an aggravation.**

DIET
Basically follow a 'paleolithic prescription', which is briefly explained on pages 225–33. Westernisation of diets is known to trigger various intestinal problems. Although a fibre-rich diet is now suggested for inflammatory intestinal diseases, I suggest refined foods such as white rice during acute bouts of diarrhoea.
Supplements
• *Efamol Marine* (evening primrose and fish oils) • *Vitamin E* • *Combined multivitamin and mineral* • *Lactobacillus acidophilus* • *Bifidobacteria* • *Lactobacillus bulgaricum*

DIARRHOEA

Description
Frequent and watery bowel motions, caused by too rapid a transit time of food through the digestive tract. This results in poor nutrient absorption, loss of fluid and minerals and may be serious, particularly in young children and the elderly. Attacks are commonly acute and accompanied by colicky pains, but it can be a long-term problem.

Causes
The cause needs to be traced. There could be a number of factors involved including viral, bacterial or protozoal infections, chemical agents, food poisoning, drugs, emotional disorders resulting in increased peristalsis, allergies or food intolerances and a number of diseases and dysfunctions.

NOTE *In severe or long-term cases, there may be mucus or blood in the stools, dehydration, anaemia and weakness. These severe symptoms require medical attention.*

Treatment

FLUID REPLACEMENT

Add to one litre of boiled, cooled water a dessertspoon of glucose powder, table sugar or honey plus a small teaspoon of salt.

The aim is to have sufficient fluid to prevent dehydration but not so much that it goes straight through. Half to one glassful sipped slowly every hour or so is usually well tolerated.

HERBS

• *Arrowroot* • *Echinacea* • *Oak bark* • *Raspberry leaf* • *Shepherd's purse* • *Slippery elm*

DIET

A bland low-fibre diet while stools are loose. Avoid irritants such as coffee, alcohol, hot spices. Other suggestions are given on pages 68–9.

Supplements

• *Lactobacillus acidophilus* • *Bifidobacteria* • *Pectin*

TISSUE SALTS OR CELLOIDS

• *Calc Phos* – for debility and poor assimilation • *Kali Mur* – regulates mucus secretions • *Nat Sulph* – for infected discharges • *Nat Mur* – balances body fluids

NOTE *Some anti-diarrhoeal drugs and antacids contain aluminium or magnesium, both of which can markedly aggravate diarrhoea. Always check labels carefully.*

DIVERTICULITIS

Description

Diverticulosis are small blind pouches or pockets in the bowel. In diverticulitis these are inflamed; there are generally cramping pains in the lower left abdomen.

Causes

Weakness in the walls of the bowel, often produced by chronic constipation, leading to the formation of pockets. The irritation and inflammation probably result from trapped faecal matter, a build up of bacteria or irritating substances.

CAUTION *Requires medical diagnosis. Large, infected pockets require professional treatment.*

Treatment

HERBS

• *Aloe gel* • *Chamomile* • *Dandelion* • *Echinacea* • *Liquorice* – not confectionery • *Oak bark* • *Senna with ginger* – if constipated • *Slippery elm powder* or *tablets* • *Yellow dock*

FROM THE KITCHEN

• *Linseed broth* – do not eat any seeds unless they are finely ground

DIET

If severe: rest, non-irritating diet, soothing herbs for one week (see Crohn's Disease, pages 86–7); then increase vegetables and fruit.

• *Whole grains* – a little to start and ensure that they are finely ground • *Carrot* and *cabbage juice* • *Sauerkraut*

Have small, regular, frequent meals. Wheat bran can be irritating.

TISSUE SALTS OR CELLOIDS

• *Calc Fluor* – strengthens body tissues

FLATULENCE
(flatus, intestinal wind, gas)

Description
Excessive formation of gases in the stomach or intestines which usually causes cramping pains or discomfort until the gas is passed or dissipates.

Causes
Eating too quickly, eating while agitated, allergies, also enzyme, pancreas, liver or gallbladder problems and a number of digestive orders.

Some foods have a bad reputation for causing flatulence, notably raw broccoli and cauliflower, dried beans, chick peas, lentils and onions.

Treatment
HERBS
Taken internally
• *Aniseed* • *Bergamot* • *Catnip* • *Chamomile* • *Peppermint* (see also Atonic dyspepsia, page 90)
Applied externally
• *Olbas* or *lavender oil* – gently massaged into the abdomen
FROM THE KITCHEN
• *Apple cider vinegar* – 1 teaspoon in water before meals • *Caraway* • *Cardamon* • *Chilli* • *Cinnamon* • *Cloves* • *Cumin* • *Dill* • *Ginger* • *Lemon* – a small quantity of fresh juice with food helps digestion • *Lovage* • *Savory*
DIET
Introduce new foods one at a time and in small quantities. Eat slowly, chew thoroughly. Always have meals in relaxed surroundings, and don't eat while working.
Supplements
• *Charcoal tablets* – occasional use only
• *Papain tablets* or *digestive enzymes*

TISSUE SALTS OR CELLOIDS
• *Mag Phos* – reduces spasms • *Calc Phos* – stimulates gastric juices

GASTRITIS

Description
Inflammation of the stomach lining. The general symptoms include abdominal pain, bloating, nausea and headache.

Attacks may be acute or chronic. Severe symptoms include diarrhoea and vomiting. Gastritis may lead to ulcers so should be treated promptly.

Causes
These include sensitive stomach mucosa, hyperacidity, excessive alcohol, coffee, aspirin or other drugs, poisonous substances, allergies or infections. Severe attacks should be referred for professional treatment and if food poisoning is suspected, seek medical advice.

Attacks may be acute (with a sudden onset and short-term) or chronic (long-lasting).

Treatment
HERBS
• *Arrowroot* • *Barberry bark* • *Liquorice* • *Marshmallow* • *Meadowsweet* • *Rosehip* • *Slippery elm*
FROM THE KITCHEN
• *Barley* or *rice water* • *Ginger* • *Thyme tea* • *Turmeric*
DIET
• *Potato broth* • *Soy milk*
Follow a bland diet initially, avoid irritants and suspected allergens. Eat small, regular meals.
TISSUE SALTS OR CELLOIDS
• *Ferr Phos* • *Kali Mur*

HEARTBURN (acid regurgitation and burning)

Description
The reflux of acid from the stomach is usually accompanied by a burning sensation in the region of the centre of the chest and a nasty, bitter taste in the mouth.

Causes
A number of possible causes, including excessive stomach acidity, nervous tension, over-eating and structural problems in the oesophagus or stomach, such as hiatus hernia.

Treatment
HERBS
• *Alfalfa* • *Chamomile* • *Marshmallow* • *Meadowsweet* • *Slippery elm powder*
FROM THE KITCHEN
• *Barley water*
DIET
Eat small, frequent meals. Avoid late suppers, chilli and highly spiced or seasoned foods.
TISSUE SALTS OR CELLOIDS
• *Mag Phos* – reduces spasms • *Nat Phos* – reduces acidity, nausea • *Silicea* – strengthens connective tissue

For other suggestions see Gastritis (page 89) and Ulcers (pages 92–3).

INDIGESTION (dyspepsia)

These are the common terms referring to digestive problems. Where the indigestion is not being caused by any serious disease, it may be useful to divide such problems into three categories:
• Atonic dyspepsia – under-functioning
• Nervous indigestion
• Over-active indigestion – as in Heartburn.

ATONIC DYSPEPSIA

Description
This refers to under-activity of the stomach muscles or inadequate gastric juices.

The types of symptoms one would expect would be a feeling of fullness that stays for hours after eating a normal-sized meal, bloating, whole pieces of food in faecal matter, nausea, belching and slow transit time.

Treatment
HERBS
• *Agrimony* • *Barberry bark* • *Chilli* • *Dandelion* • *Gentian* • *Ginger* • *Golden seal*
FROM THE KITCHEN
• *Apple cider vinegar* – 1 teaspoon in water before meals or incorporated in the meal
• *Fresh lemon juice*
Culinary herbs such as: • *Bay* • *Coriander* • *Fenugreek* • *Lovage* • *Marjoram* • *Oregano* • *Savory* • *Tarragon*
DIET
Some find that if the protein part of the meal is eaten first this stimulates the gastric juices. Don't drink any liquid with meals.
• *Charcoal tablets* – these absorb toxins; do not use if on pharmaceutical medication as the charcoal will also reduce the effects of many drugs. Charcoal is a short-term remedy.
• *Digestive enzymes*
TISSUE SALTS OR CELLOIDS
• *Calc Phos* – stimulates gastric juices

NERVOUS INDIGESTION

Description
The symptons are similar to those in Atonic Dyspepsia although the nervous origin should be fairly obvious.

Causes
Often there is intermittent diarrhoea and constipation, particularly during stressful times. When a person is emotionally upset it is better to postpone a meal.

Treatment
HERBS
• *Chamomile* • *Hops* • *Lemon balm*
• *Vervain*
DIET
If the problem is long term, then small frequent meals are better.
Supplements
• *Vitamin B complex*
TISSUE SALTS OR CELLOIDS
• *Kali Phos*

OVER-ACTIVE INDIGESTION

For excess acidity problems, refer to suggested remedies for Heartburn opposite and Ulcers (pages 92–3).

IRRITABLE COLON
(spastic colon syndrome or intestinal syndrome)

Description
Abdominal pain without internal intestinal inflammation, often accompanied by alternating episodes of constipation and diarrhoea. The pain can be constant or intermittent, often there is mucus in the stools (it looks stringy) and the patient feels anxious.

Causes
Poor handling of stress is frequently said to be the cause. The diet may contain insufficient fibre or an allergen, such as dairy foods. This problem occurs in the absence of diseases of the bowel but it is important to have this verified by a health practitioner.

Treatment
HERBS
• *Agrimony* • *Catnip* • *Chamomile*
These herbs can also be used in the form of enemas. Enemas need to be used with caution as they can damage the bowel wall and upset the bacterial balance. Don't use enemas when there is diarrhoea or inflammation. See details of administration under Constipation, pages 83–4.
• *Peppermint oil* – gives symptomatic relief but has to be in enteric-coated capsules (Mintec) and may have adverse reactions because aromatic oils taken internally are in the nature of drugs • *Psyllium* • *Slippery elm*
OTHER
Since 1984, medical researchers have wondered about the connection between an irritable mind and an irritable bowel. The *Lancet* has reported on the successful use of hypnotherapy in treating functional bowel disorders.[4] You know from your own experience that the bowel responds to stress!

I would also recommend relaxation and meditation techniques.

NAUSEA AND VOMITING

Causes
Over-eating, food poisoning, poor digestion, liver and gallbladder problems, emotional upsets, diseases and infections. Pain and some pharmaceutical drugs may also cause nausea, as may excess tea, coffee, alcohol and allergies.

Treatment
HERBS
• *Basil* • *Bergamot* • *Chamomile* • *Ginger*
• *Golden seal* • *Peppermint* • *Raspberry leaf*
DIET
Fluids should be taken frequently, in small amounts, as it is easy to become

dehydrated if vomiting is prolonged. See also Diarrhoea, pages 87–8.

Supplements
• *Vitamin B1* – if chronic or recurring
• *Peppermint* or *olbas oil* – 1–2 drops in a glass of warm water, sipped slowly, up to 3 times daily

---

NOTE **Prolonged or violent vomiting needs professional treatment. Food poisoning needs to be reported to the Department of Health by a medical practitioner.**

TISSUE SALTS OR CELLOIDS
• *Nat Phos* • *Nat Sulph*

ULCERATIVE COLITIS

Description
An inflammatory bowel disease characterised by bloody diarrhoea, lower abdominal cramps, weight loss and fever. May be accompanied by rectal fissures (cracks), abscesses or haemorrhoids. It has similarities to Crohn's Disease and requires a medical diagnosis.

Treatment
Most of the recommendations given under Crohn's Disease are appropriate. The most common food irritants are wheat and dairy products, so it is certainly worth avoiding these on a trial basis. *Psyllium* has been recommended for the routine management of ulcerative colitis.[5]

ULCERS – STOMACH AND DUODENAL

Description
A defect in the lining of the affected part of the digestive tract, so that the stomach acid is eroding the protective surface. It

may also be that excess acid is being produced by the secretory glands. Sometimes the pyloric sphincter is faulty (the ring of muscles that controls the emptying of the stomach contents into the duodenum). This leads to irritation in the duodenum. A burning or gnawing pain is felt, often in the central abdominal area. The pain often occurs about an hour after meals and at night.

Causes
A bacterium (*Heliobacter pylori*) is now thought to be a primary cause. Other causes include faulty mucous membranes (linings) and excess acidity. Sometimes there is a hereditary pattern. Worry, poor handling of stress, allergies and sensitivities, irregular eating habits, lifestyle deficiencies or excesses, such as alcohol, may contribute to the development of ulcers and then prevent healing. Ulcers are a side effect of some pharmaceutical drugs, as you will see under Arthritis (page 38) and in the *MIMS Annual*.

Treatment

NOTE **Any new remedies or foods must be tried one at a time because most people with peptic ulcers are extremely sensitive and particularly individualistic.**

HERBS
Soothing herbs: • *Arrowroot* • *Chamomile* • *Liquorice* • *Marshmallow* • *Slippery elm* – powder before meals
Antibiotic herbs: • *Echinacea* • *Garlic* • *Reishi*
Healing herbs: • *Aloe gel* • *Bayberry* • *Ginger* • *Golden seal* – not recommended if you have high blood pressure • *Meadowsweet* • *Turmeric* • *Verbena*

DIET

Eating often relieves the discomfort and pain, so small, frequent meals are suggested. Some people find that soy milk and bananas are helpful between-meal snacks.

Milk might appear to provide short-term relief, but in a four-week trial it was revealed that patients on a predominantly milk diet did not heal as well as those on a normal hospital diet. At least give soy milk a month's trial.

Cabbage juice is one of the traditional remedies; start with a small quantity and build up to 1 glass per day, diluting it with carrot juice if necessary for palatability.

A broth made from linseeds is often helpful. Ensure the diet is high in fibre and flavonoids (that is, vegetables and fruit).

Citrus fruits, coffee, alcohol and drugs may aggravate.

American herbalists recommend chilli powder, starting with ¼ teaspoon twice daily; mix chilli to a paste with a little water then fill the cup with warm water. Sip slowly. The dose should be gradually increased to 1–2 teaspoons a day. I found this hard to take at first, but got accustomed to it by adding warmed apple juice. Chilli is quite palatable combined with some herbal teas. It is certainly an effective circulatory stimulant. You could also make an infusion of a dried or fresh hot chilli.

Supplements
• *Lactobacillus acidophilus* • *Bifidobacteria*
• *Papain* • *Fish oils*

TISSUE SALTS OR CELLOIDS
• *Ferr Phos* – a good remedy to start with

OTHER

Research shows that not only do cigarette smokers have a higher incidence of ulcers than non-smokers, but their healing time is longer and recurrence is more frequent. On the other hand, *vitamin A* was shown to reduce the healing time.

Psychotherapy, regular relaxation and meditation practices are beneficial.

CHAPTER 6

FEMALE PROBLEMS AND PREGNANCY

Menstruation should not be considered as an illness although it is unusual to meet a female who does not suffer from at least a small amount of premenstrual tension, period cramping, some irregularities in the cycle or menopausal symptons. I suggest that all women should take steps to alleviate even the mildest of their symptoms, because in some cases minor inconveniences develop into more troublesome or chronic problems and, after all, we should aim for optimal health and wellbeing.

The average age for commencing menstruation is twelve and a half, but it can start at any time between eight and seventeen years. In the early stages, the cycle tends to be irregular. Most women stop menstruating at about fifty years of age; usually the periods gradually lessen in frequency and flow, but there may instead be heavy bleeding or other symptoms.

A medical diagnosis should be sought for severe pain, unusual or excessive bleeding and serious irregularities. Vaginal discharges, sores and infections should be checked by a medical practitioner because without pathology tests it is difficult to know if the condition is a STD (sexually transmitted disease). If people are too embarrassed to go to their family doctor, they can go to the nearest STD clinic: the Department of Health in each state has information on clinics and booklets about the diseases. STDs should be treated promptly to avoid complications such as infertility.

For mild symptoms, try simple remedies first. If you need to see a practitioner, never be afraid to ask questions or to seek a second opinion.

AMENORRHOEA
(absence of periods)

Description
Primary amenorrhoea
No menstruation at puberty. If the periods have not started by age sixteen then a medical consultation is required. Starting ages can vary enormously but the common age is 12–13 years.
Secondary amenorrhoea
This is cessation of periods after having menstruated. It is normal during pregnancy and lactation, and after menopause. Menstruation can stop for other reasons.

CAUTION *Always check for pregnancy.*

Causes
Primary amenorrhoea
Trauma, hormonal causes or obstruction. May be related to low oestrogen levels.
Secondary amenorrhoea
Certain drugs, including contraceptive pills and heroin. Sometimes when women stop taking the Pill they do not have periods for some months or even years. Some serious diseases, such as diabetes and tumours, may upset the menstrual cycle. Other causes include ovarian cysts, infections, emotional upsets, faulty diet, excessive exercising, anaemia, anorexia, obesity, accidents or a bad chill. Life

---

NOTE *If you are not menstruating you are probably infertile, but as you won't know when you start ovulating again, it would be wise to use some form of contraception if you don't wish to get pregnant.*

---

changes, such as overseas trips, often affect menstruation.

Treatment
HERBS
• *Aloe* • *Chamomile* • *Evening primrose oil* • *Ginger* • *Liquorice* • *Sarsaparilla*

See also the list of oestrogenic herbs, page 113. Herbalists may use some other herbs which are not available to the general public.

FROM THE KITCHEN
• *Parsley* – the simplest method is to eat a handful per day in salads • *Marjoram* – as a weak tea

DIET
Supplements
• *Vitamin B complex* or a *multi-vitamin*
• An organic iron formula

TISSUE SALTS OR CELLOIDS
• *Kali Sulph*

OTHER
• Cold sitzbath – see page 116.

CANDIDA ALBICANS (also known as monilia or thrush)

Description
Fungal infection. The fungi normally inhabit the mouth, throat, intestines and vagina. When these areas are not 'healthy', symptoms of infection occur. The mucous membranes (linings of the skin) have a patchy white colour giving a speckled look (which is why it is called thrush). Under normal conditions, useful bacteria coexist with the fungi to prevent multiplication. If the vaginal *Candida* fungi develop, there is usually a thick white discharge, sometimes looking a bit like cottage cheese, accompanied by irritation and inflammation.

Causes

Antibiotics are a common cause because they kill the useful as well as the harmful bacteria and upset the body's balance. Fungi can also multiply in alkaline conditions, especially where there is warmth and a plentiful supply of sugars. Cystitis sufferers are prone to attacks of vaginal thrush and in these cases antibiotics will usually worsen the problem. An infected partner can also pass on the infection or cause reinfection which is why *both partners need treatment*.

Semen is alkaline, whereas the vaginal mucous membranes are ideally slightly acidic so this may also be a contributing factor. Sponging after sex with diluted apple cider vinegar or diluted fresh lemon juice may help. Use about 1 teaspoon to a cup of tepid water.

Oral contraceptives are also a cause in some cases.

Treatment

HERBS

Taken internally
• *Aloe* • *Barberry bark* • *Calendula* • *Chamomile* • *Corn silk* • *Garlic* • *Golden seal* • *Lemon grass* • *Pau d'arco*

Applied externally
Douche: 6 drops of *tea tree oil* to a cup of tepid water, or use tea tree oil pessaries.

FROM THE KITCHEN

• *Thyme* – drink as a tea or use tepid, strained tea as a douche • *Apple cider vinegar* – diluted as a douche • *Pure yoghurt* – applied in and around the vagina • *Fresh lemon juice* – diluted as a douche or wash

DIET

• *Cabbage juice* has antifungal properties.
• *Olive oil* – 4–6 teaspoons a day. The easiest way to take this is as a salad oil mixed with lemon juice and herbs. While doing so you need to ensure that all other dietary fats are at the absolute minimum.

Eat a high-fibre diet with plenty of vegetables and a reasonable amount of whole grains including oats, buckwheat and millet.

No sugar or refined starches for two months (this means no white flour, white rice, white spaghetti, ice cream, soft drinks, honey etc.).

Use *culinary herbs and spices* freely in cooking, especially cinnamon, ginger, lemon balm, mustard, rosemary and turmeric.

Supplements
• *Lactobacillus acidophilus* • *Bifidobacteria*

OTHER

It is also advisable to eliminate all yeast and mould foods for a test period of at least five weeks. The list is as follows.
• *Bread* – unless labelled 'yeast-free' (Ryvita and similar biscuits are okay)
• *Mushrooms* • *Yeast supplements* • *Vegemite, Marmite* • *Cheese* • *Yoghurt* • *Buttermilk* • *Sour cream* • *Vinegar* • *Pickles*
• *Canned tomatoes and tomato products*
• *Soy products – tofu, soy sauce, miso* • *Wine*
• *Beer* • *All preserved meats – corned beef, salami, devon, etc.* • *Peanuts, peanut butter*
• *Melons – all types* • *Canned fruit* • *Dried fruit* • *Grapes* • *Olives in vinegar* • *Bought salad dressings*

Assuming the condition has cleared within this time, then small quantities of these foods can usually be reintroduced one at a time. Check vitamin supplements as some contain yeast.

Avoid perfumed soaps, talcum powder and vaginal deodorants. Don't wear nylon underwear, tight jeans or tights as the fungi like a warm, moist environment. Change underwear daily.

CANDIDIASIS

Description
The *Candida* fungus has multiplied in the body tissues and organs (systemic). As everyone has this particular fungus in their body, an over-abundance may be difficult to diagnose, but an excessive quantity causes many different problems. These include recurring respiratory and other infections, depression, headaches, swollen glands, weight gain or loss without changing diet or lifestyle, dizziness, poor handling of stress, skin eruptions, premenstrual and menstrual difficulties, digestive disorders, fatigue, intermittent diarrhoea or constipation, poor concentration and memory, 'fuzzy' thinking, food intolerances, vision disturbances, muscle pain, weakened circulation, insomnia or excess sleeping and hair changes.

Mercifully, you don't get *all* these problems.

Causes
Basically a weakened immune status allows the fungus to spread. It may be brought on by steroidal drugs, antibiotics, anti-cancer therapies where the immune system is depressed, intestinal diseases and liver malfunctioning.

Treatment
Most of the internal recommendations for Candida Albicans (opposite) are appropriate. Refer also to Chronic Fatigue Syndrome in Chapter 10 (pages 161–3) for ways of improving the immune system.

CYSTS – OVARIAN

Description
A sac containing a liquid such as fat or a semi-solid substance. Most are harmless but some cause blockages, pressure or irritation. They occasionally become infected.

NOTE **A gynaecological check is necessary for diagnosis.**

Causes
Not known. Many naturopaths relate cysts to inefficient lymph drainage or liver function.

Treatment
HERBS
• *Calendula* • *Clivers* • *Dandelion* • *Milk thistle*
The herbs listed under Liver Sluggishness (pages 144–6) can also be used.
DIET
A low-fat diet, with no alcohol or coffee.
Supplements
• *Beta-carotene*
TISSUE SALTS OR CELLOIDS
• *Calc Fluor* • *Silicea*

DYSMENORRHOEA
(period pain)

Description
When the lining of the uterus (womb) is shed each month it triggers the muscle in the uterus to contract so that the menstrual blood may be pushed through the cervix (mouth of the womb). These contractions can cause pain, which may be mild to severe, and may be accompanied by heavy or scanty periods, usually with clotting. Some women also experience

lower back pain, leg cramps, diarrhoea or constipation, nausea and headaches. It's a cold, cramp-like pain which may be why many women just want to lie down with a hot-water bottle. Generally, the pain is intermittent over the first few days of the period.

Causes

If the pain is severe, a gynaecological check is necessary because there are a number of possible causes, such as infection, fibroids, cysts, miscarriage, endometriosis, foreign bodies including IUDs, tumours, tight cervix, fluid retention, general congestion and emotional or psychological reasons. Some people think that when a woman is not having a fulfilling sex life or if she is in an unsatisfactory relationship this may also cause cramping in the pelvic region. High oestrogen levels have also been suggested as a causative factor.

Treatment

The following recommendations are not for those requiring medical attention, although they may be considered as adjunct treatments for severe cases.

HERBS
• *Bergamot*   • *Bilberry*   • *Chamomile* • *Cramp bark* • *Dong quai* • *Feverfew* • *Lemon balm* • *Sarsaparilla* • *Scullcap* • *Valerian* • *Verbena* • *Wild yam*

Generally, the results are better with a herbal consultation so that an appropriate, individual formula may be worked out. Alternatively, you may choose one or two of the suggested remedies after reading Chapter 16, 'Recommended Herbs'.

Initially you will need to take the herbs daily for two or three months, and then

a few days prior to and during menstruation.

FROM THE KITCHEN
• *Caraway* • *Ginger* • *Lovage* • *Marjoram* • *Parsley* • *Peppermint*

DIET
Constipation may contribute to the general congestion, so avoid processed foods and have a high whole-grain and vegetable diet plus an adequate fluid intake.

Supplements
• *Calcium* • *Magnesium* • *Vitamin B complex,* plus additional *B6* if there is fluid retention • *DL-phenylalanine* • *Vitamin C and bioflavonoids*

TISSUE SALTS OR CELLOIDS
• *Calc Phos* • *Mag Phos*

OTHER
• *Cold sitzbaths* (hip baths) – one a day for a few minutes, at least a week before periods • *Yoga* and *relaxation* techniques often help but they need to be done consistently; an appropriate and regular exercise programme is also recommended • Lower back and abdominal *massage* between periods • Hot *herbal foot baths* may also be helpful • Because of the liver's role in regulating hormones, I often use a strong *liver formula* in such cases

Acupuncture can also be helpful for pain. You might also like to try acupressure. One of the points for menstrual pain is found by putting your hand palm down on a flat surface and then bringing your fingers close together. Pull the thumb very close to the index finger and you will see a little bulge of muscles. In the middle of this bulge, apply pressure with your spare thumb for several minutes. There are a number of acupressure books giving other points for pain relief.

GENITAL HERPES

Genital herpes can be confused with other genito-urinary problems. If you have it discuss the problem with your partner, so that a barrier method of contraception can be used. There is some evidence that the virus can be transmitted even though the sores or discharge are not active.

CAUTION **This is a notifiable disease – you must have a medical diagnosis.**

Description
Usually starts with itchy, tender feeling. Sex is generally uncomfortable or painful. The first visible signs are small, red, raised spots in the genital area which develop into blisters and then ulcer-like sores. Some people have a mild fever, swollen glands, feel run down and have a smelly, yellow or green discharge. It is best to avoid sex when the sores are visible as they are infectious.

Cause
Virus. It is a STD (sexually transmitted disease) and may be spread by mouth also. People with cold sores on their mouths can spread the infection to their own genitals. The infectious period is uncertain. It commonly recurs and is seemingly brought on or aggravated by stress, trauma and poor hygiene.

Treatment
There is no known cure at the moment but many sufferers find that naturopathic treatments can at least reduce the number and intensity of the attacks.

NOTE **The treatment for men is the same as for women.**

HERBS
Taken internally
• *Alfalfa* • *Calendula* • *Cat's claw* • *Chamomile* • *Echinacea* • *Ginseng* • *Golden seal* • *Lemon balm* • *Linden* • *Liquorice* • *Pau d'arco* • *Reishi* • *Thuja* • *Thyme*

Applied externally
A range to choose from: • *Aloe gel* – use the fresh gel from inside the leaves or non-coloured commercial products • *Calendula ointment* – mixed to a paste with calcium ascorbate powder • *Lemon balm* – mixed to a paste with liquorice powder • *St John's wort* (Hypericum) or *chamomile oil* • *Thuja* – ointment or diluted oil

Pharmacies also have ointments that limit the spread and ease the pain.

FROM THE KITCHEN
• *Clove tea compress* – warm • Bath or wash using warm salty water or sodium bicarbonate

DIET
• Pure *apple juice* • Fresh *vegetable juice*

Diet should be high in fish, chicken, milk, cheese, lamb, beans, bean sprouts, most fruit and vegetables except peas; avoid gelatin, chocolate, carob, coconut, whole wheat and white flour, peanuts, soya beans, wheat germ.

Supplements
• *Vitamin C* (non-acidic form) and *bioflavonoids* • *Brewer's yeast* or *vitamin B complex* • *Halibut oil capsule* or *beta-carotene* • *Vitamin E* – the capsule can also be cut and used externally • *Zinc* • *L-lysine* – up to 1g per day • *Garlic* – 6 capsules per day, in divided doses after food

OTHER
• Bed rest is suggested if you have bad outbreaks • Don't use scented soaps, bubble baths, talcum powder • Take extra care with hygiene • Don't wear nylon underwear • Homoeopathic treatment or a supervised fast are recommended alternative treatments

---

NOTE *If you are pregnant and have genital herpes, you must advise your obstetrician as the virus can be transmitted to a baby during birth.*

LEUCORRHOEA

Description
A white or yellow vaginal discharge. It is a symptom of a disorder either in the reproductive organs or elsewhere in the body. The glands of the vagina and cervix normally secrete a variable amount of mucus-like fluid. Leucorrhoea is a thick, creamy-yellowish colour, not the normal white or colourless secretion.

CAUTION *Leucorrhoea requires a medical diagnosis to distinguish it from thrush and other vaginal infections.*

Causes
Often trichomoniasis, especially where the discharge is yellow, smelly and accompanied by itching. Sometimes it is related to poor nutritional status, debility, hormonal imbalances, emotional upsets, diseases and infections of the reproductive organs, including gonorrhoea, bacteria and fungi.

Treatment
Depending on the cause, it may require medical treatment.
HERBS
Taken internally
• *Barberry bark* • *Echinacea* • *Golden seal* • *Raspberry leaf* • *Thyme*
Applied externally
• *Tea tree oil* pessaries
As a douche or external wash: • *Liquorice or calendula petal tea* – cooled and strained (1 teaspoon herbs to a cup of water) • *Tea tree or sandalwood oil* – 6 drops to a cup of tepid water • *Iodine* – 2–3 drops to a cup of tepid water
FROM THE KITCHEN
• Dilute *apple cider vinegar* douche – 1 dessertspoon to a cup of tepid water
DIET
If it is known that the oestrogen levels are low use the following in cooking, as sprouts or herbal teas: • *Alfalfa* • *Aniseed* • *Fennel* • *Hops* • *Parsley* • *Red clover* • *Sage* • *Soya beans*
Supplements
• *Vitamin C and bioflavonoids* • *Garlic capsules* – 6 per day in divided doses after food • *Vitamin E* • *Zinc*
TISSUE SALTS OR CELLOIDS
• *Kali Mur*

MENORRHAGIA

Description
Excessive menstrual flow.

Causes
Pelvic inflammatory disease, fibroids, hormonal disturbances, tumours, endometriosis, malpositioned uterus and abnormal conditions of pregnancy. Sometimes the cause is not known. Excessive menstruation may lead to anaemia.

Treatment

This is another condition that requires medical diagnosis as any loss of blood, other than normal period flow, could be due to a serious condition.

HERBS

Not all the herbs used by herbalists are available at retail outlets, but the following may be helpful.

• *Bayberry* • *Chaste tree* • *Golden seal* • *Sage* • *Shepherd's purse* • *Wild yam* • *Yarrow*

Externally

A few times just prior to periods, you might try a cooled, strained *raspberry leaf tea* as a douche.

DIET

• High in green and yellow vegetables and fruit

Supplements

• *Vitamin B complex* • *Iron* – to offset blood loss until the problem is corrected

---

NOTE *If you take too much iron it interferes with calcium absorption.*

TISSUE SALTS OR CELLOIDS

• *Calc Fluor* • *Ferr Phos*

MENSTRUAL PROBLEMS GENERALLY – scanty flow, irregular periods, spotting

Causes

Cysts, fibroids, infections, tumours, hormonal disturbances. (Again, the cause can only be established by a gynaecological examination.)

Treatment

HERBS

Taken internally

Uterine tonics: • *Chaste tree* • *Ginger* • *Golden seal* • *Motherwort* • *Raspberry leaf*

Plants with progesterone precursors

You will see in Chapter 16 that these herbs have a number of different actions. They are obviously useful in cases of known low progesterone levels, such as PMT-A (page 112). • *Chaste tree* • *Fenugreek* – sprouts are more effective • *Sarsaparilla* • *Wild yam*

DIET

Oestrogenic plants

These are obviously useful during menopause.

• *Alfalfa* – best used as sprouts • *Aniseed* • *Dong quai* • *Fennel* • *Hops* • *Liquorice* – not the confectionery • *Parsley* – best used fresh; a handful daily • *Red clover* – best used as sprouts • *Sage* – as a cold tea helps hot flushes • *Soya beans* – best used as sprouts but difficult to sprout in cold weather

PREGNANCY

PRE-PREGNANCY

'The best birthday gift a mother can give her baby is a good start in life'

Dr Richard Aubry

The ideal starting point is for both parents to be as healthy as possible before conception.

• It is suspected that damaged sperm and poor quality ova may relate to birth defects. (There is still no scientific explanation for 70 per cent of birth defects.)

• Sound nutritional and lifestyle habits, including avoidance of potentially harmful chemical substances (cigarettes, alcohol, excess caffeine from coffee and some soft drinks, lead, pesticides and so on) are now being suggested prior to conception for men as well as women.

• Research suggests that there should be a new category of recommended dietary allowances for 'women in anticipation of pregnancy'. Animal studies show that low birthweight in offspring can be produced by damage to the germ cells of the mother before mating by chemicals, radiation or nutrient deficits.[1]

• Compared to mothers of normal weight babies, low birthweight mums commonly have diets that are low in protein, energy and nutrient density, that is, they eat poorer quality foods. Statistically, low birthweight babies have more health problems.

Ideally, you should put any improvements into operation *before* you intend to get pregnant, as your body needs time to adjust to your improved lifestyle and eating habits, as well as to biochemical and hormonal changes that take place during pregnancy. Additionally, some of the healthier foods may not agree with you, but during pregnancy you may not be able to distinguish food reactions from the other changes occurring in your body. If you wait until you are pregnant and you have morning sickness, you're not likely to be enthusiastic about shopping for and preparing new foods. When you're not familiar with things it always takes longer. Also, if you're not feeling great you mightn't like the healthy new foods – or even some of those you normally enjoy.

When you stop some of your bad habits (coffee, alcohol, cigarettes or excess sugary treats) you can experience quite severe withdrawal symptoms, especially if you suddenly give them up, so be prepared for this.

Physical fitness

Before pregnancy, get as physically fit as you reasonably can. Your tummy, back and legs are going to be put under pressure. After birth, your arms and shoulders need to be in good condition to breast-feed and carry your baby. Many women are concerned that their abdominal muscles are very slack after childbirth. You can't start an abdominal strengthening programme during pregnancy although it is good to do basic aerobic activities as well as some mobilising and strengthening exercises – refer to pages 107–8.

SOME SPECIFIC *PRE-PREGNANCY* EXERCISES

Generally, I recommend doing exercises you enjoy but tummy exercises and push-ups are the exception. Most people don't like doing them. Try partial sit-ups if you are unfit, or full sit-ups if you are fit (although keep knees bent to prevent back damage). Bent-knee push-ups (push-ups from a kneeling position) strengthen arms.

Avoiding environmental and ingested toxins

If you have had unusual exposure to pesticides, heavy metals, dioxins or you have lived a long time in a heavy traffic zone, before becoming pregnant you might want to contact the Foresight Association, 124 Louisa Road, Birchgrove NSW 2041, to get information and the name of a doctor near you who practises environmental medicine. You could also visit a naturopath or health farm to go on a detoxification programme prior to pregnancy.

You ought to stop all non-essential pharmaceutical and social drugs.

I should add that if we all waited until we were perfect and toxin-free before becoming pregnant, then the human race would cease to exist.

INFERTILITY

Description

Pregnancy not occurring after one year of 'normal' marital relations without contraceptives, or if the woman conceives but aborts repeatedly.

Causes

A combination of factors is common and there is a relationship to anxiety and fatigue in either or both partners.

FEMALES

Nutritional deficiencies, hormonal imbalances, infections, endometriosis – which can lead to a blockage in the fallopian tubes – tumours, developmental anomalies of the reproductive organs. It is sometimes caused by hormonal imbalances after oral contraceptives have been discontinued, although in such cases this usually corrects itself in time.

MALES

Commonly due to sperm deficiencies (low sperm count, impaired motility or other abnormalities). According to *Current Medical Diagnosis and Treatment* the male partner is 'at fault' in about 40 per cent of cases of infertility.

NOTE *A medical diagnosis is usually required to help find the cause.*

Treatment

When I first started work in a naturopathic clinic, I was amazed at the number of pregnancies in women of all ages who attended it and I am convinced that this was due to the high level of nutritional supplementation used at that clinic. Infertility is one of the few instances where I do find it beneficial to prescribe a number of supplements. When the woman becomes pregnant these are mostly phased out.

BOTH PARTNERS – LIFESTYLE AND DIETARY CHANGES

• Improve levels of fitness.
• Lose weight if obese.
• Eliminate tobacco and alcohol.
• Avoid refined carbohydrates such as sugar, soft drinks, chocolate, cakes, biscuits, white flour, ice cream and processed foods.
• Have a high vegetable intake, also fruit and reasonable quantities of yoghurt, seeds including sunflower and pumpkin, (nuts and seeds are very high in calories so these are used sparingly if there is a weight problem).
• Use whole grains, especially rolled oats and wheat germ.
• Use unheated linseed oil on cooked food and in salads.
• Take a combined multi-vitamin and mineral supplement.
• It may be necessary to treat specific health or emotional problems as well as following these general guidelines.

HERBS

Males
• *Ginseng* (Korean or Chinese)

Females
• *Golden seal* • *Raspberry leaf* • *Red clover*
• *Sarsaparilla* • *Sweet violet*

DIET

Females
• *Buckwheat* and *berries*

Supplements for males
• *Vitamin C 1000mg* • *Vitamin E 500IU*
• *Zinc 60mg* (to be taken at a different time of the day from the multi-vitamin and mineral)

Supplements for females
• *Vitamin C and bioflavonoids* (to be taken at a different time of the day from the multi-vitamin and mineral)

OTHER

Males

• It has been suggested that very tight-fitting trousers should be avoided.
• Sitting in a hot bath should be avoided.
• Another suggestion is cold sitzbaths every day for 3–4 minutes (this is simply a matter of sitting in very cold water up to hip level).

Females

Treat any infections, not only infectious diseases, but problems such as *Candida albicans*. Professional natural therapists have a range of therapies that may be helpful should the infection not be resolved by more simple remedies.

MISCARRIAGE PREVENTION

Causes of miscarriage

Chance (sometimes there is no explanation), hormonal imbalances, defective ovum or sperm, trauma, nutrient deficiencies, drugs, infections, diseases, tumours and uterus abnormalities.

Treatment

There are a few remedies which can be used for women with a history of miscarriage.

HERBS

Used prior to pregnancy to strengthen the uterus: • *Alfalfa* • *Chaste tree* • *Golden seal* • *Motherwort* • *Raspberry leaf* • *Sarsaparilla*

Raspberry leaf can be used throughout pregnancy. Many professional herbalists use other herbs which are not available at retail outlets.

DIET

• Eliminate coffee, alcohol and smoking.
• Also avoid all types of drugs unless required for life-threatening conditions.
• Increase protein intake.

Supplements

• After breakfast: a good quality combined multi-vitamin and mineral supplement plus an additional 250 IU vitamin E.
• After lunch and dinner: 1 iron supplement if your iron level is low. Some researchers advise that ferrous sulphate is not the best way to take iron supplements.

NOW YOU'RE PREGNANT!

Very soon after the sperm and the egg unite, baby's basic development plan is laid down. From fertilisation to twelve weeks pregnancy, your developing baby has increased over 2.5 million times. In nearly every case, before you know you are pregnant, the internal organs of the new baby are starting to form. From twelve weeks to full term, the developing baby's size increases only 230 times. It's obviously important to be as fit as possible and eat a healthy diet *before* the pregnancy is confirmed.

The Australian government hasn't set recommended intake levels for the forty essential nutrients, that is, those you must eat because your body doesn't manufacture them. Pantothenate, for example, has no 'official' daily intake level but it is known from animal experiments that deficiency of this vitamin leads to infertility or pathological reproduction without other symptoms in the adult. Of the nineteen nutrients with government Recommended Daily Intakes, fifteen of them have increased intake levels during pregnancy.

You can't take forty different supplements, so the first priority is to eat a wide variety of wholesome, natural foods. My definition of natural is something that looks, or at leasts tastes, like something that has grown; if it could think it would remember where it came from!

If you eat enough junk food, it will probably provide you and your baby with sufficient essential nutrients but you will also get more kilojoules, fat and salt than you need. Junk food is more likely to contain harmful food additives and unhealthy fats than unprocessed food. Basically, junk food provides more fat with fewer useful nutrients to you and your baby.

Of course, if we could all eat genuine, organically grown foods we'd be healthier. However, they're not always readily available or affordable. The next best thing is to peel everything that has removable skin and thoroughly wash all other fresh foods. Unfortunately, even in storage and shops, some fruits and vegetables are sprayed or dipped to prevent spoilage. Eat a wide variety of foods to avoid a build-up of a particular harmful chemical.

PROTEIN

The Australian Government Recommended Daily Protein Intake is 45g per day for an adult female, plus an additional 6g during pregnancy. Some doctors suggest that at least 70g is desirable to prevent pre-eclampsia (toxaemia) and to help baby's brain development – particularly in the last trimester.

Women of 25–34 years of age in Australia consume 80g of protein per day on average, so very few people (except some vegetarians) need to make a conscious effort to increase their protein intake during pregnancy. I suggest that all women eat a variety of protein foods, including vegetable protein, and reduce fat consumption.

Low-fat dairy products will give you additional protein and calcium, and so will canned fish with bones. As tuna is near the end of the food chain and thus could contain toxic waste residues, salmon and small fish such as sardines are preferable – with the oil or salty water drained out.

Vegetarians who eat eggs and dairy products should be able to get all the nutrients they need during pregnancy. Vegans and strict macrobiotic followers should discuss their diets with a health practitioner to ensure they get sufficient protein, calcium and vitamin B12 in particular.

There is no need to count and measure everything you eat. However, if you buy a book such as *Nutrition Almanac* (McGraw-Hill), which gives tables of a wide range of nutrients for about 1500 foods, you will be able to educate yourself gradually.

FOODS TO GIVE UP

• All sugary and refined foods – except for an occasional treat. Nothing offers your baby so little to grow on than refined sugar.

• Smoked seafoods and processed meats including pâté, liver sausage, devon, ham, bacon and salami. These contain undesirable preservatives and fats and are occasionally contaminated with bacteria.

• Peanuts – may contain damaging aflatoxins or pesticide residues.

• Soft cheeses such as camembert or ricotta, convenience foods and chicken may contain the *Listeria* bacteria, which affects pregnant women more than the general population. The mother may miscarry or the baby can be seriously affected although the mother may not necessarily feel dramatically ill. Dairy products can also contain this bacteria but in Australia regular checks are made for it.

• Non-dairy creamers, artificial sweeteners and additives.

Everything you eat should be nutrient-rich as opposed to high in kilojoules and low in just about everything else.

WEIGHT GAIN DURING PREGNANCY

Ideally, your weight should be within a normal range before conception. The current recommendation for weight gain is 8–14 kg. Some doctors feel that a somewhat higher gain is okay. However, excessive weight obviously makes you tired, affects your circulation and may lead to high blood pressure or other complications, as well as making a breech or caesarian delivery more difficult. Also, the unwanted fat is usually stored in the wrong places so it's harder to get back into shape after birth.

However, pregnancy is definitely *not* the time to be dieting because you don't want to deprive yourself or your baby of essentials nutrients and strength. There are stories of pregnant women doing all sorts of unhealthy things to get their weight right prior to their medical checks. Eating well should be the main priority rather than adhering to a computer-like weight-control programme.

At birth, most healthy babies weigh 2.9–3.6 kg. A junk-food diet could give you a weight gain of, say, 25 kg and a low-weight baby; a 9 kg weight gain throughout pregnancy or a nutrient-rich eating plan could give you a 3.5 kg baby.

As a guide, you will need to eat about 1250 kJ extra per day during pregnancy. This is very little and you should choose wholesome, low-fat foods as the extras.

SUPPLEMENTS

Iron is probably the most common supplement taken during pregnancy. It is often prescribed by a medical practitioner because a blood test shows that the mother's level is too low, or it may be self-prescribed for fatigue. Some forms of iron seem to make pregnant women constipated or cause nausea so you may need to try a few different forms.

Folate (vitamin B9) is increasingly being taken as it is one of the nutrients implicated in neurological disorders such as spina bifida. However, supplementation of iron and folate tends to reduce zinc metabolism.

For some other minerals, the levels inside the mother's cells may be low but the blood readings may be normal. Zinc has many biological functions such as being a vital part of growth, development and immunity.

Calcium is another commonly taken supplement and this mineral is somewhat antagonistic to iron. If you need to take both, then obviously don't have them at the same time.

Some minerals compete with others for absorption and utilisation, which is why it is suggested that a broad-spectrum combined multi-vitamin and mineral be taken at a different time of the day from a single supplement so that, overall, the body can balance the supplements.

Vitamin A (retinol) excesses and deficiencies are linked to birth defects so don't take more than 5000 IU as a daily supplement. Some researchers say that even eating liver regularly may lead to excess vitamin A. Liver has the added problem of being the major detoxification organ for both animals and humans so it is more likely to be chemically contaminated than other meats. In any event, if you eat plenty of fruit and vegetables you should easily get your vitamin A requirements.

Pyridozine (B6) is another problem vitamin: too little may cause an excessive build up of oestrogens and other difficulties and too much may cause neurological symptoms. The quantity in a multivitamin would not do any harm.

Riboflavin (B2) deficiency may not be apparent in a pregnant mother but could be the cause of low birth-weight and malformations. Good sources of riboflavin are yeast, liver, heart, rice, mushrooms, eggs, millet and soya beans. All multi-vitamins contain riboflavin.

Vitamin E is suggested as a supplement if you have a history of miscarriages. Vitamin E-rich foods include cold-pressed oils, seeds, nuts and whole grains. Some people don't recommend any vitamin supplements except for vitamin E.

Megadosing is never recommended during pregnancy. It is known, for example, that massive amounts of vitamin C supplementation are absorbed by the growing baby whose little body can adapt to this high level but immediately after birth it cannot adjust to a normal level and cases of infant deficiency have been observed under these circumstances.

FLUID INTAKE

There is no need to have additional fluids during pregnancy but you should get at least 6–8 cups of fluid per day. You will probably find that you have to urinate more than usual, especially during early and late pregnancy, but do not cut back on fluids as these are needed for circulation and carrying nutrients, to help overcome constipation, to regulate temperature, to keep the kidneys and urinary tract healthy and for baby's growth.

If you can afford it, a water filter is a good idea.

Drugs

Both prescribed and over-the-counter drugs are best avoided during pregnancy. This includes most laxatives, diuretics, pain relievers such as aspirin and so on. The Congenital Abnormalities Subcommittee of the Australian Drug Evaluation Committee has published a small booklet entitled *Medicines in Pregnancy* (AGPS, Canberra) which categorises the risk of pharmaceutical drugs during pregnancy. *MIMS Annual* contains many cautions and contraindications for the use of pharmaceuticals.

If you have to take a pharmaceutical drug during pregnancy it is doubly important to be on a super-healthy diet and I would recommend taking a broad spectrum combined multi-vitamin and mineral.

Medicinal herbs

Most professional herbalists do not recommend medicinal herbs during pregnancy but some of the exceptions are given in this chapter. Obviously if you have an infection it is better to use odourless garlic, propolis (a product of bees) or reishi (a medicinal mushroom) at the early stages rather than antibiotics. Raspberry leaf is safe throughout pregnancy as a uterus strengthener. Chicory and dandelion are coffee substitutes and mild digestive tonics.

Pregnant women should avoid cinnamon, cloves, nutmeg and sage. Other common culinary herbs are not contra-indicated in the normal quantities used in recipes.

Physical activity

• Walking, cycling or swimming – for at least 30 minutes a day.
• Mobilising and strengthening exercises,

10–15 minutes twice daily, including squatting, ankle exercises and non-strenuous yoga-type exercises.

• Use a footstool while sitting, and a high stool in preference to standing for long periods.

It is also wise to timetable periods of rest (with your feet up). I would additionally recommend that you learn a meditation technique as you are going to need heaps of patience and inner strength! Some relaxation techniques are given in Chapter 10, and a simple meditation technique on pages 124–5. Regular periods of soft, slow, rhythmic activity affect your brain in a beneficial way; your brain in turn directs your body. I don't know if this effect is passed on to your uterus but you will have observed for yourself that agitated mums often have agitated children. Enjoy your pregnancy.

PELVIC FLOOR EXERCISE

This exercise is designed to strengthen the muscles around the vagina. Muscles that are strong have the ability to stretch and contract. The aim is to give firmer support for the uterus and other organs. If your pelvic floor muscles are in good shape there is increased suppleness and muscle control during childbirth as well as a quicker recovery after birth. The exercise is also used to help urinary control, particularly in older women.

To get an idea of the muscles that require strengthening, interrupt the flow of urine and then release. Each time you finish urinating, use the muscles in the same way, that is, squeezing and releasing. To test the strength of these muscles, insert your finger in your vagina and see if you can grip around it with the vaginal muscles. Of course, it is difficult to do this immediately following pregnancy.

Should you not be able to do the initial exercise of stopping the urinary flow, you may need to start by lying down. If you can't feel the muscles working, raise your buttocks on a pillow.

With practice, you will be able to do the exercise at any time or in any position. I suggest that you do the exercise after each urination, holding for about 3 seconds, and gradually build up to about 20 contractions each time. Over-exercising will cause soreness. Do not do this exercise with a full bladder.

PROBLEMS DURING PREGNANCY

CONSTIPATION

Treatment

Generally eat a high-fibre, wholefood diet. If you're not used to these types of foods, ease into the change gradually to avoid digestive upsets. Start by adding a dessertspoon of rice, oat or barley bran to your breakfast cereal. Used dried fruits such as prunes, figs and apricots (soak them overnight). Have raw grated beetroot in a salad (don't panic when your urine and stools change colour!). Try linseed and millet meal porridge – with a few raisins added.

Have a brisk daily walk.

HERBS

• *Psyllium* • *Slippery elm powder*

Take both with a large glass of water.

NOTE **Strong herbs, irritant laxatives, abdominal massage and vigorous 'jumpy' exercises are not suitable during pregnancy.**

FATIGUE

Carrying extra kilos is fairly tiring. Are you doing too much? You may also be anaemic – have your levels of iron and vitamins B9 and B12 checked.

• *Royal jelly* can be used as a tonic – as long as you are not allergic to it • *Zell oxygen* – another good tonic

FLATULENCE

Treatment
HERBS
• Weak herbal teas such as *fennel* and *peppermint* • *Culinary herbs* added to meals
DIET
• Eat more slowly, spread three meals into six smaller ones.
• Try to relax while you are eating as tension can be a cause.
• Avoid foods that make you 'gassy' – common culprits include raw cabbage, broccoli, cauliflower, onions, garlic; also fried foods, dried beans and other legumes, cucumber and capsicum.
• Supplemental yeast often causes bloating.
Supplements – for symptons
• *Charcoal tablets* • *Digestive enzymes*

These two remedies are not recommended for regular, high-dose use because charcoal absorbs minerals as well as gases, while enzymes may depress the body's natural production.
OTHER
Tight clothes add to the pressure on your stomach – anything that puts a visible mark around your tummy is too tight. Flowing clothes look better too and are more comfortable.

HYPERTENSION

Description
The World Health Organisation definition of hypertension in pregnancy is 130/85 mmHg or higher, or a rise of 30 mmHg in systolic pressure (the first figure in the total pressure measurement) or 15 mmHg diastolic (the second, lower figure).

Treatment
HERBS
• *Dandelion* • *Linden* (lime flower)
FROM THE KITCHEN
• *Carrot, cucumber and celery juice* • Reduce salt intake
DIET
• A high vegetable intake
Supplements
Calcium, 1000 mg per day, can lower blood pressure in pregnant women who have high blood pressure.[2] It should be taken before bed. This is certainly worthy of trial at the first sign that your blood pressure is increasing – whether you are pregnant or not.

Pre-eclampsia
Pre-eclampsia (also called toxaemia) is a more serious complication than hypertension, with high blood pressure, fluid retention and protein in the urine. There is a huge weight gain in the latter stages of pregnancy, usually accompanied by blinding headaches. The cause of pre-eclampsia is unknown but there is a higher incidence in malnourished women. The protein in the urine relates to kidney function.

Many women experience fluid retention during pregnancy, especially during very hot weather.

NOTE **These problems need immediate monitoring by a practitioner.**

Treatment

Some doctors (for example, T. & G.S. Brewer in *What Every Pregnant Woman Should Know*) recommend eating all the nourishing food you want, using salt to taste and not worrying about gaining weight; others recommend strict weight control and yet others suggest a very high protein intake. What's a person to do?

Pre-eclampsia is extremely rare in vegans. If you've had a previous experience with pre-eclampsia, why not consider a major dietary change before getting pregnant next time? A well-planned vegan diet will supply you with all the essential nutrients – with the exception of vitamin B12. You may need supplemental iron and calcium too.

Vitamin and mineral supplementation, including vitamin E and vitamin A (not in high doses), has been used to reduce pre-eclampsia.

INFECTIONS

As antibiotics are best avoided during pregnancy, at the first sign of an infection use odourless garlic, propolis and vitamin C. Have more rest.

LIVER AND GALLBLADDER DISTURBANCES

Treatment
HERBS
• *Chicory* • *Dandelion* • *Ginger* • *Globe artichoke* – the fresh plant can be juiced
• *Turmeric* – tiny quantities

MORNING SICKNESS

Symptoms are variable – from a few weeks of mild nausea to prolonged and severe vomiting *(hyperemesis gravidarum)* **which requires medical attention.** Bear in mind that there are other reasons for nausea and vomiting such as food poisoning, infections, liver and gallbladder diseases as well as stomach and intestinal disorders.

Treatment
DIET
Eating something is one of the best ways of overcoming morning sickness. Most women find it more helpful to eat dry foods first but you must not become dehydrated. Water is the best drink, but you may prefer diluted pear juice or very weak tea. Sucking small, plain ice cubes may help.

Some suggest that you should have something light to eat before getting out of bed, for example, a few plain biscuits followed by weak tea – and a rest. It's a good idea if you can train the rest of the family! Have something lightish to eat before you go to bed at night, such as cold, lean chicken and a slice of wholemeal bread or a little cooked brown rice.

Avoid fizzy drinks, orange juice and coffee. Also, greasy foods and anything you find hard to digest.

Try chewing dry, rolled oats between meals and eating a small quantity of plain food every two hours. Chew everything very slowly, sip drinks and don't race around immediately after eating.

Simple foods are the least upsetting.
• Ryvita, rice, buckwheat or other plain wholegrain, unsugared, non-fatty biscuits.
• Cold stewed apple or fresh fruit (not citrus or pineapple).
• Toast with home-made apricot jam.

(Cook dried, chopped apricots in apple juice until the liquid is absorbed. If it's too tart, add some raisins.)
• Steamed vegetables or easily digestible raw vegetables such as lettuce.
• Broth or clear soup.
• Pearl barley and vegetable soup.

HERBS
• *Ginger tea* – 1 dessertspoon chopped fresh root (or 1 teaspoon ginger powder), simmered for about 10 minutes in 500 ml of water. Cool, strain and keep in fridge. Sip small quantities – cold or warm – as required. This is about two days' supply. Alternatively, use a little ginger in cooking or buy tablets if you don't like the taste.

CAUTION **It may not be wise to continue taking ginger throughout pregnancy. Midwives and others have reported that a number of Asian women have very easy births but are heavy bleeders and their newborn babies seem to cry excessively. Ginger is a 'blood thinner' and an antispasmodic; perhaps babies have a type of withdrawal after birth if their mothers have been eating excessive quantities of ginger during pregnancy.**

• *Raspberry leaf* tablets (the tea is fairly unpalatable • Weak *peppermint* or *fennel* tea
Other herbal remedies have to be prescribed by a qualified herbalist.

Supplements
A shortage of B vitamins, particularly thiamin and pyridoxine, worsens nausea so you might try a B complex formula (without yeast). If you're feeling nauseous take any supplements in the middle of a meal as your stomach may be sensitive to concentrated substances.

If you are taking an iron supplement, consider stopping this temporarily or trying another formula, as some types cause both nausea and constipation.

OTHER
Acupuncture has been used effectively to treat nausea: this has been verified under test conditions.[3] You could firstly try an acupressure technique yourself. To find the correct position, place the palm of your hand upwards, then tightly clench your fingers into a fist. Observe that two tendons become clearly visible in your lower forearm. The point to apply pressure is two thumb-widths up from the lowest crease on your wrist and between the two tendons.

Apply pressure with your thumbnail (not the ball of your thumb, the fleshy tip or the sharp point of the fingernail). Bend the thumb so that the two main joints form a right angle, allowing you to exert pressure. Press down quite firmly for about thirty seconds but don't damage the skin or cause bruising (you can either keep the pressure constant or vary it). This procedure will need to be repeated a number of times but not so many that you drive yourself crazy.

STRETCH MARKS

Gently massage your abdomen with *vitamin E, apricot kernel oil* or plain *aloe jelly.*

TEETH AND GUM PROBLEMS

Have your teeth and gums checked before you become pregnant, to avoid the necessity of X-rays or treatment during pregnancy. Cut out sugar, floss daily, brush regularly. Toothpaste that contains herbs such as sage, echinacea, chamomile and myrrh will help prevent bleeding gums and plaque build-up.[4]

VARICOSE VEINS

Treatment

HERBS

Applied externally
• *Witch hazel* – as a cold, external compress • *Calendula* extract – mixed into Sorbolene and gently massaged in with upward, stroking movements

DIET
• *Buckwheat* and *berries* should be eaten regularly.

Supplements
• *Vitamin C and bioflavonoids* – up to 1000 mg per day, but taper off gradually to zero in the last few months of pregnancy.

TISSUE SALTS OR CELLOIDS
• *Calc Fluor*

OTHER
• Rest with legs elevated • Avoid sitting with legs or ankles crossed • Don't stand still for long periods • Do ankle circling exercises and swim • Don't wear tight clothing• The problem will be worsened by excessive weight gain and constipation

PREMENSTRUAL SYNDROME (PMS/PMT)

Description

This syndrome produces a wide range of symptoms including sore breasts, fluid retention, bloating, wind, sweet or starch cravings, mood swings, depression, confusion, irritability, forgetfulness, anxiety, headaches, sinus problems, fatigue, dizziness, fainting, palpitations, weight gain and cramps.

Causes

Commonly relates to hormonal imbalances. Worsened by infections, stress, sugary foods and drinks, alcohol, smoking, coffee and excess junk food.

Researchers have categorised different types of PMT.

PMT-A

Description

Anxiety, irritability, mood swings.

Causes

High oestrogen, low progesterone. Could be related to excess milk and animal fats; possibly high copper levels and inefficient liver function. Nervous excitability generally.

Treatment

HERBS
• *Chaste tree* • *Fenugreek* • *Sarsaparilla* • *Verbena* • *Wild yam*

DIET
Reduce meat and fat; eliminate dairy products for a trial period.

Supplements
• *Magnesium* • *Vitamin B complex with additional B6* • *Vitamin E* • *Zinc*

PMT-C

Description

Sweet and starch cravings, increased appetite, insomnia, palpitations, headaches, weak and shaky spells.

Causes

Low blood sugar, prostaglandin imbalance.

Treatment

HERBS
• *Evening primrose oil* • *Motherwort*

DIET
• *Safflower oil* – 2 teaspoons per day if not taking the evening primrose oil • Small

frequent meals • Increase protein intake if on a low protein diet

Supplements
• *Spirulina* – 2 tablets three times a day between meals

PMT-D

Description
Depression, forgetfulness, crying, confusion, insomnia.

Causes
High progesterone, low oestrogen, high androgens. Occasionally lead toxicity.

Treatment
HERBS

Oestrogenic herbs
• *Alfalfa* • *Aniseed* • *Dong quai* • *Fennel* • *Liquorice* • *Parsley* • *Red clover* • *Sage* • *Soya beans* The intake of all these should be high just before the start of the PMT up to menstruation.

Other herbs helpful in depression
• *Ginseng* • *Ginger* • *Oats* • *St John's wort*
FROM THE KITCHEN
• *Rosemary*
DIET
Supplements
• *Glutamine* • *Vitamin B complex with additional B1 and B3* • *Vitamin E*

PMT-H

Description
Fluid retention, weight gain, sore breasts, abdominal bloating, fatigue. Possible allergies, high adrenal hormones.

Treatment
HERBS
• All the oestrogenic herbs above **except liquorice**.

Herbal diuretics
• *Celery seed* • *Corn silk* • *Dandelion* • *Horsetail*

CAUTION **Do not use ginseng.**

FROM THE KITCHEN
• *Celery juice* • *Cucumber juice*
DIET
• Reduce salt, coffee and tea
Supplements
• *Vitamin B complex with additional B6*
• *Vitamin E* • *Potassium*
OTHER
• Stop smoking

PMT-P

Description
Generalised aches and pains.

Causes
Possible magnesium deficiency or calcium excess.

Treatment
• *Magnesium* supplements

PMT – with migraine-type headache

Description
A throbbing headache affecting one side of the head, often accompanied by sensitivity to light, nausea. Usually lasts all day.

Causes
Believed to be related to low oestrogen, high progesterone. Might also be an allergy or circulatory problem.

Treatment
HERBS
• Oestrogenic herbs – see PMT-D

• *Feverfew* • *Scullcap* • *Wood betony*
TISSUE SALTS OR CELLOIDS
• *Calc Phos* • *Mag Phos*
OTHER
• Hot foot baths

PMT – with acne

Description
Outbreak of pimples coinciding with the pre-menstrual time (commonly 5–12 days before periods).

Causes
Probably hormonal.

Treatment
HERBS
Taken internally
• Evening primrose oil
Applied externally
• *Lemon grass oil* – diluted in water
• *Tea tree oil* – undiluted on individual pimples

GENERAL REMEDIES

These classifications are very interesting, but the main problem is that many women experience a few symptoms from each category. One of the best general remedies is evening primrose oil, which needs to be taken for 2–3 months, 6 capsules daily in divided doses. Vitamin B complex is often helpful, along with lifestyle and dietary changes.

Here are some more generally recommended remedies.
• *Kelp tablets*
• *Vitamin E,* 400 IU daily – this level was shown to benefit 30 per cent of PMT sufferers.
• *Royal jelly,* for 3–5 months, is also of

benefit as well as being a good general tonic.

NOTE ***Do not use kelp unless you can be assured by the manufacturer that the arsenic levels in the supplement or remedy are within safety limits. (Arsenic occurs naturally and as a by-product of industry; it is readily picked up by seaweeds.)***

A Canadian study showed that if women jogged about 2.5 km daily for six months this gave a significant reduction in fluid retention, breast tenderness and the overall symptoms. In cases with a complicated variety of symptoms, it might be wise to consult a trained natural therapist or a medical practitioner.

PROLAPSE – UTERINE

Description
Weakening of the pelvic tissue, allowing the uterus to drop downwards, causing pressure and discomfort, usually affecting the bladder.

The remedies suggested would not be helpful where the uterus actually protruded through the vaginal orifice.

Causes
Weak muscles, pelvic congestion, and following childbirth.

Treatment
HERBS
Internally and externally
• *Bayberry* • *Golden seal* • *Raspberry leaf*
• *Witch hazel* – ointment or douche
DIET
Supplements
• *Vitamin C and bioflavonoids*

TISSUE SALTS OR CELLOIDS
• *Calc Fluor* • *Silicea*
OTHER
• Exercises to strengthen the lower pelvic floor muscles: as suggested for Pregnancy (see page 108).

VAGINAL INFECTIONS – MINOR

Description
Itching, inflammation or discharge. Not severe or infectious conditions, which require medical diagnosis and treatment.

Causes
Excess alkalinity, poor hygiene, infection from anus or other parts of the body, emotional upsets, oral contraceptives, diabetes, antibiotics, overwork, irritating chemicals including some soaps and deodorants, faulty diet and trauma.

Treatment
• Avoid scented soaps and vaginal deodorants, nylon underwear, pantyhose, tight jeans.
• After going to the toilet, wipe yourself from front to back, and change underwear regularly.
• Remember that your partner may be infecting or reinfecting you – or vice versa.
• Refer also to Leucorrhoea (page 100) for remedies.

A report in the *Lancet* confirmed that tea tree oil pessaries were successful in treating vaginosis.[5] I would recommend self treating with this for most minor vaginal infections.

If the condition does not improve reasonably quickly you should consult a health practitioner.

ADDITIONAL INFORMATION

DOUCHES

These are used to irrigate and cleanse the vaginal area up to the mouth of the uterus (cervix). Many women find that douching relieves pain, inflammation and congestion. Ideally the vaginal area should be pink, moist and mildly acidic, as such an environment allows the correct bacterial balance. If there is too much alkalinity, then the bacterial balance is changed. This is why diluted cider vinegar, which is weak acetic acid, is suggested as a douche.

When using a douche, there are a number of important considerations.
• The equipment should be used by one person only and cleaned with boiling water and an antiseptic solution before and after use. The same equipment should not be used for an enema.
• Excessive douching can upset the bacterial balance. As a guide, three or four days consecutively and then occasional use should not present any difficulties.
• Use the solution at body heat (lukewarm or not more than 40°C).
• Test the fluid under your arms for sensitivity before using a vaginal douche.
• The solution should be gently injected into the vagina, without force or pressure. I prefer the type of equipment obtainable in kit form, which has a container, tube and catheter so that you can see that there are no air bubbles and that the fluid is running in very slowly. Don't have the container more than about 60–70 cm above the hips.
• It is generally easier to bring the knees up towards the chest while administering a douche.

• Stay lying down for about 10–20 minutes so that some of the fluid is retained for a short period. For the first few times you will find that it will run straight out and you will always lose some, which is why you need to give yourself the douche in the bathroom.

• Don't douche while pregnant.

• A healthy, non-infected vagina should not require douching; in other words it should be done only if and when required.

• A number of herbs suggested in this book are suitable for douching – such as calendula, chamomile, comfrey and golden seal. Simply make an infusion or decoction, let it cool, then strain. You will need to make about ½ cup only and you can add 2 drops of essential oil such as tea tree or sandalwood or a teaspoon of apple cider vinegar or lemon juice.

SITZBATH (hip bath)

A baby's bath is suitable for this, or you can use your own bath with about 15cm of water in it. The water should reach your navel when you sit in it.

I'm recommending cold sitzbaths for some disorders because these are stimulating. If you immerse part of your body in cold water for a short period of time, the reaction that *follows* is a rush of blood to the area. When you need something soothing, you'd be more comfortable having a full, hot bath or using a hot-water bottle.

To relieve pelvic congestion and period pain, have a cold sitzbath for a few minutes every day at least a week before your periods are due. You do not do this during menstruation.

In the cold weather, have a heater in the room or wear a jumper to keep your upper body warm.

ORAL CONTRACEPTIVES

Few naturopaths would recommend these, for a number of reasons.

• They decrease the availability of certain vitamins and minerals in the body, notably B1, B2, B6, B9, B12, vitamin C and bioflavonoids, vitamin E and zinc. Vitamin A and copper availability are increased. It is prudent for every woman on the Pill to take a multi-vitamin daily.

• They affect many biochemical systems in the body.

• It has been suggested that girls who have been menstruating for less than two years or who did not start menstruating before the age of fifteen years would be wise not to use them, because they experience more adverse effects.

There are over fifty precautions and adverse reactions listed in medical literature, including depression, fluid retention, thrush, nausea, breakthrough bleeding (spotting), period pain, skin pigmentation, breast tenderness, jaundice, itchy skin, migraine, cataracts, PMT, burning urine, nervousness, dizziness, fatigue, loss of scalp hair, increased facial hair, leg cramps, insomnia, pimples, backache, vaginitis and impaired kidney function. The warnings relating to the use of oral contraceptives include:

• greater risk of thrombotic disorders, such as stroke and coronary occlusion; heart attack risk when taking oral contraceptives is further increased by smoking, age, high blood pressure, obesity, diabetes and high cholesterol

• low dose or combination pills are not risk-free

• it is recommended that oral contraceptives be discontinued six weeks prior to elective surgery

• incidences of optic neuritis and retinal thrombosis have been reported in association with oral contraceptive use

• the link to cancer is still being debated but there is a relationship to benign liver adenomas and other liver problems

• the use of female sex hormones during early pregnancy may cause serious foetal damage; they can also cause ectopic (abnormal) pregnancies

• gallbladder disease, headaches, a decrease in glucose tolerance and hypertension are also in the listed warnings

• temporary and, occasionally, permanent infertility may occur after discontinuing the Pill.

There are a few good points, too.

• They are a reliable, convenient method of contraception and usually the periods are regular and lighter than normal.

• Often there is less period pain and premenstrual tension.

• Sometimes skin and hair improve.

If you are concerned about the long-term effects you should obtain pamphlets from your nearest Women's Community Health Centre, visit a Family Planning Centre or read *MIMS Annual* in your library.

Women who don't wish to be on the Pill should consider alternative methods of contraception, such as condoms, a diaphragm or the Billings Method, which is explained in a book of that title published by Anne O'Donovan.

CHAPTER 7

HEART AND CIRCULATION

I bet you've heard that traditional-living Eskimos don't get anywhere near the number of heart attacks that we do because of their high fish diet. Well, Eskimos bruise and bleed easily and have a high incidence of brain haemorrhages! I'm not sure whether I'd rather have a heart attack or a brain haemorrhage. What I do know is that I probably couldn't hack living near the North Pole. Eskimo people are fantastic and hardy but gnawing on raw seal meat and huddling in a confined, smoky area for months at a time doesn't appeal to me. The frozen remains of non-Westernised Alaskans have been subjected to scientific analysis and some of their health problems included atherosclerosis, chronic ear infections, gross lung pathologies and head lice. One female had calcified heart valves, pneumonia, pleurisy, harmful blood bacteria, inflammation of the heart lining and kidney failure – her death was caused by an avalanche!

'They' also tell you that the Japanese have a lower incidence of heart disease than Western societies, but did you know that Japan has the highest death rate from strokes in the world, as well as a high incidence of stomach cancer? Then there are all those stories of people in various parts of the world who live simple, long, healthy lives. One of my favourite research articles is by Z. Medvedev who studied people in the Russian Caucasus district.[1] They claimed to be 130–140 years of age but careful investigation revealed that they were only 70 or 80. They *looked* 130 because of the harsh living conditions.

This doesn't mean that you should loll around for hours looking at the television, chain-smoke, drink beer by the carton, eat as much junk food as possible or develop aggressive behaviour. It means that it is not sensible to isolate one health factor out of a whole culture and attempt to transplant it somewhere else.

CAUTION ***You cannot suddenly stop taking pharmaceutical drugs for a circulatory – or any other – problem because there can be 'rebound' effects, that is, your problem worsens dramatically. If you wish to go on a dietary and/or supplemental programme, you should be monitored so that, hopefully, the medication can be gradually withdrawn or reduced over a period of time.***

In a case of, say, mild hypertension, tell your practitioner that you wish to make lifestyle changes rather than start a pharmaceutical programme.

WHAT ARE WE DOING WRONG?

There are thousands of research papers indicating causes of heart and related circulatory problems and factors that may precipitate them. Here are some of them. Remember, though, that most people die of old age.
• Hereditary predisposition. If members of your immediate family have had heart attacks or similar problems while they were young, you should take preventive measures. The earlier you start the better.
• High blood pressure and high cholesterol.
• Obesity.
• Lack of exercise. It has been estimated that hunter-gatherers spent about fifteen hours a week collecting food and wood.

Assuming this harmonises with our genetic make-up and body structure, it is quite possible that most of us are taking too little exercise, others too much, and generally we're doing the wrong sort of activity.
• Cigarette smoking – there's even a condition called 'smoker's foot'.
• Gout, diabetes and hormonal imbalances.
• A diet that is high in red meat, salt, fats, refined sugars and alcohol.
• Coffee (especially if boiled) and caffeine-containing drinks are associated with thrombosis (clotting), increased cholesterol, high blood sugar, hypertension and heart-beat irregularities.
• Nutrient deficiencies or low levels of magnesium, selenium, vitamin E, potassium, calcium, vitamins A and C have been implicated.
• Babies with abnormal birthweights are more prone to cardiovascular diseases in adult life.
• Breastfed infants are less likely to develop abnormal cholesterol levels than bottlefed.

Type-A behaviour (ambition, aggression, impatience, etc.) was a popular culprit a decade ago, but not all studies show it is a cause. I suppose it depends on the level of enjoyment of the Type-A life and the rewards that go with it. Other studies put more emphasis on loss of social support, overwork or unemployment, sleeplessness, fatigue, hyperventilation and emotional upsets as factors in heart and circulatory disease.

The causes and distribution of heart disease are still quite puzzling. The death rate in Scotland is three times that of France; male and female death rates in Newcastle, New South Wales, are respectively 45 per cent and 95 per cent higher than in Perth; in India cardiovascular patients often have low cholesterol. In the 1920s a catastrophic rise in the occurrence of cardiovascular disease in the West began; in the last few decades the cardiovascular death rate has dropped dramatically in the USA and Australia while in some eastern countries it has increased.[2] One theory for the increase in the 1920s is that it coincided with the introduction of margarine and the use of processed (hydrogenated) polyunsaturated fats.

Margarine

Margarine was invented at the end of the nineteenth century and subsequently was promoted as a healthy form of dietary fat because of the purported link between animal fats and heart disease.

MANUFACTURING PROCESS

I visited a margarine manufacturer in Sydney and was given the following information: 'Margarine is formulated and processed in such a way that it is "tailor made" to meet the specific needs of the consumer'.

Depending on cost and availability, the oils used include sunflower, soyabean, rapeseed, safflower, cottonseed, peanut, palm, coconut and palm kernel. The oils are obtained by crushing, pressing and extracting using inert organic solvents – resulting in a darkish, smelly product. These oils are converted to 'soap' by washing with alkaline lye and water, followed by bleaching and deodorising using fine steam at very high temperatures.

The next processes are hydrogenation, fractionation and interesterification, which alter the physical properties of the oil. Hydrogenation means that hydrogen gas is bubbled through in the presence of a nickel catalyst to thicken the oil. Water is added, as well as emulsifiers, vitamins A and D, flavourings, colourings and sometimes antioxidants.

The combination of processing and heating (to 50°C) results in a high proportion of trans-fatty acids, which are found in nature in tiny quantities only; essential fatty acids are destroyed and nickel residues have been found in margarine.

When I offered the manufacturer a pile of reports I had collected showing that margarine and processed polyunsaturated oils generally were possibly doing more harm than good, the executive and his team of two scientists were somewhat taken aback. I asked, 'What evidence can you give me to refute these reports?'. About three weeks later I received one report in the mail that concluded 'trans-fatty acids have not been found to have adverse or specific effects compared to saturated or cis-unsaturated fats – provided sufficient linoleic acid is present in the diet.'

In other words, margarine is possibly more harmful than butter. What's a person to do? Well, since butter these days has all the buttermilk (with its protective factors) removed, you might consider not using either. Perhaps the labels of margarine and butter should carry the warning, *'This product may be hazardous to your health'*.

SOLUTION

Use small quantities of avocado, tahini (crushed sesame seeds), nut butters, nuts and seeds and possibly a little unheated cold-pressed oils. I don't recommend peanuts because of their aflatoxin and pesticide residue content.

I thought I'd never be able to give up the 'yellow greases' but over the years my tastes have changed and now I find them quite unpalatable.

Milk

HOMOGENISED MILK

Some USA researchers, including Dr Kurt Oster, MD, have published papers regarding the harmful effects of homogenised milk. A simplified explanation of the findings is that all milk contains a substance called xanthine oxidase. In unhomogenised milk it is broken down in the digestive system and excreted. However the process of homogenisation binds the xanthine oxidase to fat particles, and in this form it is not excreted but reaches the circulatory system and damages the tissue in the heart and artery walls. The research indicates that the regions with the highest intakes of homogenised milk are – you've guessed it – those with the highest rates of cardiovascular disease.

I wrote to the Australian Dairy Corporation, giving references, and requesting its side of the story, but did not receive a reply. When I telephoned I was told 'We've never heard of the research!'

DAIRY PRODUCTS GENERALLY

Articles with titles like 'Beware the cow' have appeared in the *Lancet*, and a *British Medical Journal* report concluded that people who drink three glasses (or more) of milk daily have four times the risk of myocardial infarction (heart attack) than that of those who drink less. For 99 per cent of human existence, dairy products were not part of the diet. There's no such thing as 'dairy deficiency', although it is a cheap, convenient source of protein, calcium and other essential nutrients.

If you're concerned about your cardiovascular system, use 'the cow' sparingly.

ANGINA

Description

A deficiency of the blood supply to the heart muscle, due to the obstruction or constriction of one or more of the heart's blood vessels. There is a range of symptoms including tight feeling in the chest, a heavy or choking sensation, pain in the central chest that can radiate to the jaw, lower neck, middle of the abdomen, sometimes to the right side and the back and more commonly to the left shoulder and arm. There may be accompanying anxiety, faintness or flatulence.

Angina occurs during or following physical exertion, overeating or stress, and sometimes in very cold weather. The attacks may be relatively mild and last for a few minutes or be more severe and prolonged which makes it difficult to distinguish from a heart attack.

Causes

Atherosclerosis, heart and certain other diseases as well as problems such as hyperthyroidism and severe anaemia. There is also some research indicating that arterial spasm may be the cause.

CAUTION *Angina requires a medical diagnosis because it can be confused with conditions such as indigestion, anxiety hyperventilation, muscle or bone pain, oesophageal spasm, gallstones, blood pressure abnormalities and heart irregularities – to name a few.*

Treatment

The standard medical treatment is usually to treat the symptoms with an anti-angina drug such as Anginine. The patient needs to look at diet and lifestyle changes, including avoiding those things that bring on an attack.

HERBS

For preventive measures or as an adjunct treatment: • *Chamomile* • *Hawthorn* • *Motherwort* • *Scullcap* • *Valerian*

FROM THE KITCHEN

• *Rosemary* – a few leaves used as a very weak tea or as a foot bath. The oil can be very soothing massaged into the scalp or over taut muscles, especially the back of the neck.

DIET

A Pritikin-type diet or Dr Ornish's programme (see pages 123–4) would be appropriate – although you can have a few whole eggs and a tiny quantity of essential fatty acids, such as 1 teaspoon cold-pressed oil daily, *or* 1 tablespoon nuts or seeds *or* ⅛ of an avocado.

Supplements

• An *antioxidant formula* • *Bromelain* • *Magnesium* • *Potassium* • *Coenzyme Q10* and *carnitine* help provide additional biochemical oxygen • EPA-DHA (fish oils) • Patients with angina tend to have low selenium levels. It is not permitted as a supplement in Australia but is plentiful in yeasts and wheat germ.

TISSUE SALTS OR CELLOIDS

• *Mag Phos*

OTHER

• Tai chi, moderate regular walking and breathing exercises (see opposite) are often helpful.

CAUTION *An exercise programme should not be started without medical approval; never undergo a stress test without warning the practitioner that you have angina.*

• No cigarette smoking.
• Regular massage is recommended.

ATHEROSCLEROSIS AND CORONARY ARTERY DISEASE

Description

Thickening of the internal surfaces of arteries due to deposits of cholesterol crystals, fats, proteins and other substances.

This internal narrowing may be in small patches or be widespread. The symptoms vary according to the degree of severity and the extent of the deposits. The patient may feel only minor cramps or tingling, or if the arteries in the brain are affected there may be dizzy attacks, slurred speech, poor coordination or strokes.

This problem can also be the cause of hypertension because of the reduced diameter of the blood vessels and it can lead to chest and arm pains, heart attacks and serious circulatory disorders.

A vertical crease in the ear does not reveal heart disease – it just happens in ageing.

Causes

A number of factors are thought to contribute, such as: faulty fat metabolism; poor diet especially in respect of excess fats; stress; cigarette smoking; lack of exercise; lead poisoning; some diseases such as diabetes and hypothyroidism. Hypertension can also be a cause because the pressure and turbulence can damage the internal vessel linings, thus precipitating plaque formation. It has been suggested that any substance (free radicals, chemicals etc.) that irritates the internal linings of blood vessels could possibly initiate plaque formation.

Treatment

A one-year study showed that people with coronary artery disease markedly improved on the following programme.[3]
• Fruit, vegetables, grains, legumes and soya bean products – unrestricted quantities.
• The only animal products allowed were egg white and one cup of non-fat milk or yoghurt daily. No meat, fish or cheese.
• No foods high in fats such as avocado, nuts, seeds, oils.
• No coffee, smoking or MSG.
• Alcohol restricted. I would suggest a maximum of 1 glass of wine or a small glass of beer a day. Always have at least one day a week alcohol-free.
• Vitamin B12 was the only supplement given on the programme.
• One hour per day of stress management techniques including stretching, breathing exercises, meditation, progressive relaxation and visualisation. Tapes were provided.
• Twice-weekly group support meetings – Americans seem to love these!
• At least three hours of exercise per week, with a minimum of 30 minutes each session. The degree of activity was within assessed target heart rates. People were encouraged to find an exercise they enjoyed.

Basically the diet aimed at a food balance of 10 per cent fat, 15–20 per cent protein and 70–75 per cent carbohydrate (mainly complex).

This dietary and lifestyle regimen would be helpful in the prevention and treatment of most heart and circulatory problems. If you were looking at a preventive programme, then you could make slight adjustments such as eating a few whole eggs and a small quantity of plant oils, nuts or seeds.

BREATHING EXERCISES

Apart from the obvious connection between the respiratory and cardiovascular systems, it has been demonstrated that performing breathing exercises can lower blood cholesterol and sugar levels.[4] Here is my basic breathing technique.
• Sit or lie in a comfortable position, with your hands resting on your upper abdomen.
• As you breathe in through the nose, let your abdomen fill up, then feel your chest expand outwards. The upper chest and shoulders are relaxed.
• Gently pull in the abdomen, then relax the chest as you exhale through the nose.

Once you've got the basic technique, then co-ordinate the breathing with very slow counting: *In, two, three; Out, two, three, four.* The aim is to make the exhalation longer than the breathing in. To control the flow of the exhalation, focus on the throat – even though you are breathing out through the nose.

Initially most people find this form of breathing somewhat uncomfortable; this is to be expected because you are improving your breathing pattern. However, it shouldn't be stressful. Start by practising for about five minutes twice daily; later you can use it as a relaxation technique for, say twenty minutes a day. What you are trying to achieve ultimately is *your* slowest, most relaxed breathing possible, with the exhalation twice as long as the inhalation.

I don't recommend holding the breath – especially if you have a heart or blood pressure problem.

MEDITATION

One of the easiest techniques is to sit comfortably, with the back straight, chin level and shoulders relaxed. Let the breath come and go gently and evenly. Silently repeat the word 'om' as you breathe in and 'om' as you breathe out.

I suggest the repetition of Sanskrit words or phrases (generally known as mantras) because if you use an English word it can become frustrating. For example, simply using the word 'one' can get boring and constantly repeating 'peace' may only reinforce the notion that you are not at all peaceful.

You can use a mantra such as '*Om shanti shanti shanti om*'. 'Om' is a sound with no actual meaning other than a Sanskrit spiritual symbol; 'shanti' means peace.

Mantras are great for lowering anxiety, impatience and blood pressure and you can repeat them at difficult times during the day instead of 'doing your block' or inwardly fuming. You can buy tapes with mantras on them but I suggest you listen to them carefully and read the explanation on the cover before using them so that you're relaxed about what you're saying.

Generally start meditating for about ten minutes a day and gradually build up to thirty minutes.

OILS

Marine lipids, MaxEPA and DHA have been promoted as being protective against heart disease by helping fat metabolism, preventing blood stickiness and lowering triglycerides and cholesterol.

However, when the blood becomes 'too thin' there's a corresponding increase in the chance of brain haemorrhages. Rather than take high doses, it would seem prudent to have no more than 1000 mg per day (1–2 capsules), or

to markedly reduce your meat consumption and have 2–3 fish meals per week instead.

Olive oil, in reasonable quantities, may also reduce the more harmful type of cholesterol circulating in the blood. Use it in cooking.

HERBS

For arterial blood flow
• *Fenugreek* • *Garlic* • *Ginkgo* • *Hawthorn* • *Linden* • *Yarrow*

For relaxing arterial walls
• *Hops* • *Passion flower* • *Scullcap*

FROM THE KITCHEN
• *Alfalfa* • *Ginger*

DIET
Follow the guidelines above.

Supplements
• *Vitamin C and bioflavonoids* – if not on a high fruit and vegetable diet • *Vitamin E* • *Brewer's yeast* – start with very small quantities as it is a common allergen and may cause digestive upsets

Some patients show signs or have pathology tests indicating low levels of minerals such as magnesium or potassium. Minerals compete with each other for absorption and metabolism so you need to be sure that a particular supplement is actually needed before taking but a broad spectrum, multi-vitamin and mineral supplement will help offset a number of damaging biochemical processes.

Avoid
• *Organ meats* • *Anchovies* • *Mussels and oysters* • *Meat extracts and gravies* • All obvious *animal fats*

EXERCISE
This has the additional beneficial effect of increasing the flexibility of the arterial walls. To get these benefits the exercise must be regular. Occasional strenuous exercise is a strain on the heart.

CHOLESTEROL – HIGH

Description
A number of signs and symptoms may be associated with high blood cholesterol such as cramps, breathlessness and hypertension. The definitive test for this is to establish the levels from a blood test.

It is now recognised that there are two forms of cholesterol, high-density lipoprotein (HDL) and low-density lipoprotein (LDL). LDL is the form that causes deposits in blood vessels.

The current Australian 'normal' levels are given in the table below.

	mmol/L
Total cholesterol	3.9–5.5
HDL cholesterol – male	0.8–1.7
– female	0.9–2.1
LDL cholesterol	1.7–4.5

If your total cholesterol is high this is not always a cause for alarm, as it may be made up of HDL rather than LDL. Also, be aware that cholesterol levels may vary within a day or from week to week.

Some people are duped into thinking that the lower the cholesterol level, the better. This is not so: low levels are associated with higher risks of stroke, cancer, depression and aggression.[5] Cholesterol-lowering and anti-hypertensive drugs have also been linked to lower coronary mortality but higher death rates from other causes.[6]

Causes
High fat diet generally, faulty fat metabolism, liver malfunction, hereditary predisposition. The whole question of dietary fats is very complex and somewhat controversial but nevertheless, if the body's circulating fats are too high, it makes sense to *lower the dietary fats in general* and to include in the diet only those fats which the body doesn't make (that is, essential fatty acids) and those that have definite benefits to the body.

Treatment
HERBS
• *Fenugreek* • *Garlic* • *Ginseng* – Korean or Chinese • *Psyllium* • *Reishi*

FROM THE KITCHEN
• *Alfalfa* • *Chicory* – as a green vegetable or a coffee substitute • *Ginger* • *Green tea* • *Prunes* • *Turmeric*

DIET
Although lowering cholesterol is somewhat controversial, if your blood levels are high it doesn't make sense to have a high cholesterol diet.

Your diet should be similar to the diet for Atherosclerosis (pages 123–4). Generally low fats and oils, no refined sugars, high fibre.

Recommended
• *Fish* – 3–4 times a week (this can be cooked in foil with finely chopped onions, cabbage or other vegetables, tomato, herbs and lemon juice and does not require any salt or butter) • *High vegetable protein* – especially soya beans, legumes and dried beans (read *Diet for a Small Planet* by Frances Moore Lappé, for tips on food combining to get complete vegetable protein meals) • High *alfalfa* and other *sprouts* • *Skim milk, low-fat yoghurt, low-fat cottage cheese* • *Garlic, onions, leeks* • *Oats, barley, rice bran* • *All whole grains* and *wheat germ* • *All vegetables* • *Fruit* – 2–4 pieces per day

Restrict
• *Alcohol* – 1 glass per day maximum
• *Eggs* – maximum 2–3 per week if not

eating any meat; otherwise use only the whites • *Butter* – 1 teaspoon (unsalted) per day • *All meat and chicken* – remove all visible fat and use more as flavouring than as main meals • *Cold-pressed oils* – 1 teaspoon per day • *Nuts and seeds* – do not use regularly if you eat meat; vegetarians can have 1 tablespoon per day • *Animal fats* – only eat a minimal amount

Avoid absolutely
• *All processed and heated fats and oils* – including margarine • *Coffee* – especially if boiled • *All refined sugars and refined carbohydrates* • *Icecream* • *All full-cream milks and full-cream yoghurt* • *Organ meats, gravies*

NOTE *If you use oils in cooking, make sure they are not excessively heated or even browned. Don't re-use oils and use only cold-pressed products.*

Supplements
• *Nicotinic acid* – other forms of vitamin B3 don't help lower cholesterol • *Vitamin C and bioflavonoids* • *Vitamin E* • *Spirulina* • *Brewer's yeast* – if your digestive system can handle it!

NOTE *Vitamin B3 can cause flushing. Take after meals. Doses higher than the manufacturers' instructions need practitioner supervision.*

OTHER
• Regular exercise; many of the suggestions given under the treatment of Atherosclerosis are also appropriate.
• Depending on the possible cause, it may be worthwhile treating the liver (see pages 144–6).
• The latest news from the USA is that chlorinated water is linked with cholesterol deposits on arterial walls. Use a filter or boil drinking water and let it stand in the fridge before use.

CIRCULATION – WEAK

Description
This can range from common, mild symptoms – such as cold hands and feet, chilblains, pins and needles – to the more serious condition known as peripheral vascular disease or occlusive disease which is accompanied by pain in the lower limbs at night or while resting, numbness, no pulses, pallor on elevation, poor healing, cramps, colour changes in the feet, the skin in the area may become smooth and shiny, the toe nails may be thickened and deformed, the legs feel cool and the feet are often dry. Extremely severe circulatory blockages can result in extensive thrombosis (clotting), external ulcers and even gangrene. The most common of the severe problems is intermittent claudication, where there is aching fatigue in the calf muscles or feet on exertion; this may develop into constant or cramping pain even after a short walk.

Obviously, all severe symptoms need professional diagnosis and treatment, and the information is given to encourage people to take steps to improve their circulation before it deteriorates.

Causes
Hereditary factors, inappropriate diet, high blood fats, cigarette smoking, insufficient exercise, arterial spasms, obesity; the more serious symptoms may relate to atherosclerosis, kidney or liver disorders, diabetes, arthritis and arteriosclerosis.

Treatment

HERBS

• *Angelica* • *Bayberry* • *Bilberry* • *Chilli, hot* • *Dandelion* • *Hawthorn* • *Nettle* • *Wild yam*

FROM THE KITCHEN

• *Chamomile* • *Ginger* • *Turmeric*

DIET

Avoiding overweight is important. Also follow the recommendations under Atherosclerosis.

Supplements

• *Vitamin B3* – both nicotinic acid and niacinamide are used • *Coenzyme Q10* • *Carnitine* • *Taurine* • *Vitamin C and bioflavonoids* • *Vitamin E*

TISSUE SALTS OR CELLOIDS

• *Mag Phos*

OTHER

• Exercise is especially important because this prevents venous congestion (the blood pooling in one area) and also leads to the development of collaterals (new blood vessel branches).

• Foot care is very important: avoid tight shoes.

• Also avoid extreme heat and cold, e.g. hot baths.

• Massage sandals may help.

• Avoid tight clothing.

• See also recommendations for Varicose Veins (page 133).

HAEMORRHOIDS (piles)

Description

These have been simply described as varicose veins in the rectum. These enlarged veins are found in the upper surfaces inside or just outside the rectum. They can cause pain, itching, discomfort and bleeding.

CAUTION **Haemorrhoids need to be medically diagnosed because, while not being dangerous in themselves, similar symptoms may be present with polyps, cancer, fissures or abscesses.**

Causes

Straining at stool, constipation, prolonged standing or sitting, poor circulation generally, obesity and anal infection. Haemorrhoids can also relate to poor liver function and they often occur during pregnancy.

Treatment

HERBS

Taken internally

• *Gotu cola* • *Horse chestnut* • *Nettle* • *Psyllium* • *Slippery elm* – powder or tablets

---

CAUTION **Horse chestnut and nettle should never be taken during pregnancy.**

Depending on the cause of the haemorrhoids, the recommended herbs for Constipation (page 82), Weak Circulation (opposite) and Liver Sluggishness (pages 144–6) may also be effective.

NOTE **Long term, it is not recommended that astringents be used internally because these tend to increase constipation. A herbalist may make up a formula that includes an astringent together with other herbs but you will need a personal consultation.**

Applied externally

• *Witch hazel* ointment – this is generally the most effective • *Calendula* or *golden seal* ointments are also helpful, particularly if there is bleeding or the possibility of an infection • *St John's wort* ointment or oil usually helps with itching and pain • A cold *sitzbath* often gives relief; it is more effective with a cooled decoction of oak, sage or raspberry leaves added to the water

DIET

Sometimes wheat bran aggravates haemorrhoids and causes itching. There are other high-fibre foods that can be used instead.

• *Millet* and *linseed meal* • *Oatmeal, oat flakes* or *oat bran* • *Rice bran* • *Buckwheat, red* and *black berries* are especially recommended because they are high in the flavonoids known to strengthen blood vessels • A small quantity of *dietary oil* may help, such as a dessertspoon of almond, linseed or olive oil. This stimulates bile flow, which in turn gives a 'slippery quality' to faeces.

Supplements

• *Vitamin C and bioflavonoids*

TISSUE SALTS OR CELLOIDS

• *Calc Fluor* • *Kali Mur*

HYPERTENSION
(high blood pressure)

Description

Excessive pressure of the blood against the walls of the arteries, as measured in mm of mercury. This measurement varies not only from day to day but within each day. It may also depend on the practitioner taking it: for example one study showed that doctors obtained higher readings than nurses. The pressure may rise with stress, excitement and as one gets older. The World Health Organisation has suggested that the upper limit of normal is 160/95. The 160 relates to the pressure when the heart is pumping (systolic) and the 95 is the resting pressure (diastolic).

Hypertension is rarely found in people under the age of twenty. It may be associated with atherosclerosis and a higher incidence of heart attacks and strokes, as high blood pressure puts stress not only on the arteries but also on the heart and kidneys.

People can have high blood pressure without noticeable symptoms, but commonly the complaints include headaches, dizziness, fatigue, palpitations, shortness of breath, failing vision, nose bleeds, anxiety, fluid retention and very taut neck and shoulder muscles.

Generally, people can have a range of blood pressures and still be considered 'normal and healthy'. In *Current Medical Diagnosis and Treatment* it is stated that in patients less than fifty years of age, the diagnosis of hypertension is not warranted unless the blood pressure exceeds 140/90 mm of mercury on a minimum of three separate occasions; furthermore, prior to the examination, the patient should have rested for at least 20 minutes in quiet surroundings. Occasional readings may be higher but this is classed as vascular hyperreactivity, not hypertensive disease, because the pressures return to normal with rest. These occasional high readings may, nevertheless, be an early indicator of sustained hypertension. People with mild hypertension should be strongly encouraged to make dietary and lifestyle changes to remedy the problem and these actions may be appropriate in moderate cases also.

The alternative to taking such measures is to go on pharmaceutical drugs, all of which have side effects. Refer to the *MIMS Annual* in your local library. Dr Mendelsohn, MD, has stated that 'Non-drug management of hypertension certainly is safer and often more effective than drug management, and it should almost always be seriously attempted as the first line of defense'.

Medical attention should be sought for severe hypertension and where there is involvement with trauma and serious diseases.

As a guide, blood pressure readings may be graded according to the level of the diastolic pressure, that is:

Diastolic pressure (mmHg)	Level of hypertension
95–100	mild
100–120	moderate
120–140	severe
140 or more	gross

An increase of more than 20 mm of mercury during pregnancy is usually considered to be hypertension and requires practitioner attention.

A 1984 article in the *British Medical Journal* suggested that there is no benefit from treating essential female hypertension unless the diastolic pressure is above 105 mm of mercury.[7]

Causes

Secondary hypertension is caused by a number of serious conditions such as kidney or hormonal disorders, atherosclerosis and some drugs and toxins.

Primary hypertension does not have a known cause in the majority of cases and has been labelled 'essential' or 'idiopathic'. The cause may be related to excess dietary salt or fats, food allergies, alcohol, poor handling of stress, obesity, insufficient rest, lack of physical exercise and is sometimes hereditary. Low levels of some nutrients are also implicated, especially calcium, magnesium and potassium. Cadmium and similar heavy metal toxicities are other possible causes.

Treatment

HERBS

• *Celery seed* • *Dandelion* • *Garlic* • *Hawthorn* • *Linden* (lime flowers) • *Motherwort* • *Nettle* • *Scullcap* • *Valerian* • *Yarrow* • *Yucca*

FROM THE KITCHEN

• *Ginger* • *Turmeric*

DIET

Step one

Eliminate all refined, processed, packaged, tinned and bottled foods. Markedly reduce or eliminate alcohol, tea, coffee, cigarettes. Instead of salt use cooked garlic, dried and fresh herbs and ginger root. More than one study has shown that regular consumption of ginger will lower blood pressure.

Instead of tea and coffee use: • *Dandelion root coffee* • *Linden tea* • *Chamomile tea* • *Peppermint tea*

NOTE ***Many people have marked withdrawal symptoms when they eliminate certain foods and drinks from their diets, particularly alcohol and coffee. These withdrawal symptoms can last up to a week. Alcoholics have additional problems.***

Step two – a short-term testing programme

Four days on fruit and vegetables only. Alternatively, a supervised fast at a health clinic. This is especially recommended if you are overweight.

Another possibility would be to have four days rest at home taking fresh vegetable juices and fresh fruit juices, both diluted 50/50 with water. The juices should not be mixed. Celery, carrot, apple, grape, cucumber are especially recommended. In cold weather you could have a broth made as follows:

variety of green vegetables
onions, leeks or shallots
1 potato
1 tomato
chopped ginger root
1 carrot
1 swede
1 beetroot
parsley and other herbs to flavour

Chop all the ingredients finely. Cover with water and simmer for 1 hour. Cool, strain and refrigerate. Drink hot, as required.

If you are on fluids only, at least 6 glasses a day must be taken, and much more in hot weather.

If, at the end of the four days, your blood pressure has dropped dramatically, this indicates that your hypertension is probably controllable through dietary and lifestyle changes.

CAUTION *If you are on drugs or have a health problem other than essential hypertension, you need to have practitioner advice before going on a liquid diet. Restricted diets are not appropriate for the frail and elderly unless professionally supervised.*

Step three – one week special diet

BEFORE BREAKFAST	½ fresh lemon juiced in hot water or ½ grapefruit and 1 glass water. If possible go for a walk.
BREAKFAST	Fresh fruit or fruit salad 1 dessertspoon lecithin and, if desired, 1–3 dessertspoons plain, low-fat yoghurt *or* porridge made from buckwheat (1 cup cooked) with apple and cinnamon and 1 tablespoon raisins *or* 1 lightly boiled or poached egg with 1–2 slices of wholemeal bread or cooked oatmeal or other whole-grain cereal such as millet (any whole-grain cereal is suitable but should be served without sugar and using low-fat dairy or soy milk) plus 1 piece fresh fruit
BETWEEN MEALS	1–2 glasses of water or a selection of the juices and drinks recommended under steps one and two.
LUNCH	Vegetable soup with 2–3 Ryvita biscuits or any low-fat, whole-grain product *or* Large raw vegetable salad, herbs to flavour (dressing: 1 teaspoon cold-pressed olive oil and lemon juice). 2 tablespoons cottage cheese can be added.

DINNER Steamed vegetables including 1–2 root vegetables
Small serving of fish (120–160g), chicken
or
1 cup savoury rice and lentils or dried beans
or
recipe from a low-calorie recipe book.
Fresh fruit

Use as wide a variety of fresh fruits and vegetables as possible. The salads should include at least one serving of sprouts, especially alfalfa. Bean sprouts may also be used. This type of diet should form the basis of your future eating habits but you should eat a wide variety of foods.

A recent large-scale study showed that 26 per cent of the meat-eating population had hypertension, compared to 2 per cent of vegetarians. To be a healthy vegetarian is not simply a matter of eliminating meat from the diet. Read *Diet for a Small Planet* by Frances Moore Lappé (Ballantine Books) and see a qualified naturopath for further advice and information.

Supplements
• *Vitamins B3* and *B6* – in addition to a *B complex* • *Vitamin C and bioflavonoids* • *Bromelain* – if on pharmaceutical drugs do not take Bromelain without practitioner advice • Possibly calcium, potassium or other minerals – depending on dietary intake and tests • *Co-enzyme Q10*

OTHER
Essential hypertension is generally helped by a progressive, regular exercise programme appropriate to age, level of fitness and joint strength and mobility. It has also been reported that patients with mild hypertension benefited from aerobic exercising for 50 minutes three times a week without drug therapy.[8]

Relaxation, meditation and visualisation techniques are often helpful in reducing essential hypertension.

CAUTION **If you are taking your own blood pressure at home get instructions from a practitioner to ensure you are doing this correctly, for example, if the cuff is above heart level, the readings are lower. Also, some equipment does not give accurate readings and all home equipment should be regularly checked against professional equipment.**

HYPOTENSION
(low blood pressure)

Description
Extremely low blood pressure may be a symptom of a serious shock, dehydration or heart failure. It is also associated with low thyroid function, some endocrine disorders and anaemia, all of which produce other symptoms.

Many people have very low blood pressure and are apparently healthy, particularly young, small-frame, vegetarian females, while others have fatigue, giddy attacks or even fainting, especially when standing for long periods or when returning to an upright posture. A reading as low as 90/60 mm of mercury is not a cause for alarm if the person is energetic and healthy. Hypotension is sometimes diagnosed as being when the diastolic blood pressure drops 10 units on standing.

Causes
Serious trauma – requiring medical emergency treatment – or one of the disorders

just mentioned. Other causes include insufficient fluid intake, inadequate diet, protein deficiency, impaired circulation and anaemia. Sometimes low blood pressure is associated with low blood sugar levels.

A report has related low systolic blood pressure and minor psychological dysfunction.[9] The authors suggested either a link between reduced blood supply to the brain or, conversely, that depression and anxiety may cause reduced blood pressure in some people.

Treatment

If the circulation is poor, refer to Circulation (pages 126–7).

If the patient is thin, tired and has a low appetite, increase food and fluid intake in conjunction with bitter herbal remedies and perhaps digestive enzymes for a few weeks. See suggestions in Chapter 5 'Digestive Problems'. To ensure good absorption, make sure food is chewed slowly. Never eat any foods that give you allergic reactions or digestive upsets.

HERBS
• *Ginseng* – Chinese or Korean • *Ginkgo* • *Golden seal* • *Liquorice* – not confectionery • *Verbena*

DIET
Supplements
• *Vitamin B complex* • *Iron, folic acid* or *Vitamin B12* – depending on blood test results

TISSUE SALTS OR CELLOIDS
• *Calc Phos*

CAUTION **Liquorice and golden seal should never be taken together.**

OEDEMA
(fluid retention)

Description

An excess accumulation of fluid in the body tissues. The oedema can be localised, for example, under the eyes, the abdomen or the ankles, or more generalised.

Causes

Poor lymphatic drainage, weak membranes around the blood vessels, varicose veins, hormonal problems, allergies, malnutrition, tumours, heart failure, kidney and liver dysfunction and various serious diseases.

Certain drugs, particularly cortisone, may cause fluid retention.

Sometimes there is no traceable cause.

Treatment

HERBS
• *Burdock* • *Celery seed* • *Dandelion* • *Horsetail* • *Juniper* • *Parsley seed* • *Yucca*

FROM THE KITCHEN
• *Celery and parsley juice* • *Corn silk tea* • *Cucumber juice* • *Green bean juice* or *broth*

DIET
You should ensure there is adequate protein in the diet, but no added salt.

Supplements
• *Vitamin B complex with additional B6* • *Vitamin C and bioflavonoids* • *Vitamin E* • *Potassium*

NOTE **People on pharmaceutical diuretics need to get professional advice before taking potassium supplements.**

OTHER
• Regular exercise and massage.

If the oedema problem is in the legs, see suggestions for Varicose Veins.

VARICOSE VEINS
(varicose symptom complex)

Description

Swollen, distended and knotted veins visible in the legs. Early signs may include fatigue in the legs, cramps, dull aching and swollen ankles. Severe cases may cause constant pain, clotting and ulcers.

Causes

Sluggish flow of blood in combination with weakened walls of the veins and faulty valves. People sometimes have a hereditary predisposition to varicose veins and the weakness is worsened by constipation or sitting and standing for long periods as the blood returning to the heart has to move upwards and this is effected by the pumping action of the leg muscles in combination with flap-like valves. Varicose veins are caused in pregnancy because the abdominal distension can restrict the free flow of blood; overweight can result in varicose veins for the same reason.

Treatment

HERBS

Taken internally
• Bayberry • Chamomile • Chilli, hot
• Gotu kola • Horse chestnut • Motherwort
• Scullcap • Wood betony

Applied externally
• Calendula • Golden seal • Witch hazel

These may be used in the form of ointments.

If the veins are swollen and inflamed, cold compresses of these external herbs, or chamomile, are more effective.

DIET
• Berries • Buckwheat • Citrus fruits
• Whole grains

If constipation is a problem, refer to Chapter 5, 'Digestive Problems'.

Supplements
• Vitamin C and bioflavonoids • Vitamin E

TISSUE SALTS OR CELLOIDS
• Calc Fluor • Ferr Phos – if the veins are swollen or inflamed

OTHER

Avoid standing and sitting for long periods (do ankle exercises constantly while sitting). When sitting, avoid crossing legs or ankles.

Check posture, especially to ensure that the circulation is not cut off at the knees. A footstool is helpful. Rest with the feet up.

Do yoga inverted postures. Go to a qualified teacher as you do not want to damage your back.

Avoid all tight clothing and tight shoes.

Apply regular, gentle massage, using upward stroking movements. Wear massage sandals or use a massage mat.

If you are overweight it may be necessary to go on a low-calorie diet.

NOTE **In some cases the problem with the veins is not entirely visible and there may be deep vein thrombosis that requires professional attention.**

CHAPTER 8

KIDNEYS AND BLADDER

The kidneys are required to function efficiently if we are to maintain good health. Their main task is to filter out of the blood the breakdown products and waste from nutrients and the body's metabolic functions; the kidneys also control the levels of fluid, sodium and potassium in the blood and adjust its acid/alkaline balance. If the filtering system of the kidneys is not operating optimally, then we may be retaining some substances that should be excreted or excreting products such as minerals and proteins that should be retained.

Both the kidneys and the liver are essential for life, so we ought to do all we reasonably can to strengthen and support them.

People often ask me how much water they should drink and it is very difficult to answer this. It depends on what you eat and drink because many fruits and vegetables have a high water content. Another factor is replacing water loss through sweating and urinating: it has been estimated that we lose about a cup of fluid per day via the skin and lungs even if we don't noticeably sweat. Obviously, if you are doing hard, physical work in hot sunshine, then you will need to drink very high quantities.

Water is no doubt the best and cheapest drink, particularly if large amounts are required. For the average adult, about 6–8 glasses of fluid per day is a reasonable estimation and although I am not sure that the body can distinguish between the water in various drinks and plain water, it would seem sensible to have at least some of that quantity as ordinary water because most other drinks have disadvantages: fruit juice is expensive, wasteful and contains fairly high amounts of sugars; coffee can be irritating to the nervous system, the kidneys and the digestive tract and so on.

Some mothers say that their children refuse to drink water and demand cordials, soft drinks or juices. This may be because of the unpleasant taste of water in many areas, and a possible way of overcoming this resistance is to use a water filter and to add a few, pure fruit, ice blocks to the water. For adults, it helps if the water is served in a long glass, with some crushed ice, mint leaves and a few slices of lemon or orange.

If you live in an area where the water has a high chlorine content, it is a good idea to at least boil the water before drinking or leave it to stand overnight in a jug in the refrigerator to allow the chlorine to evaporate.

The Australian Kidney Foundation reports that four per cent of women have urinary tract infections without realising. The main warning signs of infection are bed wetting, passing urine frequently, pain or burning when passing urine, and pain or ache in the back just below the ribs not made worse on movement. Always seek a practitioner's advice if you suspect infection.

BLADDER WEAKNESS

Description
This can take different forms. Sometimes it is manifested by constant urination during the day, and also during the night. In other cases, the weakness takes the form of incontinence where some urine escapes when the person laughs, coughs or sneezes; or it can just be a little dribbling.

Causes
There are many possible causes, some of which are: infection in the bladder, kidneys or vagina, kidney disease, nervous conditions, allergies (especially to orange juice), chills, following surgery, mineral imbalance, excess eating or drinking.

Remember that all the fluid you drink is a diuretic to some extent, so if you are drinking ten cups of coffee or tea per day, then you are bound to be urinating more than ten times per day, because in addition to the obvious fluid intake most foods contain a certain amount of water, particularly raw fruit and vegetables.

Bladder weakness may also be due to a structural or neurological fault, congenital conditions such as spina bifida, pressure of pregnancy, obesity or even constipation.

When a healthy bladder expands as it fills with urine, this triggers the nerve fibres in the bladder wall to send an 'emptying' message. Basically, anything that causes pressure or irritation can trigger the urge to empty the bladder. This also happens with nervous irritation – as you know from your own experience. In other words, it's usually very difficult to distinguish simple weakness from other causes.

Treatment
EXERCISE
An excellent exercise is one for the pelvic floor muscles, given under Pregnancy (see page 108).

Another good bladder exercise is the following. Lie on a firm surface with knees bent, feet flat, legs and feet about 20 cm apart. Lift your buttocks off the floor, without arching your back. In that position, contract your buttocks and lower abdomen muscles tightly while giving little puffs out through the mouth. Hold in that position for a count of ten. Then, still with the bottom off the floor, alternately tighten and relax those lower muscles ten times. Each time you squeeze, give a little puff out through the mouth. Lower your body to the floor, relax, and then repeat the exercise twice more.

HERBS

• *Agrimony* • *Corn silk* • *Hops* • *Horsetail* • *Marshmallow* • *Shepherd's purse*

(Other herbs that may be helpful are given under Cystitis, below).

DIET

Don't drink coffee, orange juice or pineapple juice as the problem may be related to allergies and in my experience these are common bladder irritants.

If you have to see a practitioner, it might be worthwhile collecting and measuring all your urine in a 24-hour period as well as keeping details of all you eat and drink in that period.

Supplements

• *Vitamin C and bioflavonoids*

NOTE **High ascorbic acid is an irritant to some people. If so the vitamin C is best taken in the form of sodium ascorbate.**

TISSUE SALTS OR CELLOIDS

• *Calc Fluor* • *Kali Phos* • *Ferr Phos* • *Silicea*

CYSTITIS
(inflammation of the bladder)

Description

The common symptoms are frequency and urgency of urination, usually with pain and burning. Sometimes there is a constant desire to urinate, but only a tiny amount of urine is excreted and this may cause an excruciating, burning pain. In more severe cases there may be blood in the urine, either obvious or perhaps a small quantity which tends to give the urine a pink–orangy colour. Cystitis may be accompanied by malaise, chills or fever. It can come on suddenly, or be persistent or recurring over months, and occasionally over years.

Causes

Either an ascending infection, i.e. from the exterior of the body, or a descending infection, that is, coming from the kidneys. The latter type is obviously more serious.

It may be an isolated infection, or it can be a result of some other physical condition such as urinary retention, stones, tumours or a neurological problem. In females it can also be caused by sexual activity. I have seen cases of mild, long-term burning urine that were apparently caused by orange juice, either an allergy to it, or simply drinking too much acidic juice.

The more complicated types of cystitis are often accompanied by other health problems, but in any event it is always wise to have a medical diagnosis because you are not otherwise able to treat the cause; for example, it may be caused by a chronic vaginal infection.

Cystitis may also be related to, or be worsened by, too little fluid intake, incorrect use of toilet paper (don't wipe towards the front), inadequate personal hygiene, bacteria transferred from tampon string, nylon underwear, tight jeans, scented soaps, talc, dirt or other substances transferred to the urethral area from fingers during love making and it has also been linked to fungal infections. Chlorine in swimming pools may be an aggravating factor for some people.

Treatment of uncomplicated cystitis

The first step is to have a very high fluid intake – some people suggest as much as 4 litres per day. This at least dilutes the urine and flushes out irritants. If it is extremely painful to urinate, one suggestion is to urinate while sitting in a basin with some tepid water in it.

FLUIDS

Drink water, preferably distilled, boiled or mineral water, at least 1 large glass every hour for 3–4 hours, with ⅓ teaspoon sodium bicarbonate added for the first 3–4 glasses. Then endeavour to have a drink every hour, selecting from water, vegetable broth, celery juice, green bean juice, cucumber juice, barley water or one of the herbal teas below.

For the first day, fluid only is recommended.

HERBS

• *Alfalfa* – tea, tablets or sprouts
• *Burdock* – tablets, decoction or extract
• *Catnip* – tea • *Chamomile* – tea
• *Clivers* – juice or extract • *Corn silk* – infusion or extract • *Echinacea* – extract
• *Fennel* – tea • Garlic – capsules, 6 per day • *Golden seal* – tablets or extract
• *Marshmallow* – tea or extract • *Sandalwood oil* – 3 drops three times daily for 1–2 weeks • *Slippery elm* – tablets or powder

Uncomplicated cystitis is treated very successfully by qualified herbalists, who stock a number of herbs such as *buchu* and *uva ursi* that are not often available at retail outlets.

DIET

No coffee, ordinary teas, alcohol or citrus fruits during an attack. Following one day on fluid, for a few days restrict the diet to vegetables (raw and cooked), brown rice, buckwheat and millet. Sugars and high protein intake are inappropriate during an attack. Plums and obviously acidic fruits may be aggravating; large quantities may even cause burning urine.

Pure cranberry and blueberry juices are helpful for treating and preventing urinary tract infections.[1] I recommend a high intake of all *red* and *blue berries*. Bilberry is now available as a herbal extract.

Supplements
• *Vitamin A* • *Vitamin B6* • *Vitamin C* – this should be taken in the form of calcium ascorbate or sodium ascorbate
• *Zinc*

TISSUE SALTS OR CELLOIDS
• *Ferr Phos* • *Mag Phos* • *Nat Mur*

NOTE **In cases where cystitis is constant or recurring, it is worthwhile considering allergies and Candida.**

A 1992 article advised that antibiotics can adversely affect the outcome of urinary tract infections.[2] If necessary, courses should be short – three days for acute cystitis. The article warned against improper, repeated and prolonged courses of antibiotics, which may result in long-term complications without resolving the problem.

KIDNEY STONES

Description

Hard or hardish desposits of varying sizes and types that may form in part of the kidneys or in the urinary tract. These deposits may be so small that they are classed as 'gravel', or medium-to-large in varying shapes.

It is not uncommon for there to be no symptoms, but if there is an obstruction there will be pain in the back, sides and abdomen, depending on the locality of the stone. Often this pain is in the form of severe colic and the patient may be doubled up in agony, or the pain may be dull or constant.

There may be nausea, vomiting, abdominal distention and blood in the urine. When the blockage is lower down the urinary tract, the symptoms may be similar to acute appendicitis and diagnosis is necessary. If there is an infection, there will be chills and fever as well as irritability of the bladder, usually with cloudy or discoloured urine. During an attack, the patient will be, understandably, agitated and anxious.

Causes

Metabolic, inherited or congenital disorders, excess acidity or alkalinity, failure of kidneys to empty due to cysts or some other obstruction, abuse of antacids, injury causing immobilisation, infection (bloodclots or clumps of bacteria may serve as a nucleus for stone formation), hyperparathyroidism and other endocrine disorders, excess vitamin D or excess calcium.

Certain groups of foods may be an aggravation for particular types of stones: an American study showed that excessive dietary protein contributes to the formation of kidney stones.

Treatment

The treatment is complicated because there are different types of stones. Unless you know the type of stones you have, the wisest course of action is to follow the advice given to you by a qualified practitioner; in any case you should always discuss with your practitioner the support remedies you wish to use.

GENERAL MEASURES

Ensure a high fluid intake, particularly water. This usually means about 2–4 litres per day but depends on levels of sweating and type of diet. In some areas the water is very high in certain chemicals, minerals or even heavy metals, and it is suggested that if you live in such a hard water area filtered or pure spring water would be preferable.

Eat a sensible, balanced diet, with plenty of variety. You should have minimal tea, coffee and alcohol.

POULTICES

A hot poultice or hot compress often helps to relieve kidney pain. Refer to Chapter 1, 'Using the Remedies'.

HERBS

The herbs suggested are those that can be obtained from at least some retail outlets or easily collected.
• *Aloe* – below laxative dose • *Bergamot*
• *Burdock* • *Corn silk* • *Dandelion* • *Juniper*
• *Shepherd's purse* • *Yellow dock*

A number of natural therapy books recommend parsley.

With a problem as serious and painful as kidney stones I would recommend that people seek the assistance of a qualified herbalist who prescribes therapeutic doses and has access to herbs not available at retail outlets.

NOTE **In all cases of kidney problems any accompanying infections need to be treated with practitioner advice.**

CALCIUM OXALATE STONES

Over 50 per cent of urinary stones are composed of pure calcium oxalate or calcium oxalate mixed with phosphate. These are associated with a high urinary pH (i.e. the urine is too alkaline).

Treatment

Calcium restriction is no longer recommended for kidney stone patients because this may lead to problems, such as osteoporosis and hypertension. However, no one suggests they have high calcium diet, and calcium supplementation should not be used by them without medical advice.

DIET

• Low protein • High intake of *vegetables* and *complex carbohydrates* • *Rice bran* – 1 dessertspoon per day • *Pumpkin seeds* • Not excessive calcium and vitamin D (milk, cheese, butter, margarine, fats, carob, sesame seeds, brewer's yeast) • No foods high in oxalates (cocoa, tea, rhubarb, spinach, chard, beets, sorrel, chocolate) • No kelp supplements; no molasses • Low salt, nuts and seeds

Supplements

• *Ascorbic acid* – ½ teaspoon powder in juice twice daily • *Fish oil together with evening primrose oil* – 1000 mg of each twice daily • *Vitamin B complex, plus additional vitamin B6* • *Magnesium citrate* – 100 mg twice daily

OTHER

Avoid aluminium compounds and alkalis; these are used in some antacids and anti-diarrhoeal medications.

MAGNESIUM AMMONIUM PHOSPHATE STONES

These are treated as Calcium Oxalate Stones.

URIC ACID STONES

These are commonly associated with gout and low pH (excess acidity). Occasionally there is a link with high levels of lead in the blood.

Treatment

It is suggested that the urine should be slightly above pH 6.5.

DIET

Foods to include in the diet:

• *Alfalfa sprouts* or *tea* • *Almonds* • *Black cherries* – whole, fresh or as unsweetened juice • *Buckwheat* • *Buttermilk* • *Coconut* – small quantities • *Corn* • *Fresh fruit* – especially *apples* • *Fennel* • *Garlic* • *Globe artichoke* • *Millet* • *Sweet potatoes* • *Vegetables* – generally • *Yams*

A vegetarian diet, or at least a very low red meat intake, is generally beneficial. Foods to avoid in the diet: • *Alcohol* • *Anchovies* • *Brains* • *Coffee* • *Fish roe* • *Herrings* • *Kidneys* • *Liver* • *Meat extracts and gravies* • *Mussels* • *Sardines* • *Sweetbreads* • *Tea* • *Yeast supplements*

Citrus juices and apple cider vinegar may cause an aggravation.

Supplements

• *Vitamin B9* (folic acid) • *Calcium ascorbate*

CYSTEINE STONES

These are associated with a low pH, so the treatment involves trying to keep the urine alkaline.

Treatment

HERBS

• *Echinacea* • *Golden seal*

DIET

Drink 3–4 litres fluid per day. Include some *alfalfa tea* and diluted *vegetable juices*.

Follow the dietary advice given under Uric Acid Stones, above. Also reduce methionine-rich foods (soy, wheat, dairy products, fish, meat, dried beans, mushrooms, nuts).

Supplements
• *Vitamins B6, B9, B12* • *Sodium ascorbate*

STRUVITE STONES

Treatment
It is suggested that attempts be made to keep the urine below pH 6.5 (acidic).

DIET
Follow the dietary advice under Calcium Oxalate Stones.

Supplements
• *Ascorbic acid* – 3g per day in divided doses

NOTE **If you are considering a treatment that crushes kidney stones, ask about possible side effects as I have seen cases of permanent lung and organ damage resulting from this.**

NOCTURIA

Description
Having to get up during the night to urinate. This has a number of disadvantages, including causing fatigue due to broken sleep.

Causes
Generally nocturia is due to an accumulation of fluid during the day and increased kidney excretion when lying down. During sleep the kidneys, normally and ideally, function to concentrate the urine.

Anything that causes pressure, including constipation, and irritants such as infections, upsets and allergies, can be a cause.

Treatment
HERBS
• *Celery and juniper tablets* – use these after breakfast and after lunch, the aim being to increase the urinary flow during the day.

NOTE **Juniper is not recommended as a continuous, long-term remedy.**

Horsetail • *Valerian*
Other sedative/relaxing herbs can be used.

DIET
• Check for allergies • *Linseed oil* – 1 tablespoon per day • Reduce all other fats

Supplements
• *Magnesium* • *Potassium* • *Zinc*

OTHER
If the problem is associated with nervous problems some of the remedies given in Chapter 10, 'Nervous and Immune Systems', may help.

Some find that the problem is helped by having a teaspoon of bicarbonate of soda in half a glass of water before bed.

Most people find it is better not to have any fluids after dinner and to avoid large, late evening meals.

PROSTATE ENLARGEMENT – BENIGN

Description
A common complaint in men over fifty years of age. Usually the early signs are that the urinary flow is not as forceful as

it once was and the bladder never feels really emptied. There may be hesitancy, straining, urging to empty the bladder during the night and sometimes blood in the urine.

Often there is pain or discomfort in the lower abdomen.

NOTE **This condition requires a medical diagnosis.**

Cause

The enlargement is due to a metabolite of testosterone (a male hormone). The enlargement may be malignant or the gland itself may be inflamed.

Because of the position of the urinary outlet (urethra), enlargement of the prostate interferes with the normal flow of urine from the bladder.

Treatment

Some practitioners use massage per rectum to reduce the enlargement and increase urinary flow.

CAUTION **Complete blockages of urinary flow require urgent medical attention.**

HERBS

• *Clivers* • *Couch grass* • *Ginseng* • *Hops* • *Horsetail* • *Nettle* • *Saw palmetto* – this herb has given good results in ten trials.[3]

Professional herbalists have access to other herbs that are not generally available from retail outlets.

DIET

• *Alfalfa, soya bean* and *red clover sprouts* – all types of sprouted seeds, whole grains and legumes are suggested because of their beneficial hormonal content

• *Beans* – green string and red kidney (soaked and well cooked) • *Beetroot* • All plants in the *cabbage family* • *Celery and cucumber juice* • *Fennel* or *aniseed* – as a tea, vegetable or flavouring • *Fish* • *Onions* • *Parsley* – a handful a day • *Pumpkin seeds* • *Sage* and *hops* – as weak teas

Some people find that a raw vegetarian diet is helpful.

Avoid: • *Beer* • *Wine* • *Yeast* • *Smoking* • *Animal fats*

Supplements

• *Bee pollen* • *Evening primrose oil* (or one tablespoon of linseed oil) • *Garlic* • *Vitamin E* • *Zell oxygen* • *Zinc*

PROBLEMS WITH CERTAIN DRUGS

Prescription and some over-the-counter drugs can damage the kidneys. The following is a list of some specific drugs that can harm healthy kidneys and aggravate existing problems.

Actifed	Amoxil	Aprinox
Aspirin	Bricanyl	Bufferin
Butazone	Chlotride	Clinoril
Colchicine	Dalmane	Digest-eeze
Digesic	Eromycin	Flagyl
Gantrisin	Inderal	Indocid
Lasix	Lithicarb	Midamor
Moduretic	Moxacin	Mylanta
Naprosyn	Steclin V	Streptomycin
Tagamet	Theo-Dur	Tranxene
Tryptanol	Voltaren	Zyloprim

This is by no means a comprehensive list but a selection of the more commonly used drugs. A Japanese study showed that taking spirulina in addition to pharmaceutical drugs generally reduces kidney toxicity. However, some spirulina from Mexico has been shown to contain mercury so I would suggest you buy organic products or get verification from the manufacturer that its product is free of excess heavy metals.

Australians spend around $60 million a year on analgesics which are well known for their potentially damaging effects on the kidneys; both over-the-counter and prescription drugs can also adversely affect the kidneys, particularly in large, prolonged doses. In normal circumstances, an occasional use of painkillers is not harmful although a healthier course of action might be to find out why you are getting headaches or other pain and see if there is a completely harmless method of overcoming the problem, such as stress management or biofeedback. If you have to take analgesics keep them minimal and take a vitamin C supplement to counteract some of their harmful effects (aspirin blocks the uptake of ascorbic acid into the blood platelets).

A study indicated that a dose of 30 mg of aspirin per day was as effective as a dose of 283 mg in preventing death from vascular disease and non-fatal myocardial infarction (heart attack) in a group of patients who had previously had a transient eschaemic attack or minor stroke.[4] *However, there were 40 episodes of major bleeding out of 1555 patients, including both gastro-intestinal haemorrhage and haemorrhagic stroke.*

Media reports of the benefits of aspirin tend to give only the benefits without the risks. A major trial of USA medical practitioners who used aspirin for some years was widely publicised without reporting that the doctors actually used Bufferin, not plain aspirin, and they also took beta-carotene. The trial was discontinued after three years of its projected five-year study. A British study failed to support the American findings: of 3429 British doctors who took aspirin, 148 died of heart attacks or strokes, while of 1710 who did not take aspirin, 79 succumbed of the same causes.

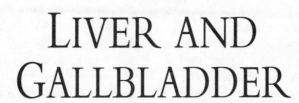

CHAPTER 9

LIVER AND GALLBLADDER

If you have a serious liver malfunction or disease then you are markedly and obviously ill; this book is not intended for such conditions, but rather for the many problems that can arise from partial malfunctioning or underactivity. Before looking at some of the disorders related to liver functioning, it is worthwhile listing some of the main functions of the liver, so that you can appreciate why such a wide range of problems can be associated with it.

FUNCTIONS OF THE LIVER

STORAGE
• The liver stores glycogen (glucose) which is needed by the body for energy.
• Fats, vitamins (such as B12) and minerals (such as iron) are stored in the liver.
• Large amounts of blood can be held within the blood vessels of the liver.

CONVERSION AND SYNTHESIS
• The liver can convert protein and fats to glucose; it also converts excess sugar into fat and sends it to other parts of the body for storage.
• The liver makes proteins for various purposes.
• It produces clotting substances.
• It converts different types of sugars to glucose.
• It forms a large amount of the body's cholesterol requirements, and many other important biological compounds.
• It produces bile, which is then stored and concentrated in the gallbladder. Bile has a number of functions, the main one being to aid the digestion and absorption of fats and oils.

BLOOD CIRCULATION SYSTEM
• About 1500 ml of blood flow through the liver each minute. The liver breaks down worn-out blood cells, utilising

some components and sending others through the bloodstream for disposal by the kidneys.

• The liver also removes bacteria and foreign bodies from the blood.

DISPOSAL OF TOXINS

• By various mechanisms, the liver neutralises poisons, drugs and a whole range of metabolic by-products.

HOMOEOSTASIS

• The liver performs a number of 'balancing' functions in the body, such as disposing of excess female sex hormones in males, and vice versa.

In view of the many vital functions carried out by the liver, it is not surprising that a number of naturopaths and herbalists include a liver remedy in their treatments, particularly when you consider the numerous chemicals throughout the food chain and in our atmosphere which place an added burden on the liver's detoxification processes. It is known that some chemicals, such as DDT and carbon tetrachloride, can adversely affect the liver's detoxification system.

NOTE *Always use liver and gallbladder remedies at a low dosage initially because maximum doses may activate the organs to the extent that they cause nausea, vomiting or headaches.*

LIVER SLUGGISHNESS OR UNDERFUNCTIONING

Description

It may be difficult for an untrained person to arrive at a diagnosis, and the general underfunctioning I am referring to would not necessarily show up in a liver function test.

In the absence of another explanation, the following symptoms may indicate liver sluggishness; it would be unlikely that an individual would have all of the symptoms but a number of them might be present at one particular time.

• Feeling of fullness or tenderness below the right ribs • Fatigue even after rest; often with excessive yawning and sighing • Constipation, or some diarrhoea • Poor appetite • Flatulence and other digestive problems • Headache • Irritability and general malaise • Coated tongue • Bad breath • Allergic-type reactions to oranges/eggs • Skin problems

Causes

Environmental and food toxins, pharmaceutical and social drugs, alcohol, microorganisms, poor diet and hygiene, intestinal permeability (leakiness) and, possibly, allergies. People with long-term liver diseases are often deficient in specific nutrients, such as vitamin E and some of the vitamin B complex, but this may not have caused the problem.

Treatment

HERBS

• *Barberry bark* • *Dandelion* • *Fenugreek* • *Garlic* • *Gentian* • *Golden seal* • *Hops* • *Milk thistle* • *Yellow dock*

Professional herbalists might use some of these but they also have access to other herbs that are not commonly available at retail outlets.

FROM THE KITCHEN

• *Chilli, hot* – small quantities are stimulating; very large amounts are harmful • *Ginger* – fresh ginger root used in cooking is helpful to the digestion, generally stimulating and helps to lower cholesterol levels • *Globe artichoke* • *Horseradish* – very small quantities are stimulating • *Turmeric* • *White radish* – the large type, used in Asian recipes (I grate it into salads)

CAUTION **Do not take hot spices in large quantities or on an empty stomach.**

DIET

If possible, use as many organically grown products as you can because these do not contain pesticides or other chemicals which put added strain on the liver; by reducing the levels of toxins in the diet the liver is freed for other metabolic processes. Also, avoid alcohol and all non-essential drugs and chemicals; the reasons for this are expanded later in this chapter.

Drink one or two juices per day, preferably freshly made, and selected from:
• *Apple* • *Beetroot* • *Carrot* • *Celery* • *Cucumber* • *Grape* • *Green bean* • *Lemon* or *grapefruit* • *Pear*

NOTE **In my clinic I have observed that some people get yellowing of the palms of the hands if they drink more carrot juice than their bodies can handle. This may be due to a weakened liver or excess juice.**

Juices are helpful where there are problems of assimilation and absorption because they provide a concentrated, easily digested form of nutrients. It is easier for the digestion to have the juices singly, although two fruits or two vegetables can be combined to make a juice more palatable.

Some people do not tolerate orange juice and they may be allergic to it; however, if this is not the case, then it can help stimulate the digestive juices.

Eat generous servings of all vegetables, preferably in salads or steamed. Vegetables especially recommended include cabbage, celery, chicory, small quantities of dandelion greens, endive, fennel, globe artichoke and watercress. Sprouts are very nutritious and should be served regularly. Bean sprouts may be used in soups and casseroles; don't cook them but stir them in at the end of the cooking time instead of a thickening agent.

Use a wide range of whole grains (preferably organically grown). Select from barley, brown rice, buckwheat, millet, oats, rye and wheat. These grains are now available from health food stores in many forms, such as flour, flakes and meal (roughly ground). Regularly include in the diet well cooked and pre-soaked dried beans, especially soya beans; also lentils and other legumes.

Protein is needed for rebuilding and fish is the most recommended food in this category (2–4 servings a week; not shellfish). Nuts and seeds should be used sparingly. Eggs and dairy may not be well tolerated and should be eaten in small quantities; use low-fat dairy products.

Cold-pressed olive oil – 1–4 tablespoons – plus half that quantity of lemon or grapefruit juice often stimulates the liver and gallbladder, especially if used in conjunction with liver herbs. The oil and lemon juice can be used in a salad of grated raw beetroot, chopped cabbage, tomato and parsley. This quantity of oil would not be eaten daily.

NOTE **People with certain liver pathologies would not be able to assimilate the oil.**

Supplements
• *Vitamin B complex* • *Vitamin C* • *Vitamin E* • *Carnitine* • *Choline* • *Lecithin* • *Magnesium* • *Methionine* • *Taurine*

There are some lipotrophic and anti-oxidant formulae on the market which combine some of the above supplements.

Specific foods to avoid
• All animal fats, such as red meat, butter, full-cream milk • Processed oils and margarine.
• All refined and processed foods. This is especially important where the appetite is poor because when only small amounts of food are eaten, it is vital to have them in a form that gives as many nutrients as possible, with the least amount of chemicals such as preservatives or pesticides.

TISSUE SALTS OR CELLOIDS
• *Nat Sulph* • *Kali Mur*

OTHER
In 1987 a doctor reported a case of cirrhosis with severe ascites (abdominal fluid retention due to advanced liver malfunction).[1] A diuretic drug was not adequate. Using a modified spa bath, the patient sat for two hours with 35°C water up to his neck. His weight dropped 2 kg in a day and the effect lasted for six days with a diuretic. Further 'water therapy' again produced rapid weight loss (8 kg) and the patient was left with no fluid retention in the abdomen or limbs.

In a home situation, I would suggest sitting upright in a deep bath for about half an hour at 35°C once or twice weekly to get a similar but less dramatic reduction in abdominal fluid. Undergoing a massive change in internal fluid requires supervision – don't do it if alone. You also need to take care to keep warm after these types of baths.

GALLSTONES

Description
These are present in many people, but they may not have any obvious symptoms. Gallstones range between numerous small stones in the gallbladder, or a few medium-sized ones, or even one enormous stone. The very tiny stones and the very large ones may not cause as many problems as the medium stones because one of the main complications is when a stone is dislodged and gets caught in the bile duct.

The liver produces bile, which is mostly stored and concentrated in the gallbladder and secreted into the intestine after meals via the bile duct. Bile is needed for the breakdown and absorption of fats as well as for correct intestinal and excretory functions.

The pain caused by obstruction of the bile duct is extreme, and may be accompanied by fever and jaundice. Flatulence is a common symptom of gallstones along with fat intolerance, but many digestive problems may be present, including nausea and vomiting. The pain may be fairly constant or sudden, and often it radiates to the shoulder blade and the back.

In a few cases, the duct may become inflamed and infected and, like the appendix, it can rupture.

Causes
Obesity, infections, some drugs, pregnancy, oral contraceptives, excess dietary fats, excess dietary sugars, liver malfunctioning and a familial predisposition.

There is a relationship between oral contraceptives, hormone replacement therapy and gallbladder problems.

Treatment

Here is an old naturopathic treatment.

Don't eat anything after midday (water and juices are permitted). At about 6.30 in the evening start taking pure cold-pressed olive oil followed by pure, freshly squeezed lemon juice. Every 15 minutes take 4 tablespoons of the oil, immediately followed by 1 tablespoon lemon juice. Finish the treatment with a lemon juice dose.

Total quantities: 500 ml olive oil and the juice of 8–10 lemons – depending on how juicy they are.

I suggest you use a straw to take the lemon juice as pure juice in this quantity may irritate the lips. You may need to use a lip salve also.

The treatment is to be continued until all the oil and lemon has been ingested, even if vomiting occurs. Surprisingly, very few people experience vomiting, although some get discomfort and colicky abdominal pains. People who do not complete the procedure may run the risk of after-effects a few days after.

When all the oil and lemon juice is taken there have been quite remarkable results, with the stones passing out. To my knowledge there have not been any cases of stones lodging anywhere in the system when the instructions have been followed precisely.

It is suggested that the next day all the bowel motions should be collected in a receptacle, such as an old colander; tap water should be run over these. There are quite amazing stories of the types and numbers of stones collected in this way, commonly numerous greenish stones about the size of a split pea; sometimes there are large, soft ones.

People who didn't fancy collecting their faeces in this way reported hearing the stones land in the toilet bowl. The bowel motions are usually quite messy following the treatment. Some naturopaths report that in certain cases all of the stones come out in liquified form.

CAUTION **This procedure should not be undertaken by young children, pregnant women, frail or elderly people. It is not suitable for people who are experiencing pain, nausea or vomiting, or whose gallbladders are acutely inflamed.**

Although this particular naturopathic treatment may seem heroic and extreme, I know of hundreds of people who have used it successfully. In my experience, the worst thing that can happen is vomiting.

One would expect that this type of procedure could precipitate a blockage of the bile duct, but in all the cases I know of, not one emergency operation has been required.

The people who first introduced this method maintained that the stones do not cause blocking because they are softened. However, I would suggest that this treatment should not be followed without the advice of a practitioner who knows your medical history.

For people with a family history of gallstones, and who have signs of liver and gallbladder sluggishness, this treatment can be considered as a preventive measure, because there is no doubt that it is a means of completely flushing out the gallbladder and the intestines. I rarely recommend it as a preventive measure for anyone under the age of thirty, however, because the individual indications do not warrant it.

There are two less heroic versions of the above.

• 25 ml cold-pressed olive oil followed by 120 ml fresh grapefuit juice every morning for two weeks.

• 2–4 tablespoons cold-pressed olive oil, in equal or smaller quantities of fresh, unsweetened lemon juice. Take daily as a drink or in salads, or mixed in with other food (but not heated), for a period of 3–4 weeks.

With these two methods I have not found that the stones can be collected; such milder treatments work better with herbal support.

Some Canadian practitioners use the following method.

Drink 4 large glasses of pure apple juice per day for two weeks. Then, on a non-working day, take ½ cup olive oil blended with ½ cup freshly squeezed lemon juice and 1 teaspoon Epsom salts. The patient then lies down on his or her right side with the right leg up to the chest for half an hour. This causes a strong contraction of the gallbladder which expels any sludge or stones. Another teapoon of Epsom salts is taken in the evening.

One practitioner has treated over 3000 patients with this method without a stone getting stuck. If necessary, the treatment can be repeated in a couple of weeks.

These treatments may seem heroic, but in some cases the only alternative is to have the gallbladder removed. There are number of reasons for avoiding this operation if at all possible. First, any operation carries an element of risk. Second, the gallbladder stores and concentrates bile, and without it the patient may find

that: the liver will take over the total function and there will be no apparent subsequent problems; or the liver will *not* adequately cover the gallbladder's function and the person will suffer from mild to severe abdominal discomfort, particularly following meals with an obvious fat content, and there may be bloating and other digestive problems; or there will be an excess of bile from the liver to the small intestines and this can cause irritation and diarrhoea, both of which can lead to further problems.

According to a British medical report, there is an increased risk of developing colon cancer for those whose gallbladders are removed.

Strong pharmaceuticals can dissolve the stones and lasers can shatter them, but these are not without risks either. However, I admit naturopaths have a somewhat 'jaundiced' view of medical treatments because we see mainly the bad results of medical treatments.

HERBS

Those listed under Liver Sluggishness (pages 144–6) plus • *Vervain* • *Wild yam*

There are some specific herbs for gallstones but these have to be obtained from a practising herbalist, as they are not available in health-food stores.

DIET

Eat a *high-fibre diet* – use a variety of whole grains and avoid all processed and refined foods. Include plenty of vegetables, fruits, dried beans and legumes.

1 glass *beetroot juice* per day is recommended, with a small quantity of juiced parsley. (Do not use the green tops of beetroot.) Pear juice is also recommended. Take a little lemon juice in hot water first thing in the morning.

Alternative juices are given under Liver Sluggishness.

Avoid
• *Fried foods, oils and fats* • *Cooked cheese* – use low-fat products • *Eggs* – use the whites only • *Oranges* – these may aggravate some cases of gallstones • *Coffee* – increases the amounts of circulating fats • *Milk* – use skim milk or low-fat yoghurt • *Cream* – substitute buttermilk You should cut to a minimum • *Seeds* and *nuts* • *Red meat* • *Alcohol* and *tobacco* – but it is best to avoid both.

A report has also associated the problem with a high sugar intake.[2]

Supplements
• *Vitamin B complex* – 1 tablet a day should be sufficient in most cases • *Vitamin C* – ¼ teaspoon powder twice daily in a pure juice • *Vitamin E* – 500 IU maximum • *Lecithin* – 2 tablespoons per day.

TISSUE SALTS OR CELLOIDS
• *Nat Sulph*

OTHER
Generally, the remedies under Liver Sluggishness (pages 144–6) are appropriate for a congested, underfunctioning gallbladder. Another general recommendation for gallbladder problems is to work on reducing the levels of cholesterol: further information on this is given in Chapter 7, 'Heart and Circulation'.

For some related problems, such as flatulence, symptomatic remedies will be found in Chapter 5, 'Digestive Problems'. It is worth noting that bitter-tasting medicinal herbs reflexly stimulate the digestive organs, including the liver and gallbladder.

HEPATITIS

Description
In early stages the general symptoms are: malaise (generally tired and feeling unwell), lack of appetite, headaches, chills with flu-like symptoms, nausea, vomiting, diarrhoea or constipation, tenderness around lower right rib cage, constant upper abdominal pain, lymph nodes (glands) may be enlarged, aversion to smoking.

Next stage symptoms (usually 5–10 days after onset of the above symptoms): whites of eyes yellow, dark urine, pale bowel motions.

The convalescent stage follows. In some cases it may take several months, or even longer, for the patient to completely recover. There can be a relapse, for example, after drinking alcohol. Very occasionally the condition may persist, or it can lead to chronic liver disease.

Causes
Hepatitis may be secondary to disorders such as amoebic dysentery, cirrhosis and glandular fever; generally, it is a viral infection transmitted via the mouth or rectum through direct contact or contaminated foods or drinks. Serum hepatitis is transmitted via the blood and is a particular problem with heroin users and other illegal drug addicts. Hepatitis may also be caused by or related to alcoholism, and is a side effect of a number of pharmaceutical drugs, for example, the anti-depressants Laroxyl and Marsilid and some arthritic medication. All drugs are detoxified by the liver. A stressed liver is obviously more prone to disease than a healthy one.

Precautions
Strict isolation is not normally advised at home but it is recommended that the patient's linen, soap and eating utensils be kept separate. Thorough handwashing is necessary after going to the toilet and

when other members of the household handle the patient's personal effects. Maintaining a high level of hygiene and general cleanliness is recommended. Ensure that the person affected gets plenty of rest, as well as other members of the household, because people who are tired and run-down are more prone to catching infections.

Treatment

Absolutely no alcohol. Adequate fluid intake and rest are the first essentials.

HERBS

• *Echinacea* • *Milk thistle* • *Reishi*

Take herbs in tablet, capsule or powder form.

NOTE **Never use herbs that are preserved in alcohol if you have a liver problem.**

DIET

Some naturopaths recommend a completely raw vegetarian diet, including wheatgrass and other juices. Soups and broths (without fats or oils) are other options.

Protein is required for rebuilding the damaged liver tissue but the hepatitis patient will not tolerate fats and will usually have a low appetite.

Try brown rice, fish, lean chicken or low-fat soy milk flavoured with fruit. A protein supplement or whey powder can be incorporated into some of the food or juices tolerated by the patient. It may be necessary to use a combined multi-vitamin and mineral supplement.

Supplements

• *Vitamin C* • *Lactobacillus acidophilus*
• *Bifidobacteria*

OTHER

Chinese or *Korean ginseng* is a useful convalescent tonic, as tablets or capsules.

The dietary and general recommendations given throughout this chapter should be useful, always being sensitive to the needs and tastes of the particular patient.

JAUNDICE

Description

Yellowing of the skin and the whites of the eyes, usually noticed first in the eyes. It may occur quite suddenly or come on so gradually that it is not obvious. Depending on the cause, the jaundice may be accompanied by other symptoms such as itchy skin, digestive problems, steatorrhoea (fatty and smelly stools), nausea, abdominal pains, fatigue and malaise. The urine may be dark and the stools pale.

Some people have yellowing of the eyes without having any apparent liver or gallbladder problems; also some people have yellowing of the palms of the hands that does not always relate to the liver or gallbladder, nor is it always connected to excess or poorly metabolised carrot juice.

The yellowing of skin in jaundice is caused by an excess of bilirubin (a colouring agent in the bile). It escapes into the bloodstream instead of being broken down and excreted, and then causes the yellowing.

Causes

Jaundice is not a disease but a symptom of a number of disorders of the liver, gallbladder and blood. it can reflect a relatively minor condition such as drinking excess carrot juice or indicate a serious problem, for example: a gallstone obstructing the bile duct, exposure to toxic substances, a drug side effect or an infection such as viral hepatitis. Jaundice can also relate to anaemia, alcoholism, congenital disorders, cancer or any disease affecting the liver and gallbladder.

CAUTION ***Jaundice requires a medical diagnosis, because some types of hepatitis are dangerous and highly infectious. Gallbladder obstructions can be life-threatening.***

Treatment

To a large extent, the treatment depends on the cause, but the general guidelines given for Liver Sluggishness (pages 144–6) are appropriate in most cases.

TISSUE SALTS OR CELLOIDS

• *Ferr Phos* • *Nat Sulph*

EFFECTS OF ALCOHOL, DRUGS AND CHEMICALS

ALCOHOL

In Australia, alcoholism is the fourth major public health problem. An intake of two glasses per day is probably not harmful for most people, but over that quantity there may be minor, initially imperceptible, brain damage – according to some researchers.

The liver converts alcohol to energy; this is energy without the benefits of other nutrients, and the surplus energy is stored as fat. Many alcoholics are not overweight because they get most of their kilojoules from the alcohol and therefore don't feel hungry; in other cases these people cannot adequately absorb the food

they eat as the alcohol has so irritated the stomach and intestines.

Alcohol can produce harmful effects in all the body's organs, particularly the liver, which can become fatty, or develop hepatitis or cirrhosis. Although the liver has significant powers of regenerating itself, there is a point at which damage becomes irreversible.

Animal studies show that lecithin may protect against cirrhosis and reverse early stages of the disease.

DRUGS – LEGAL AND PHARMACEUTICAL

There is a drug, prescription or over-the-counter, for practically every kind of ailment, real or imagined, and ultimately these have to be broken down by the liver and excreted, with the help of the kidneys.

If you have a life-threatening condition and need a particular drug to stay alive then you should consider reducing all other drugs, toxins and chemicals you take, so that the liver and kidneys are not overburdened.

If your condition is not serious, then you should read *MIMS Annual* to see the potential danger of that drug for yourself. Then you will be able to ask questions, get a second professional opinion and make a judgement for yourself as to whether the drug's benefits outweigh the risks. Obviously, it is not practical for individual medical practitioners or other concerned individuals to make completely informed decisions, because of the vast amount of material and its enormous complexity; according to an American report, one chemical recently put forward for approval as a drug required 20 000 pages of data, five years of research and a budget of $55 million dollars, so you will appreciate why no one person can be a watchdog.

In spite of all the tests, there are some commonly used prescription drugs that print statements such as 'exact site and mode of action unknown' or 'safety of continuous long-term therapy has not been established'; a few examples in this category are: Aldecin, Beconase, Capoten, Inderal, Normisan and Norgesic.

A few commonly prescribed pharmaceutical drugs that should not be taken when there is liver damage, or which may cause damage to the liver are:

Aldomet	Migral
Arterioflexin	Minipress
(Clofibrate)	Murelax
Brufen	Pethidine
Butazolidin	hydrochloride
Dantrium	Premarin (and
Dilantin	other hormonal
Eromycin	drugs)
Heparin	Quinine bisulphate
Imodium	Serepax
Librium	Valium
Lomotil	

The above is simply a random sampling taken from *MIMS Annual* and is by no means a comprehensive list; I did not include whole groups of drugs such as the anti-neoplastics, cardiac drugs and corticosteroids.

In *Current Medical Diagnosis and Treatment*, edited by Drs Chatton and Krupp, there is a section entitled 'Drug and Toxin Induced Liver Disease' which states that there has been an increase in many types of toxic reactions due to the introduction of new pharmaceuticals. The diagnosis of liver damage caused by therapeutic agents is not easy because of the wide range of drugs involved. Practitioners need to be aware of this possibility and to question patients carefully about medications. The drugs concerned are listed under various categories including direct hepatotoxic group, viral hepatitis-like reactions, cholestatic reactions, chronic active hepatitis, fatty liver and granulomas. Compromising the liver is only one of many, even hundreds of, possible side effects from prescription drugs. Articles in *Progress in Liver Diseases* provide some evidence that a liver disease may get progressively worse – even after the offending drug has been discontinued.

Iatrogenic illness is the term used to describe drug-induced damage – a new epidemic. Always ask your doctor, 'Is this prescription really necessary?' A report found that only 30–50 per cent of patients expected a prescription for every symptom, while 80–90 per cent of doctors believed that a drug was sought.[4]

CHEMICALS

Peanuts

Peanuts are not really true nuts because they grow under ground. Peanuts contain a naturally occurring mould called aflatoxin. Aflatoxin is a potent liver toxin and a real carcinogen. Over the years government testing has shown that the aflatoxin levels in peanuts and peanut butters are diminishing.[4] However, the National Health and Medical Research Council concluded that 'any level of aflatoxins is cause for concern and no provisional tolerable weekly intake has been assigned by the World Health Organisation'. Although the latest Australian survey showed that only one of 33 samples tested was contaminated with aflatoxin, infants were shown to be ingesting more than they had previously.

Then there are man-made toxins: from 33 samples of raw peanuts, two exceeded the allowable cadmium limit; from 32 samples of peanut butter, seven exceeded the allowable cadmium level. Nine out of 33 peanut samples contained alpha-BHC and beta-BHC (nasty chemicals related to DDT); 2 samples contained chlorpyrifos and were in violation of the Food Standards Code as this pesticide is not permitted to be used on peanuts. Likewise for peanut butter, there were 11 violations of the Food Standards Code involving the pesticides alpha-BHC, beta-BHC and pirimiphos methyl which have no residue limits for use in peanuts and therefore should not be used.

I'm not particularly 'down' on peanuts but am using them as an example because many people are under the impression that they are 'healthy'. An article in *Science* entitled 'Ranking Possible Carcinogenic Hazards' gave the same hazard ranking to a cup of comfrey tea and a peanut butter sandwich.[5] Comfrey was placed on the Poisons Schedule some years ago in Australia as it was considered to be highly dangerous. Politics and commercial interests aside, it is quite likely that some individuals may be extremely sensitive to aflatoxins (and comfrey).

Pesticides

You're probably familiar with the reasons why the use of DDT and similar chemicals was discontinued in agriculture and horticulture. Although most pesticides in current use are not as persistent in the environment and in the body, many can affect the liver, digestive system and blood as well as producing reactions in the skin and nervous system.

I know from my experience as a horticulturist that some people are more sensitive to pesticides than others. There are plenty of stories about shaky and sick horticulturists: here's a true one. I worked part-time in a nursery where the owner used to mix pesticides and fungicides with his hands and happily sprayed without any protection or thought. His skin was always itchy. Some of the staff weakly complained about headaches and nausea caused by the smell from all the pesticides stored under the work-bench. A few blue-tongue lizards lived under this storage area. When their babies emerged, I crept over to look and was horrified to see that one of the infants had only one eye. From that day onwards, the nursery was galvanised into action. All old products were taken away, full protective gear was purchased and pesticides were stored in a separate, lock-up shed.

Here's what you can do to avoid potentially hazardous pesticides:
• wash or peel all fruits and vegetables, or buy organically grown products
• avoid using all chemicals as far as possible (there are thousands of home gardeners and an increasing number of commercial growers who never use chemicals)
• join your local organic growing society – addresses are given in organic gardening magazines.

CHAPTER 10

NERVOUS AND IMMUNE SYSTEMS

The idea that the mind affects the body is not new. In 1884, a doctor wrote in the *British Medical Journal* that 'depression of spirits at these melancholy times [bereavement] disposes them to some of the worst effects of chills'. Modern research can now pinpoint emotional changes at a cellular level. Psychoneuroimmunology is the science of the connection between your emotions or thoughts and the functioning of your nervous and immune systems.

Of course what happens to your body also affects your mind. If you get a serious disease or have a nasty accident, this can make you understandably anxious and depressed. So can stress.

People have always been stressed in various ways. Primitive hunter–gatherers would have worried about where their next meal was coming from. I doubt that any of them would have given a thought to being a few kilos overweight or any of the common modern anxieties.

It has been estimated that on average traditional hunter–gatherers spent about 15 hours a week collecting food.[1] They would have had other jobs to do as well – like making spears. In other words, their work was probably around four hours a day of moderate physical activity and there would have been a fair amount of lolling around. Other evidence tends to support the notion that many of our ancient relatives were very prone to bashing each other.

Stress hormones are used in physical activity. Most of us in today's world need to get more physical activity or find new ways to work off stresses. If you're angry or upset, your computer screen does not provide stress relief. You can't pick up the nearest object and biff a colleague over the head, either. Nor is it always appropriate to laugh or cry – especially these days when jobs are hard to come by. The alternative is to train ourselves to think more nobly and effectively: to turn frustrations into challenges, to appreciate that people are not perfect, to accept that life without difficulties would probably be insipid and to realise that we are only 'visiting' the planet.

For at least 5000 years, sages in various cultures have been telling us to improve our thinking. Obviously, if we all loved one another, a large proportion of our stress would disappear. If we gave up pleasure seeking, another block of stress would go (the more most people get, the more they want; as Buddha said: 'Even a rain of gold would not satisfy their desires'). If we had a deep spiritual belief, another mound of stress would be non-existent.

'Oh yeah,' you say to yourself, 'I know all that', or 'Quit dreaming'. So, you either know what is right but don't act on it or you don't believe it.

Much of human behaviour is inexplicable. We can't or won't do what is good for us. Perhaps that's what makes us so interesting. When life is full and exciting, we say, 'Give me peace and quiet.' When life is calm, we say, 'I'm bored.' Stress gives us energy. Without it we might become stagnant. But we need to cope with it, or transcend it, or it can cause problems.

In 1983, the National Heart Foundation of Australia published a booklet entitled *A Profile of Australians*. One of the findings was that 11 per cent of men and 17 per cent of women gave answers that indicated they were severely psychologi-

cally disturbed, while a total of 25 per cent of men and 30 per cent of women were mildly to severely disturbed.

Each year in Australia there are almost 10 million prescriptions written for tranquillisers, antidepressants, hypnotics (drugs for insomnia) and sedatives. When you drug your mind, you drug your senses and your thoughts. The Australian government has a great deal of information on a whole range of pharmaceutical and social drugs, including alcohol, coffee and cigarettes. Your local Department of Health is able to provide pamphlets and information about counselling services.

I appreciate that there is a need for anti-psychotic drugs and medication to help prevent suicide and mutilation. Also, during major trauma, many people need more than comfort (or platitudes). But, generally, the less you use drugs the better it is for your body and mind. Even the so-called 'minor' tranquillisers cannot be discontinued abruptly, so it's better not to get on them in the first place.

The suggestions in this chapter do not relate to psychiatric disturbances or severe psychological problems but are aimed at helping with everyday stresses before they lead to serious complications.

If you could suddenly switch to noble thinking then most of your earthly problems would disappear, or at least seem trivial. However, you – and I – do not have the disposition of a Buddhist monk; so we need remedies and suggestions to help us cope.

Homoeopathy, Bach Flowers and aromatherapy are especially helpful for nervous and emotional problems. Chapter 2, 'Explaining Some Natural Therapies', will tell you how they're used.

ALOPECIA (falling hair)

Description
This does not refer to hereditary male baldness or the normal and somewhat variable loss that occurs when combing and shampooing; but, rather, when the loss is fairly sudden and obvious, and the hair comes away in clumps.

Causes
Severe illnesses, certain pharmaceuticals, extreme anxiety, hormonal imbalances and faulty nutrition are common causes. Hair loss is also associated with rapid weight loss, following surgery, childbirth, and any major change or stress.

Treatment
HERBS
• *Bayberry*   • *Chamomile*   • *Horsetail*
• *Nettle* – internally and also the cooled infusion used as a rinse and scalp massage
FROM THE KITCHEN
• *Olive oil* – a little massaged into the scalp before washing hair • *Rosemary, sage* or *cedarwood oil* – small quantities massaged into the scalp

When the scalp is being massaged, use a reasonable amount of pressure to move the skin rather than rub over the hair. If the scalp is very dry, *evening primrose oil* is an alternative remedy, for use before shampooing (cut open a capsule).
DIET
Check for adequate protein and vitamins (especially A and Bs). Eat seaweed products. Females may be helped by using the oestrogenic herbs listed on page 113.
Supplement
• *A combined multi-vitamin and mineral with additional PABA and biotin*
TISSUE SALTS OR CELLOIDS
• *Silicea* together with *Calc Fluor*

ANOREXIA NERVOSA

Description
Loss of appetite relating to emotional states.

Causes
Anxiety about weight gain, psychiatric disorders, fears.

CAUTION Anorexia usually needs professional counselling and treatment; if untreated it can lead to malnutrition and other life-threatening conditions. Sometimes the problem may be hidden, for example, patients may eat and then make themselves vomit directly after meals (bulimia).

Loss of appetite can also relate to loss of smell and taste, or poisoning, for example, lead toxicity.

Treatment
HERBS
To stimulate the appetite: • *Burdock*
• *Centaury* • *Gentian*
Nutritives: • *Alfalfa* • *Fenugreek* • *Rosehip*
• *Slippery elm powder*
Culinary herbs to stimulate appetite and digestion: • *Cardamon* • *Ginger* • *Lovage*
• *Savory*
DIET
Small, frequent, appetising meals.
Supplements
• *A combined multi-vitamin and mineral*
• *Zinc* • *Biotin*
One researcher has related anorexia nervosa to subclinical pellagra (vitamin B3 deficiency).[2] Particularly for vegetarians, additional vitamin B3 is suggested. All anorexic patients might also benefit from a fish oil supplement.

Of course, people with anorexia lack many essential nutrients so specific supplements should be taken at a different meal from the combined multi-vitamin and mineral supplement.

ANXIETY

Description

The dictionary describes anxiety as uneasiness, concern, apprehension or feelings of dread. These feelings will sound familiar to a lot of readers and are quite normal if you are changing your job or sitting exams, if someone you love is ill or in similar circumstances. Occasional bouts of irrational anxiety are experienced by most of us and this, too, may be considered fairly normal, as long as we are still able to carry out our usual day-to-day activities.

Recognising when the anxieties need attention may be helpful in avoiding deeper and more long-lasting psychological problems, and some early indications are recurring headaches, chronic insomnia, compulsive behaviour such as overeating, refusing to eat, thumb sucking or nail biting.

Anxiety and tension often lead to additional problems such as lifeless hair, falling hair, skin aggravations (especially itching and rashes), nervous dyspepsia, gastric ulcers, diarrhoea or constipation, recurring infections or constant coughs and colds. The nervous conditions may also be accompanied by anti-social behaviour, hyperventilation, withdrawal, aches and pains.

When the anxieties are constant or not traceable to any cause, and you cannot carry on with normal everyday activities, then it is necessary to seek professional help.

Causes

Poor handling of stress, illness, hormonal imbalances such as hyperthyroidism, overwork, lack of interests, insufficient exercise, nutrient deficiencies, fluctuating blood sugar levels, excess coffee, alcohol, drugs, possible heavy metal toxicity (lead and mercury are two examples), personal and financial concerns, and also an inherited predisposition that may have been reinforced by upbringing or the environment.

Treatment

HERBS

• *Chamomile* • *Cowslip* • *Linden* (lime flowers) • *Valerian* – do not use if fatigue is also one of the symptoms

BACH FLOWERS

• *Agrimony* • *Aspen* • *Elm* • *White chestnut*

AROMATHERAPY

• *Basil* • *Marjoram* • *Melissa*

DIET

Avoid eating when emotionally upset. If the problem is constant, then small, frequent meals are better for absorption and digestion than large ones. Eat a well balanced diet, with plenty of variety.

Supplements

• *Vitamin C* • *Vitamin B complex*

OTHER

• Seek out sympathetic friends or family members for support.

• Get professional advice from your practitioner, the Department of Health or one of the many welfare associations listed in the Yellow Pages and the Community Help and Welfare section at the front of the White telephone directory.

• Find some interesting activities. If you ask around or look in your local paper you will find that there are many adult learning centres offering a wide range of courses.

• If you hyperventilate so that your chest feels tight and full, try to swallow when breathing out. The other recommendation is to breathe into a paper bag – but you might not have one handy!

• Do some things for other people. Many community organisations rely on volunteers.

• Many naturopaths use Bach Flower remedies for emotional problems. This is preferable to resorting to alcohol, social or pharmaceutical drugs; the last should be reserved for extreme cases.

• Try a course of meditation, yoga, tai chi, stress management or something similar. Don't be discouraged if the first course you do does not suit you; keep trying until you find something to your liking because you will learn something from each experience and meet people who are also interested in improving their health.

• Coffee and alcohol tend to give a temporary lift but the overall, long-term effect is that these substances tend to increase anxieties. Recent research indicates that high doses of caffeine (also found in some soft drinks) appear to induce anxiety states in both normal and panic patients.

• Treat yourself to a few luxuries.

• Try at least some of the exercises given at the end of this chapter (pages 167–70), especially rhythmic abdominal breathing.

BAD TEMPER AND IRRITABILITY

Description

Over-reaction or violent reaction to stimuli.

We are all justifiably angry at times but when our anger loses friends, alienates us from our colleagues at work and our families, then it is time to sit down and consider self-assessment, perhaps with the help of a professional counsellor. For example, it is unreasonable to lose one's temper if the car ahead of us is a little slow at the traffic lights. Using up energy on such trivial matters is exhausting and puts stress on the whole body. It can lead to chronic fatigue, or is perhaps concurrent with it.

Causes

Pressures of work or family, feelings of insecurity, low self-image, envy and sometimes habit or chronic fatigue. Hormonal disturbances, pain and physical problems can also make you cranky.

Treatment

Self-examination, possibly expert help, yoga, tai chi, stress management course, appropriate exercise and lifestyle adjustments.

HERBS

• *Hops* • *Linden* • *Motherwort* • *Scullcap* • *Vervain*

BACH FLOWERS

• *Cherry plum* • *Holly* • *Impatiens*

AROMATHERAPY

• *Chamomile* • *Lavender*

DIET

Avoid coffee and alcohol. Reduce red meat.

CONCENTRATION AND MEMORY PROBLEMS

Description

These problems may be part of the general state called nervous debility. People may feel that their thinking is 'woolly' and they may also suffer from headaches, dizzy spells and a general malaise.

Causes

Lack of interest or stimulation, hearing impairment, lack of sleep, inadequate nutrition, accidents, psychological factors, allergies and metal toxicities such as aluminium or lead.

Aluminium has been linked to memory loss and more serious brain problems. There is some evidence that aluminium in aerosols, toothpastes, deodorants, tobacco smoke and other sources is absorbed into the circulation through the lungs and the skin and lodges in the brain. You also ingest tiny quantities from food, cooking pots and water. Relatively high amounts are found in some antacids.

Lead is said to be the greatest environmental threat to human intelligence.

Slimming diets produce concentration and memory problems as they may not provide your brain with sufficient glucose for optimal functioning. Dietary carbohydrate is needed for the nervous system to operate normally.

Alcohol and other drugs may also adversely affect the memory and concentration.

A certain amount of memory loss is quite normal as one gets older, particularly short-term memory – for example, going to the kitchen and forgetting what you went there for. Many people experience this and don't consider it a problem because this slight loss is offset by a lifetime of experience and learning. Physical exercise, learning new skills, reading and doing courses seem to keep the mind more active. Brains are like muscles – if you don't use them, you lose them.

If you tell yourself you cannot remember things, you won't make an effort.

Treatment

HERBS
• *Ginkgo* • *Ginseng* • *Gotucola* • *Oats*
• *Rosemary* • *Sage*

BACH FLOWERS
• *White chestnut*

AROMATHERAPY
• *Rosemary* • *Sage*

DIET
Supplements
• *Glutamine* • *Vitamin B complex with zinc*
• *Vitamins C and E* • *Zell oxygen*

DEPRESSION

Description

A morbid state of sadness or melancholy, as distinguished from a normal state of grief resulting from a personal loss. Sleep patterns are often disturbed.

Causes

Often difficult to assess. Can be brain chemical imbalances, thyroid malfunctioning, oral contraceptives and other hormonal treatments, pain, physical problems, low kilojoule diets, family, work or environmental circumstances and low self-esteem. May be related to boredom, sometimes to allergies, low blood sugar, anaemia and certain drugs.

---

*CAUTION **Severe depression, especially where there are self-destructive tendencies, requires professional help.***

Treatment

HERBS
• *Ginseng* • *Maté* (not long term) • *Oats*
• *Rosemary* • *St John's wort* • *Vervain*

BACH FLOWERS
• *Gentian* • *Gorse* • *Mustard* • *Olive*

AROMATHERAPY
• *Jasmine* • *Rose*
DIET
• *Glutamine* • *DL-phenylalanine* • *Vitamin B complex*

EXCITABILITY AND HYPERACTIVITY

Description
In this context, I am using the terms to mean conditions that are excessive, uncontrolled or prolonged, sometimes to the extent that others consider the behaviour to be anti-social, too aggressive or damaging.

Causes
Family, hereditary and environmental factors. Allergies, excess sugar and milk in particular. Occasionally, hyperactivity relates to heavy metal toxicity, such as lead and mercury. The cause may also be insufficient exercise, inadequate diet or simply lack of discipline.

Treatment
HERBS
• *Catnip* • *Cowslip* • *Chamomile* • *Evening primrose oil* • *Hops* • *Passion flower* • *Valerian* • *Wild lettuce*
DIET
Eliminate refined and processed foods. Check for allergies, especially to milk, gluten, food additives and colouring agents.
Supplements
• *Vitamin B complex with extra B3* – in the form of niacinamide • *Vitamin C* • *Glutamine* • *Zinc*
BACH FLOWERS
• *Vervain*

AROMATHERAPY
• *Chamomile* • *Lavender*
TISSUE SALTS OR CELLOIDS
• *Kali Phos*

FATIGUE AND EXHAUSTION

Description
Fatigue results when waste products resulting from oxidation are not removed from the blood. This may follow intense exertion and a build up of acids in the tissues. The muscles become inefficient and generally the whole system is under strain.

Recuperation comes through rest. If rest does not restore the energy level, then the fatigue is said to be chronic and if this persists for a length of time then you may accept this low energy as normal.

It may be difficult to establish whether the exhaustion starts as a physical or a mental problem.

It's a vague and subjective condition and individuals have different capacities and expectations. A simple description of fatigue could be a reduced ability to react or to function.

Causes
Continued stimulation or excess activity. Overwork is not a common cause unless the job is frustrating; boredom is a common cause.

The possibility of a disease and liver or kidney problems should be considered; also anaemia and faulty nutrition. Constant stress or pain are also causes unusual fatigue. The underlying problem must be treated as well as the fatigue.

Treatment

HERBAL TONICS
- *Alfalfa* • *Chilli* • *Fenugreek* • *Ginseng*
- *Golden seal* • *Lemon balm* • *Maté* • *Oats*
- *Rosehip*

BACH FLOWERS
- *Hornbeam* • *Olive* • *Wild rose*

AROMATHERAPY
- *Basil* • *Jasmine* • *Rose geranium*

FROM THE KITCHEN
- *Ginger*

DIET
Eat a well-balanced diet with plenty of variety.

Supplements
- *Vitamin B complex* • *Royal jelly*
- *Vitamin E* • *Zell oxygen*

Digestive enzymes may be required if there are problems of digestion and absorption; people who suspect this should obtain practitioner advice.

OTHER
As far as possible, do something to trace and eliminate the cause of the fatigue. Take steps to conserve your energy, perhaps practise relaxation techniques, meditation or even take a holiday.

CHRONIC FATIGUE SYNDROME

This is known as ME (Myalgia Encephalomyelitis) and Post-viral syndrome, among other names. The syndrome is difficult to diagnose as fatigue is a symptom in many serious diseases and dysfunctions as well as psychological disorders.

Description
Chronic fatigue lasting for months, extreme weakness, recurring sore throats, low-grade fever, swollen glands, head-aches, muscle and joint pain, diarrhoea or other digestive system problems, anxiety, depression, lack of concentration, mood swings, vision difficulties, changes in sleep patterns (too much sleep or insomnia), hyperventilation and food sensitivities.

According to some researchers, during relapse periods the red blood cells lose their shape and elasticity.

Dr Peter Nixon, a British doctor, said it was 'one of the commonest conditions in the 1930s; only the labels have changed'. He recommends a treatment that includes emotional arousal, breathing exercises, balance between rest and effort and improving self-esteem.

Causes
Viral (some of us have the same viruses in our bodies but don't become ill), weakened or disordered immune functioning, physical and mental stress that can lower resistance and energy, poor intestinal functioning, chemical overload – especially mercury, lead and aluminium – allergies, candidiasis and nutrient deficiencies.

Dr H. Nieper, a German doctor, has suggested that catalytic converters in motor cars (which are supposed to make motoring 'green') are a cause of chronic fatigue syndrome because they emit dangerous free radicals that are subsequently inhaled.[3]

A poor oxygen supply to the body is another possibility. Many people are habitual shallow breathers.

Treatment
Treatment is in three stages. First comes a basic naturopathic detoxification programme, which you should follow for about one month.

HERBS

These will help stimulate the liver and digestion: • *Barberry bark* • *Dandelion* • *Golden seal* • *Milk thistle*

DIET

A wholefood diet, avoiding all additives, added chemicals and processed foods (as far as practicable). Ensure it is high in vegetables and fruit – mainly raw. Eat small, regular meals. Drink filtered or spring water.

If you're overweight, go on the diet programme suggested under hypertension (see pages 129–31).

Supplement

• *Bifidobacteria and lactobacillus acidophilus* – one course at the maximum dose.

The basic programme for the second stage treatment.

DIET

Supplements

• *A combined multi-vitamin and mineral formula* plus an additional *magnesium* supplement – to be taken at a different meal from the multi • *Evening primrose and fish oil* (such as Efamol Marine) – 4 capsules twice daily for three months

When you take such high dose fish oils, add a *vitamin E* supplement to each dose; that is, 100 IU of vitamin E twice daily.

If you can't afford the evening primrose and fish oil supplement, use 1 tablespoon linseed oil per day and have two or three fish meals per week. All other fats and oils are kept to a minimum.

OTHER

Exercise – brief sessions two or three times daily work better than one long session. Gentle yoga and walking are ideal.

Relaxation and *meditation* techniques help as long as you don't attempt too much. Start with exercises you can do lying down. Use *breathing* techniques – as described on pages 167–70 and under Atherosclerosis (pages 123–4).

Consider counselling, laughter therapy, the transcendent factor, Bach Flowers, homoeopathy and aromatherapy.

Vitamin B12 injections increase well-being and energy in about 50 per cent of those with chronic fatigue.

It helps provide the cells with more oxygen. When cells don't get enough oxygen (as in unaccustomed exercise) the muscles don't work efficiently, there's a build up of lactic acid and the muscles feel sore. Emotional problems, such as anxiety, also result in high levels of lactic acid. That's how you can get a sore neck and upper back when you're upset.

Specific remedies for persistent or recurring infections

HERBS

• *Clivers* • *Echinacea* • *Garlic* • *Lemon balm* • *Nettle* • *Reishi* • *St John's wort*

DIET

Supplement

• *Vitamin C*

Specific remedies to improve muscle and brain oxygen supply

HERBS

• *Ginkgo* • *Ginseng* (Siberian)

DIET

Supplements

• *Coenzyme Q10* • *Zell oxygen*

For the third, recuperative stage of the programme I have found that *Chinese* or *Korean ginseng* is the best remedy for preventing relapses of chronic fatigue. Generally, I suggest that ginseng be taken for two months, then have a break and use it intermittently if necessary.

OTHER

Medically, IVIG (intravenous immuno-globulin treatment) was shown to help 43 per cent of patients in an Australian study but no improvement was seen in a US study; there were side effects ranging from phlebitis (55 per cent) to constitutional symptoms (82 per cent).[4]

One US study showed that a fairly high proportion of people complaining of chronic fatigue were psychiatrically disturbed.

FEARS

Description

Fears become a health problem when they prevent us going about our normal activities. They can be related to symptoms such as dizziness, palpitations, phobias, diarrhoea, difficulty swallowing and gastro-intestinal problems such as spastic colon. Insomnia may also follow from excessive fears.

Causes

Often unknown; sometimes hereditary or trauma. Depending on the severity and complexity of the problem it may be necessary to obtain professional counselling.

Treatment

HERBS
• *Chamomile* • *Rosemary* • *Scullcap*

BACH FLOWERS
• *Aspen* • *Cherry plum* • *Mimulus* • *Red chestnut* • *Rock rose*

AROMATHERAPY
• *Chamomile* • *Lavender*

HEADACHES

It is not possible to describe all the many types of headaches in one chapter but two types will be covered – tension and migraine.

TENSION HEADACHES

Description

These are usually recurring, lasting, constricting, affecting both sides of the head with associated tender neck and shoulder muscles. They can be accompanied by poor concentration, pain behind the eyes, ear and tooth pain, dizziness and bad temper.

Causes

Worry, physical and mental trauma, bad posture or muscle strain. Sometimes poor lifestyle habits, lack of exercise and faulty nutrition are factors.

Other causes include digestive problems, constipation, sinusitis, infections, eye problems, allergies, hormonal imbalances, trauma, neuralgia, depression, high blood pressure, circulatory disturbances, teeth and jaw problems, lack of sleep, extremes of temperature, certain drugs, various diseases and very serious conditions such as meningitis and tumours.

Any treatment should involve endeavouring to find, and then remove, the cause.

Treatment

Tranquillity doesn't come in a bottle, of course, but you usually need something to help settle you down and ease the discomfort so that you can then consider your lifestyle.

HERBS
- *Chamomile* • *Hops* • *Lemon balm*
- *Motherwort* • *St John's wort* • *Scullcap*
- *Valerian* • *Vervain* • *Wood betony*

A five-minute, hot foot bath may be beneficial, especially using chamomile, lavender or lemon balm. This is usually most effective if done at the first sign of a headache.

DIET

Supplement
- *Vitamin B complex*

TISSUE SALTS OR CELLOIDS
- *Calc Phos* • *Mag Phos*

MIGRAINE

Description

Usually recurring, affecting one side of the head, throbbing, with visual disturbances and light sensitivity, and often accompanied by nausea and vomiting. May last all day. The patient invariably prefers a quiet, dark room.

Causes

Not always known. Often brought on by allergies to chocolate, coffee, monosodium glutamate, aerated drinks, added salt, refined sugar, cheese, alcohol; also emotional upsets, low blood sugar levels or menstruation. There is usually a constriction of the blood vessels in the head, followed by a reflex dilation that brings excess blood to the area, causing throbbing and tenderness.

Treatment

Remove cause, if known.

HERBS
- *Chamomile* • *Feverfew* • *Ginkgo* • *Lemon balm* • *Linden* • *Wild yam*

To avert an attack, or reduce its severity, try a five-minute foot bath, as hot as possible, using yellow jasmine flowers, one of the above herbs or an aromatic oil. This needs to be done at the first suspicion of an attack.

FROM THE KITCHEN

Ginger has been used to treat migraine.[5] At the first sign, one patient took only 600 mg (slightly less than ¼ teaspoon) of powdered ginger in water to abort an attack. As a preventive, use a small quantity of ginger daily in food or herbal teas. I suggest a daily dose of ¼–1 teaspoon.

BACH FLOWERS
- *Vervain*

DIET

Write down the foods eaten prior to an attack to see if you can trace any allergies.

Supplements
- *Vitamin B complex with extra B2* • *Vitamins A and E* • *Calcium* • *Magnesium*

TISSUE SALTS OR CELLOIDS
- *Mag Phos* • *Nat Phos*

OTHER

Regular massage, acupuncture, homoeopathy, mobilising and posture improvement exercises (see Arthritis, pages 47–51) and relaxation therapy.

INSOMNIA

Everyone has an individual sleep pattern – not all of us are blessed with the capacity to fall into a sound sleep within minutes of putting the head on the pillow.

Some of us may function better with more sleep than we are getting. A study of American college students, who normally spent eight hours in bed, showed that when given the right conditions they actually slept for nine hours *and the extra sleep gave them improved alertness during the day*. However, more sleep may not provide you with more energy because there are lots of things that cause fatigue. The amount *you* need may be specified as being enough to make you alert and energetic during the day. It is a myth (I hope!) that everyone should wake up feeling instantly on the ball.

Description

Insomnia falls into two kinds. Some insomniacs have difficulty getting to sleep. They take their troubles to bed with them; the general pattern is to have conversations in the mind, something analogous to a broken record – going over the same thing again and again.

Other insomniacs wake constantly or very early in the morning. Some experts relate this to depression; it can also relate to fears and anxieties; sometimes to excitement or alcohol.

Insomniacs usually feel tired, irritable and incompetent, especially if they dwell on how little they slept the night before. One of the worst things is worrying about not sleeping – remind yourself that there are thousands of people who are seemingly quite healthy on a few hours' sleep a night.

Causes

Insomnia often starts with an emotional crisis. Following a period of stress, during which there has been difficulty in sleeping, a fixation may occur and you become convinced that you cannot sleep.

Many things cause or worsen insomnia, including allergies, asthma and other respiratory disturbances, bladder or kidney dysfunctions, coffee, colic, constipation, depression, drugs, fasting and slimming diets, guilty conscience, high altitudes, hormonal imbalances, hospitalisation, hypertension, hypochondria, inappropriate exercises, indigestion, jet travel, lack

of positive experiences, low blood sugar, muscle tension, nightmares, pain, setting unrealistic goals, shift work, trauma, worrying and so the list goes on. One of the latest theories is that chronic insomnia indicates an internal clock (circadian rhythm) that is 'out-of-kilter'.

Treatment

HERBS
• *Catnip* • *Chamomile* • *Cowslip* • *Hops*
• *Passion flower* • *Scullcap* • *Valerian*
• *Vervain* • *Wild lettuce*

BACH FLOWERS
• *Agrimony* • *Vervain* • *White chestnut*

AROMATHERAPY
• *Hops* • *Lavender*

Both these herbs are useful in herbal pillows and as foot baths.

DIET
Restrict tea, coffee, alcohol. Do not eat a heavy meal within three hours of going to bed, if possible. Don't eat foods which cause flatulence.

Limit after-dinner drinks to a small cup of herbal tea or warm milk.

TISSUE SALTS OR CELLOIDS
• *Calc Phos* • *Mag Phos* • *Kal Phos*

OTHER
• Emotional and nervous problems are not the only causes of insomnia. Sinus infections, digestive problems, constipation and pain can also prevent sleep. In other words, where the cause is known it should be treated.
• Some people are highly sensitive to colours. For example, yellow can be stimulating to the mind; orange and red are also stimulating. Green is generally neutral, while the best colours for sleep inducement are blues, violets and mauves. Try sleeping in a blue room.
• There are those who can't sleep at all unless their heads are facing north; others

are all right as long as their feet are not facing north.

• Most people sleep better if they have plenty of physical activity, although if you get over-tired this will cause muscle and joint pain.

• Gentle stretching exercises about an hour before bed usually help sleep, but avoid vigorous activity late at night. Satisfying sex is an 'insomnia cure' for many people.

• Too much lolling around during the day alters your body's internal clock. Your brain also likes daily exercises. If it is not stimulated during the day, it might seek activity at night.

• It is useless to lie in bed if you cannot sleep. Instead get up and read or look at television (use headphones so you don't disturb other people). You can record something on cassette to listen to – I prefer Eastern philosophy such as extracts from the Upanishads, with meditation music in the background. If you don't want to make your own there are cassettes you can purchase, but with a little practice your own voice may work better for you. Alternatively, every night learn a verse of poetry (perhaps from the Bible) and repeat it to yourself.

• Don't use the bedroom as a thinking place. If you are a worrier try allocating a specific time of day for worrying, e.g. 10.00–10.30 a.m.

• Don't *try* to relax or sleep because this usually acts as a trigger to stop you sleeping. After 40 years of insomnia, I can now trick myself into sleeping by saying to myself 'I want to learn this verse and then think about the meaning behind it' or something similar. I find that the worst thing you can do is say to yourself that you want to look good and feel bright the next day.

• Do not go to bed until you are feeling drowsy. Going to bed later than usual but getting up at the same time is a mild form of sleep deprivation that can improve sleep quality and patterns. Gradually you should be able to go to bed earlier. In any event, if you sleep only six hours each night, what do you gain by going to bed at 10 p.m. and getting up at 7 a.m.?

• As far as practicable, follow a regular sleep schedule. Get up at the same time each morning – even after a night of poor sleep.

• Don't nap or lie down during the day unless you're ill or very elderly.

• 'Owls' may be able to re-set their internal clocks by having exposure to bright lights between the hours of 6 a.m. and 9 a.m. You can buy 'full spectrum' lights that mimic sunshine to use in your house on dark mornings.

• Learn relaxation or meditation. It isn't an instant cure but works in the long run and has other benefits. Try acupuncture, hypnotherapy or homoeopathy – one at a time. Individuals respond differently to various therapies.

• Be comfortable: your mattress should not be hard as a board, nor saggy. The pillow should provide soft support for your neck. Your body temperature falls when you sleep so you may need an extra blanket. A recommended sleeping position is to lie on your right side (then you won't be so conscious of your heart beating), right leg straightish, left knee bent.

• If practicable, select a partner who has approximately the same sleep requirements as yourself. It is extremely irritating for an insomniac to have a partner who goes to sleep within a minute of hitting the pillow, and then breathes loudly and peacefully – or, worse still, snores.

• If all else fails, join the night people. If possible, work different hours or have more evening social activities, but always allow for a wind-down period before going to bed.

Insomniacs have one common trait. They spend an excessive amount of time thinking and talking about sleep. Dwelling on the problem makes it worse. It's also boring or incomprehensible to many people.

Drugs for insomnia should be considered as a last resort and used for short periods only. One of the main drawbacks of sleeping pills is that you do not get REM (Rapid Eye Movement) sleep, that is, you don't have the dreaming state that is necessary for the brain to sort through your daily frustrations and anxieties.

BREATHING EXERCISES AND RELAXATION TECHNIQUES

BREATHING EXERCISES

There are certain breathing techniques that not only help some respiratory problems – because shallow breathing may cause tension in the chest – but also improve general health, for every cell in the body needs a good supply of oxygen to function optimally. In addition, deep breathing ensures that the diaphragm acts as a pump for the venous and lymph circulations. Most importantly, it can be used as a technique for relaxation and meditation.

If you are not accustomed to deep breathing, or you practise excessively to start with, you might hyperventilate and feel dizzy or even faint, so it is a good idea to begin the exercises lying down.

Breathe in through the nose, not the mouth, because this filters the air and helps to control the temperature and moisture content in the respiratory passages.

The following is a basic yoga breathing technique.

1   Lie on your back on a firm surface. You might be more comfortable with a pillow under your knees and a soft pillow under your head.

2   Place your hands lightly on your diaphragm, fingers just touching.

3   When you breathe out, suck your abdomen in. (Imagine that your navel is touching your spine; this action also strengthens abdominal muscles.)

4   As you breathe in, your abdomen expands and your fingers come apart.

Practise for a few minutes each day to start, perhaps when you wake up and before sleep. After a few days' practice, try to make the breathing slow and rhythmical – counting slowly to yourself, 'In, 2, 3; out, 2, 3'. Later, you will be able to do the breathing while sitting or standing; it will be deep and relaxed at the same time.

As you become more proficient in deep breathing, you can expand the chest also, but do not lift the shoulders. Breathe in: on the count of 1 the abdomen fills, on 2 the rib cage expands and on 3 the air flows into the upper chest. Everything is slow and rhythmical. The out-breath is needs to be controlled and even. Imagine the control taking place in the throat centre, even though the air is actually going out through the nose. When you're doing this correctly, you will have the impression of gentle sighing. As you breathe out the abdomen goes down first to the count of 1, then the lower rib cage relaxes to the count of 2 and the upper rib cage relaxes to the count of 3. It is important to keep the flow of air even and relaxed, always breathing in through the nose.

When you have mastered this technique, you can use it for relaxation and to start meditation. After a short period of deep breathing, you should then let the breath come and go naturally and just focus your attention on the breath, or you can count to each breath. The best way to do this is to say to yourself, 'In 1, in 2,' etc., in an unhurried way.

There are a number of other techniques that can be used in conjunction with the breathing.
• If you are feeling jittery or upset, repeat to yourself the word 'calm' as you breathe in and 'peace' as you breathe out.
• When you are tired or depressed, imagine that you are breathing in a warm, soft colour such as gold, orange or pink, and as you breathe out visualise that the colour you are focusing on is being sent throughout your body.
• During a time of agitation, try to visualise breathing in a cool, calming colour such as blue or mauve.
• Another technique is to visualise a colour, such as a soft green. Breathe in that colour and, as you exhale, imagine that it is going to any part of the body where you feel discomfort, tension or pain.

Walking and breathing
First thing in the morning go for a walk, or use the following technique on your way to work.
1 As you walk, for about 3–5 minutes imagine that you are breathing out grey smoke – this represents all your negative feelings. Following that, spend a period of time visualising little, soft silver stars

and as you breathe in your body is being filled up by them; they are filling your mind and body with positive feelings and lightness.
2 Depending on your state of mind, you might then like to repeat a positive affirmation to help you through the day. It could be a few words to boost your self-esteem, to help you in your work or personal life. Two examples are:
• my mind is clear and calm;
• my body is light and strong.

RELAXATION TECHNIQUES

Relaxation and meditation instructions are available on cassette tapes. Most people have to try a number of different methods before finding something that suits them.

You will have better quality relaxation if you do some stretching exercises first. Some simple exercises are given under Arthritis (pages 47–51).

Another good pre-relaxation exercise is alternate nostril breathing as this helps settle you down mentally.

Alternate nostril breathing
1 Sit with back straight, shoulders relaxed.
2 Place your right index and right middle finger between your eyebrows. Your ring finger is placed lightly over your left nostril, and the thumb lightly over the right nostril.
3 Lift the thumb and breathe in calmly and slowly through the right nostril, then close the thumb over the right nostril.
4 Lift the ring finger and breathe out through the left nostril. Then breathe in through the left nostril; close the nostril.
5 Lift the thumb and breathe out through the right nostril, then in through

the right nostril, next close the thumb over the right nostril.

Repeat steps 4 and 5 for twenty or more breaths. You can use the left hand to support the right elbow. Once you are familiar with the technique, you should establish a deep, even breathing rhythm, such as 6–8 slow counts in and 6–8 counts out.

Detailed relaxation technique

I suggest that you put the next exercise on cassette. It is usually better to read it very slowly, with pauses between each phrase or sentence. I like to have soft classical music in the background when recording, or to have music in one largish segment towards the end. Once you have done one tape, it is relatively easy to make others to your individual requirements.

1 Lie on your back on a firm surface, using pillows if necessary to make yourself comfortable. Take a few deep, diaphragmatic breaths.

2 Take a deep breath in as you point both toes down and tighten the muscles in your legs. Breathe out as you relax your legs and feet.

3 As you breathe in again, pull your toes back towards your body, hold, then breathe out and relax.

4 Have your heels slightly apart and let your feet drop to one side.

5 On an in-breath, tighten the buttocks and the lower abdomen, hold, then breathe out and relax.

6 Breathing in, arch your upper back, pushing your chest upwards; breathe out and relax.

7 Lightly press your lower back into the floor and curl the shoulders forward. Then relax.

8 Make fists with both hands as you breathe in, then lift your arms up off the floor as you tighten all the muscles in the arms; hold, breathe out and relax the arms and hands. Then stretch the fingers.

Now place your relaxed arms a few inches out from the body, palms facing upwards, fingers slightly curled.

9 Take another breath in, stretch your chin up towards the ceiling, hold, then breathe out as you move your chin back. Gently turn your head to each side and down to the chest.

10 Breathe in, close your eyes very tightly, purse your lips, puff your cheeks out, then breathe out and let your face muscles relax. Open your mouth and give a big yawn. Then let your head rest comfortably with the chin level.

11 Close your eyes, take a few deep breaths, then let your breath come and go naturally.

For the next part of the exercise the aim is to let each part of the body relax as you breathe out. The breathing should be natural, gentle and regular. Remember to keep the eyes closed. Go through the exercise very slowly, with a pause between each phrase. Say the following to yourself.

1 Right foot relax. My right foot is soft and relaxed and gently dropping to the side. Right leg relax. My right leg is melting into the floor.

2 Left foot relax. My left foot is soft and relaxed and gently dropping to the floor. Left leg relax. My left leg is melting into the floor.

3 Buttocks relax. Lower abdomen relax.

4 My breath is gently flowing in and out.

5 Middle of the back and upper back

relax. My chest is soft and relaxed. My whole body is melting into the floor.

6 I breathe in calmness, I exhale peace. (Repeat 3–4 times.)

7 Right hand relax. My right palm is facing upwards, my right fingers are gently curled. Right arm relax. My right hand and right arm are melting into the floor.

8 Left hand relax. My left palm is facing upwards, my left fingers are gently curled. Left arm relax. My left hand and left arm are melting into the floor.

9 I breathe in calmness, I exhale peace. (Repeat 3–4 times.)

10 Shoulders relax, back of the neck relax. Back of the head relax.

11 Throat relax, muscles of the face relax.

12 My breath is coming gently and evenly. My lips are slightly parted, tongue heavy and relaxed.

13 My eyes are relaxed and feel like soft, black velvet.

14 My forehead is smooth, calm and peaceful.

15 I breathe in calmness, I exhale peace. (Repeat 3–4 times.)

At this stage of the relaxation you can use one of the techniques given in the first breathing exercises, that is, focus on an appropriate colour, breathing silver stars or repeat to yourself some positive affirmation. Some people like to memorise a sentence or small verse from a religious philosophical text to use here. Alternatively, you can record a segment of appropriately relaxing music and simply enjoy that experience.

To wake yourself up

1 Think of an energising colour such as red or yellow, take three or four deep breaths, visualising that you are breathing in that colour and sending it throughout the body as you exhale.

2 Start wriggling the feet and hands.

3 Puff the cheeks and screw the eyes tightly together.

4 Open the eyes, yawn, and give the whole body some thorough stretches.

5 Slowly sit up, then stand, do some more stretches, take a few deep breaths and lastly do a few gentle swinging exercises.

6 Splash your face with cold water and have a short walk in the fresh air.

CHAPTER 11

RESPIRATORY SYSTEM

Some people can catch a relatively minor infection and take months or years to get over it (for instance, see Chronic Fatigue syndrome, pages 161–3). If you don't treat a head cold or a sore throat, it will usually get better by itself, but there's also a possibility that the infection will spread and you'll end up with a really bad cough. In addition, there's plenty of evidence that natural remedies can speed up the recovery process and prevent reoccurrences, even though they may not be actual cures.

The treatments are not harmful nor outrageously expensive. Many of the recommendations have other advantages too. For example, aniseed is a traditional remedy for irritating coughs and it also helps with flatulence and other digestive problems. Garlic has antibacterial properties and is also useful for 'thinning the blood'. Brief, cold showers prevent colds and stimulate the circulation.

Some herbal respiratory remedies work by reflex action, that is they are not directly absorbed into the respiratory tract but may sedate or stimulate one area of the body and thereby affect the head or chest. Other remedies may have a drawing or counter-irritant effect, such as poultices and foot baths.

It is often stated that it is not wise to sedate the cough reflex because this is the means by which the air passageways are maintained free of foreign matter, excess or tenacious mucus. However, when constant coughing causes exhaustion, sleeplessness and irritation, then soothing remedies are called for. It is not surprising that constant coughing uses a lot of energy when you consider that the large airway passages (bronchi and trachea) are so sensitive to foreign particles, chemicals and other irritants that the air in the lungs may be expelled at velocities as high as 120–160 kilometres an hour.

Old natural therapy books often referred to mucus as if it was something to be avoided at all costs. However, the linings of the human respiratory and gastro-intestinal systems, the mouth and all the canals and cavities in our bodies are covered with a specialised membrane that secretes mucus. Ideally, this membrane is light pink, moist and covered with a thin layer of protective mucus.

If there is no mucus secreted, then the particular area does not function properly and a great deal of discomfort and other problems are experienced, as in the case of a sore, dry throat. The opposite problem is an excess of mucus. Infectious or sticky, tenacious mucus prevents normal functioning. (I have chosen to use the word mucus but in respiratory problems it may be more correct to describe it as mucoid sputum, phlegm, muco-purulent sputum or viscid mucus.)

Cigarette smoking aggravates respiratory problems and it is not only the smoker but sometimes a non-smoking member of the family who is affected, such as an asthmatic child. Any smoker who is not aware of the hazards of this addiction should contact the local Department of Health for literature.

As far as practicable, people with respiratory disorders should not work in inappropriate environments; for example, it would be detrimental for an asthmatic to work hunched over a machine all day, and people with chronic bronchitis would hinder their recovery while working in a smoky or dusty atmosphere.

It is very difficult to set a treatment time because you would expect a cold to be cured within a week but chronic bronchitis may take some months. In my own clinic, I always try to give a time span within which a marked improvement should be effected. I often use a number of approaches at the same time, such as a herbal formula, dietary

improvements, a supplement, celloid or tissue salt, as well as regular massage – if the patient can afford this.

There are specific massage techniques that, if done regularly, are beneficial to many respiratory problems. For home use a vibrator used to massage the back and chest may be helpful – at least it feels comforting. I suggest that a towel be placed over the bare skin when using a vibrator. Regular breathing exercises are often helpful, and some of these are outlined in this and other chapters.

One remedy by itself may not be sufficient, for example, with chronic bronchitis you would not expect one cup of aniseed tea per day to make an improvement. However, too many remedies at once may upset your gastric system! With a little practice most people can evaluate what is right for them.

A particular caution when treating respiratory problems is that something that is safe when rubbed on the chest or inhaled is not necessarily safe if ingested, nor does it always have the same effect.

Preventive measures

People with recurring coughs, colds and respiratory infections may like to try the following as a means of preventing the problem. If the problems occur only in the winter, start the programme in autumn and continue through until after the start of spring because, for some people, seasonal changes apparently trigger viral attacks.

• *Cod liver oil* – 1 capsule daily • *Garlic* – 2 cloves per day in cooking (or 2 capsules) • *1 combined multi-vitamin and mineral* • *Vitamin C* – ⅓ teaspoon powder in fruit juice once or twice daily (calcium ascorbate, ester C or sodium ascorbate can be used if ascorbic acid irritates the stomach) • *Echinacea* – 15 drops per day (or 2 capsules) • *Lemon juice*

Although some scientists will say that these are unproven remedies I am amazed myself how many people find that even one or two of the above have made a marked improvement in the incidence and severity of recurring respiratory problems. Some of the scientific tests have not used sufficient quantities to make the test valid, for example, giving 250 mg vitamin C per day for two weeks. From my own research, I would estimate that 2000 mg per day for some months should be the minimum for testing purposes.

A ten-year study on Norwegian lumberjacks who had no colds during the time they spent in the mountains, but who became susceptible when they returned to valley life, indicated that vitamin C may have been the protectant. The lumberjacks applied isotonic sodium ascorbate to the mucous membranes of the nose in order to reduce the danger of irritation by toxic substances emanating from pinewood that was burned in their cabin stoves. The prevention of colds was a favourable side effect.

The writer of an article in the *Lancet* decided to try it at the first sign of what seemed to be 'an especially nasty cold'.[1] He put some ascorbic acid powder up each nostril and sniffed in hard to get it to the back of the nose and palate. Within fifteen minutes the accumulated mucus turned liquid and had to be blown out. He then repeated the treatment and went to bed. After half an hour he felt queasy. Matters improved during the night and in the morning he repeated the treatment twice. By lunchtime he was fine, with little trace of a cold.

My experience is that this treatment is effective as a cold preventive and mucus dissolvant. Use sodium ascorbate for this purpose because ascorbic acid stings. Simply put a little powder on the end of your little finger, insert it not more than 0.5 cm up a nostril, hold the other nostril closed and sniff up. This may also help hayfever and sinus problems by strengthening the mucous membranes, but you have to do it twice daily for at least a month and stop if it irritates.

Although it should go without saying, a basic preventive measure for all respiratory conditions is to avoid known allergens and irritants as far as practicable.

ASTHMA

Description, causes, dietary factors, treatment and general information on adult asthma are basically the same as given in Chapter 4, 'Common Childhood Ailments'.

CAUTIONS **It is particularly important for asthmatic sufferers to know that any sudden discontinuing of medication could result in a rebound effect, that is, the condition could dramatically worsen.**

Asthmatics can be extremely sensitive and anything new needs to be tried cautiously. Royal jelly, for instance, is an excellent general tonic but one case of a fatal allergic reaction to it has been reported.

Additional treatment

The recommendations given below are not intended for acute attacks but rather for mild, chronic conditions or as support therapy.

HERBS

• *Aniseed* • *Chamomile* • *Chilli* • *Garlic*
• *Ginkgo* • *Horseradish* • *Linden* • *Liquorice*
• *Reishi*

Some stronger herbs used by professional herbalists are not available at retail outlets.

FROM THE KITCHEN

• *Onion juice* – sipped before exposure to irritants • *Apple cider vinegar* – 1 teaspoon in warm water, sipped slowly • Hot *foot baths* – marjoram and mustard are two examples • *Ginger* • *Green tea* • *Turmeric*

DIET

In one study, 92 per cent of asthma sufferers showed a significant improvement on a vegan diet but this took 4–12 months. Grains were restricted or eliminated and the following were avoided completely: meat, fish, eggs, dairy products, soya beans, green beans, apples, citrus fruit, tap water, coffee, tea, chocolate, sugar and salt. The people in the study had been on pharmaceutical drugs for an average of twelve years.

Most people need help (and dedication) if they wish to become *healthy* vegans. With restrictions on so many foods, some nutrient supplementation is required.

TISSUE SALTS OR CELLOIDS

• *Kali Phos* • *Mag Phos* • *Calc Phos*

These need to be taken for at least six months.

AROMATHERAPY

• *Chamomile*　　• *Hyssop*　　• *Lavender*
• *Melissa*

Inhale the vapours or use as hand or foot baths.

OTHER

Regular massage by a qualified person is frequently beneficial; this can incorporate European-type massage, with pounding and cupping, or shiatsu. A massage that may be done at home uses a vibrator over the back for about ten minutes daily; put a towel over the bare back.

Read Chapter 4, 'Common Childhood Ailments', for information on allergies and other remedies. Negative ionisers, swimming, singing and hypnosis have also helped many asthmatics. Yoga is an ideal treatment because it combines physical mobility with breathing. A basic breathing technique that may help is given under Atherosclerosis (pages 123–4).

Aspirin and some anti-arthritic drugs (NSAIDs) increase the incidence of asthma. Some asthmatics are also sensitive to alcohol.

BRONCHITIS

Description

Bronchitis can be chronic or acute. An orthodox definition of chronic bronchitis is 'coughing most days for a period of three months over two consecutive years'. Initial symptoms include morning coughing with mucus. There is often a gradual increase in symptoms, which may include thick, coloured mucus, possibly with some blood in it, breathlessness and later there can be cardio-vascular involvement with high blood pressure and fluid retention.

In acute bronchitis there may be fever, chills, infected mucus (yellow-green coloured), wheeze, heavy coughing, cyanosis (bluish discoloration on lips and skin) and chest pain.

Causes

Hereditary predisposition, cigarette smoking, inhaled irritants, and viral or bacterial infections.

Treatment

NOTE *Any treatment must include cessation of cigarette smoking.*

Mild coughs should be treated in the initial stages to avoid them getting worse. Persistent coughing needs to be medically screened. It could be a nervous cough or a more serious problem, so you need to find out.

HERBS
• *Angelica* • *Aniseed* • *Echinacea*
• *Eucalyptus* – externally • *Hyssop*
• *Liquorice* • *Marshmallow* • *Peppermint*
• *Red clover* • *Sweet violet* • *White horehound*

FROM THE KITCHEN
• *Caraway* • *Chilli* • *Cloves* • *Garlic*
• *Ginger* • *Lemon* – the oil is also helpful as an inhalation • *Linseed* • *Rosehip*
• *Thyme*

DIET
Avoid dairy products and chocolate.
Supplements
• *Vitamin C* • *Vitamin A* or *beta-carotene*

TISSUE SALTS OR CELLOIDS
• *Ferr Phos*

OTHER
A vaporiser is likely to be helpful where the cough is croupy, the throat is dry and the chest feels tight and sore (in some cases the dampness aggravates the respiratory system).

Some pharmacists hire vaporisers on a weekly basis so you can give them a short trial period. A few drops of essential oil in the vaporiser may help: I generally suggest lemon oil for this purpose. Most people prefer to keep the vaporiser in the bedroom.

Inhalations, herbal pillows and poultices also provide relief. Massage, negative ionisers and breathing exercises are also recommended.

THE COMMON COLD

Description
Often starts with feeling tired and unwell, mild fever, headache, watery nasal discharge and sneezing. The discharge becomes purulent (thick and discoloured), the nose feels blocked and the throat may become dry and sore. The glands around the neck may become swollen.

Causes
A viral infection. Some people disagree that the actual cause is viral and place the cause on the individual. This argument can become somewhat academic but if the cause was solely viral, then one would expect everyone in a particular area to be stricken to a greater or lesser degree.

In my experience it seems that a cold often follows some stressful situation or an emotional upset. It is almost as if the viruses were waiting for a small chink in our immunological armour before getting a toehold.

Treatment
There is no medical cure for the common cold. In traditional natural therapy teaching, it has been suggested that one should not suppress a cold as this is a form of elimination but, as anyone who gets heavy, prolonged colds knows, it would be quite hard to imagine that a human head could contain so much that needed eliminating. One must therefore conclude that it is the body's reaction to these viruses that is causing the discharge and not toxins stored in the body waiting for some catalyst to release them.

Probably the best thing to do is spend

a day or two in bed, or at least resting at home. However, this is often not possible with young children to be cared for, work commitments and so on, so you need to consider ways to reduce the length of time and severity of the infection and to give you energy to carry on.

TO SPEED UP THE RETURN TO GOOD HEALTH

• *Ascorbic acid, ester C* or *sodium ascorbate powder*

Take 1 teaspoon in pure apple juice every half-hour until you get watery stools; then lower the dose until you have no more diarrhoea or intestinal colic. Continue on a high dose for two more days, then gradually reduce the amount over the following few weeks.

TISSUE SALTS OR CELLOIDS

• *Ferr Phos* • *Kali Mur*

Take one of each every half-hour for 4 hours; then every 2 hours for the rest of the day; then three times daily for at least a week.

If both vitamin C powder and tissue salts are taken at the first suspicion of infection, the cold may be avoided altogether.

FOR NASAL CONGESTION

• *Eucalyptus* or *peppermint essential oil* – as an inhalation • *Sodium ascorbate* powder – sniff up a little 2–3 times daily

HERBS

• *Elder* • *Fenugreek* • *Horseradish* • *Hyssop*

FROM THE KITCHEN

Mustard foot bath: mix a tablespoon of mustard powder to a paste and put it in a large basin with enough hot water to cover the feet. It really does ease the congestion in the head but you need to have the water as hot as possible and go to bed immediately afterwards to get the full benefit.

An alternative is to use one or two teaspoons of hot *chilli* powder in a foot bath.

If you're one of those people who prefers to go to bed to 'sweat it out' try chilli powder in a hot bath before bed; mix it to a paste first otherwise it floats on the water and makes you sneeze.

FOR A SORE THROAT

• *Sage tea* – as a warm gargle; add a few buds of cloves and a teaspoon of glycerine if the throat is dry • *Apple cider vinegar* as a cold compress

See also under Sore Throat (pages 180–1).

TO PREVENT THE INFECTION SPREADING TO THE CHEST

• *Aniseed* • *Echinacea* • *Garlic* • *Lemon* • *Thyme*

TO PROMOTE SWEATING

• *Catnip* • *Peppermint* • *Yarrow*

TO STIMULATE CIRCULATION AND PROVIDE ENERGY

• *Composition powder*

This is a traditional herbal remedy, a simplified version being to mix together:

4 teaspoons ginger powder
1 teaspoon hot chilli powder
1 teaspoon cinnamon powder
1 teaspoon cloves powder

This makes 28 doses.

Mix ¼ teaspoon with a little cold water, then add a cup of hot water or a herbal tea such as rosehip. Sip slowly. For most people even this small quantity is very strong initially but if you persevere a little at a time, it is markedly warming and stimulating. 2–3 cups a day is recommended.

Some old natural therapy texts give several quite heroic treatments for colds and to me these seem disproportionate to the illness. Fasting, enemas, emetics and hot mustard packs are a few examples and I would especially caution people not to use these techniques on small children and the elderly.

DIET

Supplement

• *Zinc* – a controlled clinical study, using an active form of zinc, shortened the duration of symptoms from 6.1 days to 4.9 days (8 lozenges, each containing 5.26 mg zinc, were consumed each day).[2]

OTHER

A German trial over a six-month period showed that cold showers can reduce the incidence of the common cold by 44 per cent. For the first three months, however, no change was noted – presumably while the body adjusted to the shock! The procedure was: first week, a five-minute warm shower (36–40°C) followed by a thirty-second cold shower to arms and legs (18–24°C). Second week, five-minute warm shower followed by thirty-second cold, whole body shower. Third week, five-minute warm shower followed by thirty-second cold shower, slowly increasing over a period of two to three weeks to a two-minute cold shower. The cold showers were taken five times a week.

People who take cold showers often say they never get colds, so perhaps an even longer trial would have given better results. Personally, I'd rather have a cold once a year than have the cold showers, but if I were prone to recurring or persistent colds then I'd give this a go.

COUGH

This is a very common symptom of respiratory diseases. It may be produced by disturbances from the nose, throat, the sinuses, or the terminal air passages in the lungs.

Description

When you cough, nerve impulses pass from the respiratory passages to the brain and then there is an automatic sequence of events. First, about 2.5 litres of air is taken in, the epiglottis (the flap at the back of the throat that covers the top of the air passages during swallowing, to prevent food entering the lungs) closes, the vocal cords shut tightly to keep the air in the lungs; the abdominal and chest muscles contract strongly and the pressure in the lungs rises. Then the vocal cords and the epiglottis suddenly open widely so that the air under pressure in the lungs 'explodes' outwards. The compression of the lungs collapses the main airway passages so that the exploding air actually passes through bronchial and tracheal slits and the rapidly moving air usually carries with it any foreign matter or excess mucus. Because coughing has this clearing function, which at times is lifesaving, many naturopaths are reluctant to suppress it in any way. But incessant coughing can be exhausting and irritating (for example, in tracheitis) and, furthermore, coughing may occasionally be brought on by an irritation in another part of the body or nervousness, so there are times to use treatments to dampen the cough reflex just as there are times to increase expectoration (excretion from the respiratory passages).

Causes

Viral, bacterial and other infections, 'nerves', cigarette smoking and other inhaled irritants and pollutants. Also allergies, lung abscesses, inhaled foreign bodies, tumours and other serious diseases such as tuberculosis, bronchiectasis and aneuryism, to name a few.

Treatment

HERBS

See under Bronchitis (pages 174–5) and Influenza (opposite).

Some general cough formulae:

1 *⅓ teaspoon thyme*
   ⅓ teaspoon crushed aniseeds
   1 teaspoon peppermint tea leaves
   Pour over 1 cup boiling water, 2 teaspoons fresh lemon juice and a little honey if required. Sip slowly. Take 2–3 cups per day.

2 *1 onion, finely chopped, covered with honey*
   Stand for a few hours, then strain resulting liquid. Sip half a tablespoon at a time.

3 For an irritating cough:
   1 teaspoon dried horehound
   1 teaspoon crushed aniseeds
   1 teaspoon liquorice powder
   1 teaspoon chamomile flowers
   juice of 1 lemon
   2 teaspoons raisins
   Mix together, then simmer for 10 minutes in 500 ml water. Stir in 2 teaspoons of honey until dissolved. I like to add a tablespoon of brandy too. Stir well, strain. Keep in fridge. Warm before taking; sip half a cup at a time – 2–4 times daily.

NOTE *A medical explanation should always be sought for a persistent cough.*

TO HELP WITH SLEEP

• *Valerian* • *Wild lettuce*

Here is a recipe for a hot chest poultice.

Simmer a small cup of linseed meal for 5 minutes in just enough water to keep it from sticking. Thicken with bran if necessary.

Wrap hot paste in a towel and place on the chest over another towel. Keep the poultice warm with blankets or a partially filled hot-water bottle.

Keep it on for 15–20 minutes before going to sleep.

NOTE *Use poultice as hot as possible but take care not to burn the skin. An aromatic chest rub before the poultice will add to the benefit.*

HAYFEVER
(allergic rhinitis)

Description

Watery nasal discharge, sneezing, itching eyes and nose; linings of nasal passages are boggy and pale, eyelids are often red and swollen.

Causes

Allergic or hypersensitivity reactions to inhaled substances, commonly pollens and sometimes environmental pollutants.

Treatment

Homoeopathic or medical desensitisation is sometimes beneficial, the aim being to normalise reactions to the known allergens. A report in the *Lancet* showed that a homoeopathic, mixed-grass pollen desensitiser was more effective than a placebo.[3] Suspected allergens, and those from skin or blood tests, should be related to the symptom pattern, especially with foods – some people conscientiously avoid certain foods for years but this does not necessarily improve the condition. Trials and avoidance of certain allergens are quite complicated and best done through a qualified practitioner because you need to know all the sources of the suspect allergen and the type of reactions to expect.

Some naturopaths suggest starting with a detoxifying programme as outlined under Chronic Fatigue syndrome (see pages 161–3).

HERBS
• *Aloe* • *Dandelion* • *Eyebright* • *Liquorice*
• *Reishi*

FROM THE KITCHEN
• *Ginger* • *Turmeric*

DIET
Rotational-type eating plan, that is, not eating the same things every day.

Supplements
• *Vitamin A* • *Sodium ascorbate powder* – a small quantity sniffed up the nose twice daily

TISSUE SALTS OR CELLOIDS
• *Nat Mur* • *Mag Phos* • *Silicea*

INFLUENZA

Description
Often starts suddenly with fever, nasal discharge and stuffiness, chills, headaches, muscle and joint pain, sore throat, a non-productive cough, fatigue and sometimes nausea. Can be mild to severe, and may lead to secondary bacterial infections and more serious complications. It normally lasts about a week.

Causes
Viruses transmitted via the respiratory tract, commonly in autumn and winter in epidemics.

Treatment
Bed rest in the early stages, a light diet and plenty of fluids are the most effective treatments. It is worth resting and treating the condition to avoid feeling tired for a long time afterwards and then getting a series of minor infections (see also The Common Cold, pages 175–7).

HERBS
• *Boneset* • *Echinacea* • *Garlic* • *Golden seal*
• *Lemon balm* • *Peppermint* • *Yarrow*

FROM THE KITCHEN
1 teaspoon chopped garlic
1 teaspoon chopped ginger root
2 teaspoons raisins
juice of 1 lemon

Simmer all ingredients in 1 cup water for 15 minutes. Add a little honey if preferred. Strain, and sip warm with a few sprigs of peppermint leaves on top.

(There are many variations of this, such as adding elder flowers, liquorice powder, rosehips, thyme or a herbal tea.)

DIET
• *Vitamin C* • *A combined multi-vitamin and mineral* – if the diet is not excellent

TISSUE SALTS OR CELLOIDS
• *Nat Sulph* • *Ferr Phos* • *Mag Phos*

SINUSITIS

Description
The symptoms are similar to a head cold but generally more severe. There is usually a headache with frontal and facial pain, and swelling; the nasal discharge is obstructive and infected (discoloured) and an ache is felt between and behind the eyes.

Postnasal drip may cause a sore throat and a cough. The teeth may ache or 'feel long', and there is invariably tension in the upper back and neck. When the problem is long-standing there may be exhaustion and emotional strain.

What happens during an attack is that the linings of the sinuses become red and swollen and the openings from the sinus cavities into the nose become partially or completely blocked; the accumulations in the sealed-off sinuses cause pressure which results in the discomfort.

Causes

Often occurs during a respiratory infection; may also be a complication of teeth infection, allergy or infectious diseases. Other causes include air pollution, diving and underwater swimming, extremes of temperature, dampness in the environment and structural defects in the nose and sinuses.

Sometimes the cause is unknown and may be an over-reaction of the immune system.

Treatment

As the infection can spread to the ears, throat and chest, it is recommended that diagnosis and treatment be started immediately.

HERBS

Taken internally
• *Chilli* • *Elder* • *Eyebright* • *Fenugreek* • *Garlic* • *Golden seal* • *Horseradish* – always take with food as it can be irritating to the stomach • *Hyssop*

Hot foot baths to decongest
• *Chamomile* • *Marjoram* – these are both physically relaxing
• *Hot chilli powder* • *Mustard* – these are both stimulating

Inhalations
• *Aniseed* • *Eucalyptus* • *Tea tree* – all as essential oils

Ointment rubbed over painful area
• *Phytolacca*

Nasal irrigation
Weak salty, warm water – the yogis use a Neti Pot but a dropper or breathing the water in from the cupped hand may be adequate.

DIET

Some foods may aggravate, especially dairy foods and chocolate. 1–2 days on fresh fruit and vegetable juices may be helpful.

Supplements
• *Vitamin A* • *Vitamin C* • *Papain* or *bromelain* tablets

TISSUE SALTS OR CELLOIDS
• *Ferr Phos* • *Kali Sulph* • *Nat Mur*

OTHER
• *Negative ioniser*

SORE THROAT
(laryngitis, pharyngitis)

Description

Laryngitis is where the lower part of the throat is infected, inflamed, swollen and sore and the voice is affected (the voice is produced in the voicebox, or larynx, hence the word laryngitis). It sometimes occurs alone but usually is in association with a respiratory or other infection.

Pharyngitis involves the upper part of the throat and it usually occurs as part of an upper respiratory tract disorder that may also affect the nose, sinuses, larynx and the trachea. The throat usually feels dry, the mucus is thick and sticky. There may be a cough and accompanying fever, fatigue and difficulty swallowing.

Breathlessness and a rasping sound on inspiration are more serious symptoms and need practitioner treatment, as does any persistent sore or troublesome throat.

Causes

Bacterial or viral infection, measles, influenza, inhalation of irritants, cigarette smoking, vocal abuse, violent weeping, sinus problems, allergies, foreign bodies such as fishbones, tumours and other serious diseases, such as diptheria and secondary syphilis, that require medical diagnosis and treatment.

Treatment

Although many sore throats will respond with rest, treatments generally shorten the duration and severity of the condition, and may prevent the infection spreading.

HERBS

• *Echinacea* • *Golden seal* • *Propolis* – sipped slowly • *Slippery elm powder*

FROM THE KITCHEN

• *Chilli,* hot • *Garlic,* cooked • *Sage* • *Thyme*

Sipping undiluted *lemon juice* can be very effective, although the first few sips might make you gasp. *Onion juice* and *chilli tea* are other home remedies – but not for the faint-hearted.

INHALATIONS

(Refer to Chapter 1.) These can be very effective for throat conditions, especially using one or two of the following essential oils: • *Eucalyptus* • *Lemon* • *Peppermint* • *Tea tree*

GARGLES

CAUTION **All gargles should be at tepid temperatures.**

• *Sage* and/or *thyme tea*

NOTE **This gargle can be drying if used too often so add a teaspoon of glycerine.**

• Warm *salt-water* gargles

For voice problems

Gargle with *cabbage* or *celery* juice.

For removing tenacious mucus, hot *chilli* is a helpful additive to a gargle. The amounts tolerated are variable from ¼–1 teaspoon powder. Always mix it to a paste first before adding a cup of warm water or herbal tea. I combine mine with fenugreek tea. It is not as heroic as it seems, although the first few mouthfuls may make you cough. Take a few sips first to get accustomed to it.

NOTE **Some people are allergic to chilli; others may have such sensitive skins and mucous membranes that they can not tolerate it. Obviously, this remedy is not suitable for children.**

COMPRESS

• *Cold water and apple cider vinegar*

My personal experience is that cold compresses are the most helpful for sore, swollen throats, although some people swear by small, hot poultices.

DIET

Juices, broths and blended foods are the most appropriate while the throat is red and sore. Avoid hot foods and drinks. Dairy foods may aggravate.

Supplements

• *Vitamin A* • *Vitamin C* • *Zinc*

TISSUE SALTS OR CELLOIDS

• *Calc Phos* • *Ferr Phos*

NOTES **Non-specific organisms can cause a septic throat and this seems to happen when the resistance of the individual is lowered for one reason or another. In Australia, some summer sore throats are linked to certain beaches and swimming pools.**

Some of the above remedies may be helpful for tonsilitis.

GENERAL DIETARY GUIDELINES DURING RESPIRATORY ILLNESSES

Foods to avoid

All refined, processed, packaged, tinned, bottled and frozen foods, alcohol, coffee, tobacco. My reasons for suggesting the avoidance of processed foods are that they contain less nutrients but usually about the same kilojoules as the whole foods.

In many cases dairy products seem to aggravate the problem, although some people may tolerate a little yoghurt.

SOME MILK SUBSTITUTES
• *Fruit juice* over cereals.
• *Almond milk* – 30g crushed or ground almonds blended with 1 litre water. Can be flavoured with a little honey or raisins. Strain.
• *Soy* or *rice milk* – there are a number of different types available in retail stores.

You can simmer 30 g ground almonds in 1 litre soy milk. The simmering and added almonds improve the taste and calcium content. Depending on how you want to use it, some carob powder can be added for flavour and to improve the nutrient content.
• *Coconut cream* in cooking instead of cream.

Foods to eat

Generally a light diet is recommended; many naturopathic books suggest juices, raw fruit and raw vegetables. However, not everyone feels like munching their way through raw food when they are feeling weak and miserable; vegetable soups are a good alternative.

Fluid intake is very important, especially if the person has been sweating a lot. This can be in the form of water, fruit and vegetable juices, herbal teas, broths and barley water.

Here are some light meal suggestions.
• Soups, especially onion and leek; also carrot, pumpkin, broccoli, lentil, rice and other vegetables.
• Raw, finely sliced fennel root with grated carrot.
• Omelette with mushrooms and chives.
• Stir-fry vegetables with fish or chicken – use only tiny quantities of oil.
• Vegetables steamed with lemon and fresh thyme.
• Grated beetroot and apple salad.
• Green beans (lightly steamed and cooled) with tomato and herbs.
• Grated carrot with chopped oranges.
• Red cabbage and oranges.
• Bean sprouts and corn (lightly cook the corn, then remove from the cob).
• A salad dressing: blended avocado, lemon, culinary herbs.
• Nuts blended with fruit juices and poured over fruit salads, then topped with sesame seeds and sultanas.

BREATHING EXERCISES

All people with respiratory problems should do a selection of breathing exercises on a daily basis as part of a preventive and treatment programme. A qualified yoga teacher can give more details about breathing techniques and appropriate exercises.

EXERCISE 1
1 Sit or stand, back straight, shoulders relaxed.
2 Place your fingertips lightly on your shoulders. As you breathe out, bring your elbows to the front until they meet.
3 As you breathe in, take the elbows up and back, with your head and shoulders

moving in the same direction.

Repeat four or five times.

EXERCISE 2

1 Sit with your back straight, shoulders relaxed.

2 Breathe in deeply, evenly and slowly, completely filling your lungs. Holding your breath as long as you can, tap all over your chest with the fingers of both hands. Start from the lower part and work up.

3 Stop tapping, breathe out.

Repeat this sequence three or four times. When you are more experienced, try to have the in-breath to a slow count of 8, the held breath to 16 and the out-breath to 8. The number should be increased or decreased according to individual capacities. This exercise can also be done with the hands gently closed into soft fists and a gentle pounding action.

EXERCISE 3

1 Sit with your back straight, shoulders relaxed.

2 As you breathe in, place your left hand on your right shoulder blade, palm of the hand facing out.

3 Take your right hand back over your right shoulder and grasp your left hand.

4 Hold as long as comfortable with the chest fully expanded.

5 Slowly release the hands as you breathe out.

Repeat three times with each arm. If one side is less flexible, do twice as many on the weak side. If you can't reach the hand initially, use a handkerchief.

EXERCISE 4

1 Stand with legs apart.

2 Breathe in deeply, bringing the arms up sideways to shoulder level, to a slow count of 6.

3 Hold the breath in for a slow count of 6.

4 Breathe out, bringing arms down to a slow count of 6.

Repeat four times.

EXERCISE 5

1 Lie on the floor on your tummy.

2 Interlock your fingers behind your buttocks with palms towards your feet.

3 Breathing in deeply, raise the head and shoulders off the floor, keeping the feet on the floor and lifting your arms up as high as you can.

4 Lower yourself down, breathing out slowly.

Repeat twice.

EXERCISE 6 *(The Cobra)*

1 Lie on the floor on your tummy.

2 Put hands under your shoulders, palms on the floor, chin on the floor.

3 Breathing in, slowly lift your head and shoulders up. Push down with your arms, keeping your hips on the floor, legs and feet heavy and relaxed. Come up as high as you can without undue force or strain, thrusting your chest out and keeping your chin level. Don't try to straighten your arms.

4 Breathing out, slowly lower yourself down, keeping your head straight and your chest out until the very last.

Repeat twice.

EXERCISE 7 *(The Cat Pose)*

1 Kneel on your hands and knees.

2 Breathing out, drop your head forward and pull your abdomen in as far as you can, humping your back upwards.

3 Breathing in, lift the head up and look at the ceiling as you fill the abdomen with air, arching your abdomen downwards.

EXERCISE 8 *(The Bee)*

This exercise will help you relax, especially before going to bed.

1 Sit with your back straight, shoulders relaxed.

2 Breathe in fully through both nostrils.

3 Close your ears by plugging them gently with your index fingers (if your fingernails are long, then put your hands firmly over the ears).

4 With your teeth slightly apart and lips together, exhale slowly making a humming sound like a bee.

Do at least six repetitions.

EXERCISE 9

1 Lie on back, knees bent, feet flat on the floor, arms by your sides.

2 As you take a deep breath in, slowly raise your right hand and take it over your head to the floor; feel expansion in the right side.

3 Breathing out, slowly take the arm back to the starting position.

Repeat three times each side.

EXERCISE 10

1 Lie on back, knees bent, feet flat on the floor, elbows bent, arms at right angles, palms facing upwards.

2 Breathing in, slowly push the abdomen and lower chest out, then expand the middle and upper chest (don't lift the shoulders).

3 Breathing out, squeeze the abdomen in and relax the chest.

OTHER

A report in the *Lancet* supported the notion that voluntary control of breath is a useful adjunct in the treatment of bronchial asthma.[4] The researcher suggested a 1:2 inspiration:expiration ratio.

I recommend that you start with the breathing and counting technique given under Atherosclerosis (pages 123–4). Over a period of time, gradually lengthen the out-breath until it is double the count of the inspiration. Remember that although you are breathing out through the nose, during the out-breath you focus on the throat so that the air flow is controlled and slow.

Controlled, slow, rhythmic breathing has many benefits, both physical and mental. At first you will experience some discomfort and strain but this should reduce after a few weeks of daily practice; if it does not you must moderate the technique or get help.

A yogic belief is that we are not given so many years of life but so many breaths, so don't squander them with rapid, shallow breathing. Focusing on the breath can in itself be a method of relaxation. Alternate nostril breathing is helpful for balancing the nervous system as well as for clearing and relaxing the nasal passages. This technique, together with other breathing and relaxation exercises, is given in Chapter 10, 'Nervous and Immune Systems'.

CHAPTER 12

SKIN AND RELATED PROBLEMS

The skin is not just a covering of the body; it is an organ supplied by nerves, blood and lymph. It shares in the role of elimination and so is related to the kidneys, lungs, liver and bowels. A problem in one of these organs is frequently reflected in the others. This is why some skin problems are not helped by external applications. For example, if the kidneys are not filtering the blood effectively, then this places an additional burden on the skin's eliminative function and the result may be skin eruptions.

My main recommendation is to do something at the first sign of any skin problem because a relatively minor problem can spread and intensify. See if you can relate the outbreak to a particular activity or food, perhaps something different in the diet, or something in excess. Were you exposed to a particular plant, chemical or drug? Did you use a different washing powder, wear something new, have too much exposure to the sun or come in contact with a possible infection?

Skin cancers require referral to a skin specialist. From my own experience and observations, I would urge people to have suspect lumps and discolorations diagnosed as soon as they are noticed. If they are allowed to continue, these small, benign 'spots' can develop into more serious problems; they may be subjected to irritation or aggravated by shaving or injuries.

Sunlight is healthy and necessary but a little is good and a lot harmful, so for the sake of your skin avoid sunbathing and working in strong sunlight without protection.

There are hundreds of skin diseases, many of them being difficult to diagnose and treat, and, frequently, a remedy that works for one person will not be effective for another, or might be an aggravation. Even dermatologists may have difficulty diagnosing particular skin diseases; diagnosis may be further complicated by a secondary infection or a fungal overgrowth.

Certain conditions do not need treatment, apart from a soothing or moisturising cream, but require the removal of an irritant. A number of skin problems are worsened by stress and, as a simple illustration of this, you may notice that many people scratch their arms, chest or head when they become irritated or upset.

When treating skin problems, you need to have some patience, because improvement is rarely dramatic and I would recommend continuing with the treatment for a reasonable period following the disappearance of the lesions. Where a skin disease has persisted for many years, a rough guide to treatment time is one month for every year suffered. I use the word suffered because we need to be reminded of the embarrassment, poor self-image and sometimes physical restrictions and pain brought about by skin diseases.

I am hoping that you will be encouraged to take an active interest in your health but I am also relying on your common sense. For example, when using external applications, try the remedy on a small test patch first, under the arms being a particularly sensitive area. Serious skin diseases and infections should be professionally diagnosed and treated.

Where the problem matches the example given in this chapter then the recommended remedies may well suit you, or you might prefer to get confirmation from your practitioner that one or more may be the most appropriate for your particular case. In my own practice, when treating skin problems, I commonly use a herbal formula, plus a supplement, and invariably suggest dietary and lifestyle improvements.

Throughout this chapter, you will notice that food and environmental allergies or sensitivities can be an impediment to a healthy skin. In Chapter 3, 'Arthritis and Other Joint and Muscle Problems', I outlined the link between a permeable (less selective) intestinal wall and sensitivities. Fragments of substances that should stay in the intestines and be excreted can end up in the bloodstream, joints and other organs. Some of these 'toxic fragments' even resemble parts of your body structure or microorganisms. Considering all the truly unnatural chemicals in our food and environment, it's hardly surprising that your body may become confused and many skin problems may be a result of such toxic fragments.

If your skin problem is obstinate, I suggest a 'full-on naturopathic' treatment of a short fast or special diet, avoidance of all chemicals (within reason), special baths, wholefoods and a month or two on high-dose, quality Lactobacillus acidophilus and Bifidobacteria supplements. Then you may be more responsive to remedies.

Dry skin brushing

The basic aim of dry skin brushing is to help elimination via the skin by removing the upper layer of dead skin and other debris, and also to improve circulation. As you sweat, the skin removes metabolic wastes and it follows that if the whole surface area is eliminating there is less likelihood that one area, such as the face, will be over-burdened with a concentration of toxins.

Dry skin brushing is not recommended over areas covered with rashes or infected skin conditions as it would cause irritation.

Soaps
Unless otherwise indicated by the manufacturer, soaps are alkaline.

Ideally, the skin should be slightly acidic so if you have a skin problem it may be wise not to use any soap for a trial period of about four weeks. If the problem clears in that time it may be that you have an allergy to something in the particular soap you have been using, or your skin does not return to the desired acid level after washing and so this leads to a bacterial imbalance. Using diluted apple cider vinegar or diluted fresh lemon juice as external skin toners will help restore the acid balance.

You can now buy soaps that are pH (acid) balanced or neutral.

Some alternatives to soap are:
• Sorbolene cream – apply, gently rub in with water, then rinse off (this can also be used for shaving)
• any edible oil – apply, tissue off, then splash skin with warm water
• rolled oats – place in a stocking with the top tied, let hot water run on it, allow to cool; splash on face or use water as a bath
• plain water – using a cleansing cream first.

Sweating
Sweating is good because it cools your body and eliminates toxins of various kinds. However, the sweat is alkaline and some people's skin does not readily revert to its ideal slightly acidic state after sweating. If you have a skin problem mainly in areas where you sweat heavily, try the recommendations under Soaps (above). I also recommend that you use aluminium-free deodorants.

Elimination crises
Sometimes when a strict naturopathic diet, lifestyle and supplemental programme is commenced a skin condition can get worse. This unfortunate effect is called an elimination crisis. It also occurs fairly commonly when fasting. Although some of these programmes may be a good way of starting a healthier lifestyle, you may not be able to handle a skin outbreak!

I generally try to avoid an elimination crisis by making dietary and other changes over a period of time and introducing supplements one at a time in smallish quantities.

Aromatherapy
I have suggested some treatments using specific aromatic oils in this chapter. Make sure you do apply a little as a test patch first because allergic reactions are fairly common. If the skin problem is widespread, you may need to dilute these oils in water, Sorbolene or similar cream, glycerine or almond oil.

You may think it is useless to treat the skin externally because this rarely focuses on the cause, but some problems relate to external irritants or a skin metabolism problem. Also, aromatic oils actually penetrate the skin and enter the bloodstream.

ACNE

Description
Inflammation of the sebaceous glands and hair follicles, commonly on the face, neck and shoulders. Starts with roughened skin, then a pus spot that forms and bursts. Accompanied by blackheads; there

are often large pores and the lesions may leave visible scars.

The problem is a combination of trapped oil, bacteria and thickened skin (keratinisation).

Causes

Commonly hormonal, starting at puberty and usually clearing in early twenties. Faulty diet, poor hygiene and stress may be aggravating factors.

Treatment

There are different forms of acne and the following suggestions generally apply to all of them.

Acne rosacea is accompanied by redness. It is often helped by taking a *vitamin B* supplement and avoidance of allergies. Anything that stimulates heat or flushing should also be avoided – such as alcohol, coffee, hot spices. A few drops of *lavender oil* on acne rosacea may help, but keep it away from the eyes.

HERBS

Taken internally

• *Burdock* • *Echinacea* • *Evening primrose oil* • *Fenugreek* • *Garlic* • *Lemon grass* • *Red clover* • *Sarsaparilla*

Applied externally

• *Calendula* • *Golden seal* • *Tea tree oil* – apply undiluted on the lesions (the *Medical Journal of Australia* reported that even a 5 per cent strength was beneficial)[1]

NOTE *All thick, greasy ointments should be avoided as they tend to suppress normal skin functioning.*

For prevention of scarring use pure *aloe gel* or *vitamin E oil*.

FROM THE KITCHEN

• *Fresh lemon juice* – dabbed on affected areas • *Fresh cabbage juice* – applied externally • *Sage* – the cold tea may be patted on as an astringent; it is mildly antiseptic and has a drying effect

Facial *steam baths* using any of the pleasantly aromatic herbs or eucalyptus leaves can help.

DIET

High in vegetables, fat-reduced soy products and fish. Low in fat and salt. Avoid all refined foods.

Use filtered water for drinking if possible. Water is nature's flushing out agent, but don't overdo it.

Supplements

• *Vitamin A* • *Vitamin C* • *Zinc*

TISSUE SALTS OR CELLOIDS

• *Calc Sulph* • *Ferr Phos* • *Kali Mur*

OTHER

• *Acupuncture*

ATHLETE'S FOOT
(tinea pedis)

Description

A chronic, superficial fungal infection of the skin of the foot, frequently located between the toes and on the soles. There is visible scaling, splitting, wasting of tissue, itching and swelling; often with blistering and redness. It may be secondarily infected.

Causes

A fungal infection that may be aggravated by allergies, poor diet, profuse sweating, stress and other factors.

Treatment

HERBS

Taken internally

• *Corn silk* • *Echinacea* • *Red clover* • *Thyme*

Applied externally
• *Aloe* • *Calendula* • *Comfrey* – decoction of root as a foot bath; use at tepid heat
• *Sandalwood oil* • *Tea tree oil*
FROM THE KITCHEN
• *Garlic powder* – externally

CAUTION **Garlic will aggravate broken skin.**

• *Thyme* – soak feet in a cooled, strained infusion • *Diluted apple cider vinegar* – this is especially helpful if there is itching and redness • *Sage* – soak feet in a cooled, strained infusion; this remedy helps where there is excess perspiration
DIET
In severe cases: avoid all yeast and mould foods for a trial period of five weeks (bread, mushrooms, Vegemite, cheese, yoghurt, soy products, wine, beer, preserved meats, peanuts, peanut butter, dried and canned fruits, vinegar, melons, grapes, olives and salad dressings). Some vitamin supplements also contain yeast. Eliminate sugar from the diet.
TISSUE SALTS OR CELLOIDS
• *Kali Sulph* • *Mag Phos*
OTHER
Dry feet properly after washing, keep feet dry, avoid nylon socks and stockings, avoid getting feet overheated, use clean and dry footwear. Wear thongs in public showers, at swimming pools and gyms.

BRUISES

Description
Blotchy, superficial discolorations due to haemorrhage into tissues from ruptured capillaries beneath the skin surface, with or without the skin itself being broken.

Causes
Injuries, weakened blood vessels, blood cell abnormalities.

CAUTION **Seek practitioner advice for unusual or persistent bruising and, of course, for any serious injuries.**

Treatment
HERBS
Applied externally
As a compress or ointment: • *Arnica* • *Calendula* • *Witch hazel*

CAUTION **Do not use arnica if there is broken skin.**

FROM THE KITCHEN
Crushed *ice* – in a small towel.
For mild injuries, rest and cold applications are generally advisable in the first instance; later, alternate applications of hot and cold help speed recovery. Refer to Chapter 1, 'Using Natural Remedies', for details.
Cabbage poultice – the bruised, fresh outer leaves, with the main stem removed, applied in layers. See Chapter 16, 'Recommended Herbs', for more information on cabbage.
DIET
Eat foods rich in *vitamin C and bioflavonoids*, i.e. chilli, capsicum, parsley, cabbage, broccoli, Brussels sprouts, watercress, cauliflower, berries, paw paw, spinach, citrus fruit, turnips, mangoes. Also eat buckwheat.
Supplement
• *Vitamin C and bioflavonoids*
TISSUE SALTS OR CELLOIDS
• *Calc Fluor* • *Ferr Phos* • *Kali Mur*

COLD SORES (herpes simplex)

Description

Recurring, contagious, itching, burning or stinging blisters; usually in small clusters around the mouth but can be on other areas. They typically become weepy, crusty, then disappear.

CAUTION **Genital sores need a medical diagnosis.**

Causes

They are caused by the *Herpes simplex* virus. The problem commonly recurs because the virus persists in nerve tissue.

An attack may be brought on by minor infections, stress, sun exposure, fatigue, windburn, menstruation and mental or physical trauma; therefore take protective action as far as practicable.

Treatment

HERBS

The severity and frequency of attacks may be reduced by herbal and other means but the treatment has to continue for at least six months and you may need to see a practitioner as some of the remedies used are not available at retail outlets. However, there are some remedies that may be helpful.

Taken internally

• *Aloe gel* • *Echinacea* • *Garlic* • *Ginseng* • *Golden seal* • *Lemon balm* • *Pau d'arco* • *Reishi* • *St John's wort* • *Thuja*

Applied externally

• *Aloe gel* – if you can grow aloe, the gel inside the plant is beneficial to treat the lesions and as a preventive measure. Aloe is also available as a lip salve; it works well in combination with jojoba.

• *Comfrey* – the best results are from freshly juiced root.

• *Essential oils* – a little of one of the following, undiluted, applied directly on the sores (if it stings too much dilute in water or an ointment): *calendula, clove, peppermint, tea tree.*

• *Calcium ascorbate powder* – mixed to a paste with an ointment such as calendula, comfrey or golden seal.

• *Thuja* and *lemon balm* are external antiviral herbs.

• *Vitamin E oil* – cut open a capsule and apply undiluted.

FROM THE KITCHEN

• *Alfalfa* • *Thyme*

Applied externally

• *Cabbage juice* – undiluted, applied on the lesions • *Cold tea bags* – as a compress

A little crushed ice in a washer may relieve the pain; ten minutes on, five minutes off.

NOTE **External creams, treatments etc. will be far more effective if they are used frequently when the initial itching or pain is noticed (in the first 24 hours).**

DIET

Drink pure apple juice and fresh vegetable juice.

Eat meals high in fish, chicken, milk, cheese, lamb, beans, bean sprouts, most fruit and vegetables, except peas. The diet should be low in wheat.

No gelatine, chocolate, carob, coconut, white flour, peanuts or wheatgerm.

Supplements

• *L-lysine* – 1g per day for six months, then reduce dose • *A combined multivitamin and mineral*, plus additional *zinc* taken at a different time

TISSUE SALTS OR CELLOIDS
• *Kali Sulph* • *Kali Mur* • *Ferr Phos*
OTHER
In serious cases a supervised fast may be the best action to take. A brief explanation of fasting is given in Chapter 14, 'Fasting'.

CYSTS – SEBACEOUS

Description
Benign swellings that contain and retain the fatty secretions of a gland. They are usually soft and movable within their sacs, but sometimes they are solidified. They occur singly or in clusters in various parts of the body.

Causes
Usually malfunction of the gland, but possibly a fault in fat/liver metabolism with associated poor circulation.

Treatment
HERBS
Taken internally
• *Calendula* – weak infusion • *Dandelion*
  See also Liver Sluggishness (pages 144–6).
Applied externally
• *Calendula* ointment
FROM THE KITCHEN
• *Chilli* • *Ginger* • *Turmeric*
DIET
A low-fat diet.
  There are some lipotropic formulae on the market that can be taken as supplements. These are capable of decreasing fat deposits in the liver and helping fat metabolism.
TISSUE SALTS OR CELLOIDS
• *Silicea* • *Calc Fluor* – when the cysts are hard

OTHER
Gentle, regular massage sometimes helps but this should not be done if the cyst is painful or infected. If the cyst is not causing any problems and is not being irritated by clothing it may be best to leave it alone.

DANDRUFF
(seborrhoeic dermatitis)

Description
A scaly material from or on the scalp. If not checked it may spread to eyebrows, ears and neck. In extreme cases it may cause other skin problems.

Causes
Various, possibly fungi – usually worsened by emotional stress and poor diet.

Treatment
HERBS
Taken internally
• *Dandelion* • *Evening primrose oil* • *Tea tree oil* • *Valerian* – for nervous system
Applied externally
• *Aloe* – in astringent form, or the pure gel massaged in before shampooing hair
• *Nettle tea* – as a rinse or massage • *Rosemary oil*
FROM THE KITCHEN
If the hair and scalp are dry: *olive oil* – massage a little into scalp and hair, wrap in a hot towel or plastic wrap before shampooing.
  If the hair and scalp are oily, or if the problem is worsened by sweating: *diluted apple cider vinegar* or *lemon juice* – massaged in or used as a rinse after shampooing.
DIET
No sugar, no refined foods. High in vegetables and soya beans. Take 1 tablespoon

linseed oil per day – minimal or no other fats or oils.

Supplement
• *Vitamin B complex*

TISSUE SALTS OR CELLOIDS
• *Kali Sulph* • *Nat Mur*

DERMATITIS

Description
The simple meaning is 'inflammation of the skin' and it manifests in so many ways that it is not possible to be more definite. It may be accompanied by swelling, scales, itching, dryness, suppuration or scabs.

Causes
Many different causes, such as a disorder of an internal organ (usually in respect of the gastro-intestinal tract or kidneys), internal or external irritants and allergies. There is often a relationship between dermatitis and nervous or emotional tension.

NOTE **The treatment should involve acing possible causes.**

There are some specific types of dermatitis, for example *dermatitis herpetiformis*, which is controlled by a gluten-free diet and supplementation with PABA (one of the B vitamins). Some people have other allergies as well as to gluten.

Treatment
• *Vitamin E oil* – cut open a capsule or buy the pure vitamin E and dab on

HERBS

Taken internally
• *Aloe* • *Clivers* • *Gotu cola* • *Lemon grass*
• *Yellow dock*

Applied externally
• *Chamomile tea* – as a wash or bath
• *Chickweed* • *Comfrey* • *Nettle* • *Witch hazel*

NOTE **Some lanolin-based ointments aggravate skin diseases. Sorbolene is a suitable base to make herbal ointments from as it is a good moisturiser. However, it sometimes aggravates sensitive skins.**

FROM THE KITCHEN
Bran or oatmeal baths (see page 201).

DIET
Check for allergies. Try a gluten-free diet for two months.

Supplements
• *Vitamin A* • *Vitamin B complex*

OTHER
If the hands are affected, use cotton-lined rubber gloves when working, washing dishes or if in contact with chemicals.

ECZEMA (atopic dermatitis)

Description
Inflammation of the skin with a variety of appearances.

Found in all ages, from babies to the elderly. May be dry or with a watery discharge. Can be acute or chronic but in

---

NOTE **The distinction and terminology of the various types of eczema and dermatitis are very complex and I have simplified them into two categories: dermatitis relating primarily to irritants and eczema linked to hereditary traits. A professional diagnosis is required for exact identification.**

---

nearly all cases requires patience as the treatment is generally long-term. There is often associated itching, burning and pain; sometimes secondary infections.

Causes

Varied, often hereditary and linked to asthmatic constitutional types. Worsened by stress, allergies, chemical irritants and some food additives and colourings. Dust mite and environmental substances may be causes.

Treatment

Refer also to Chapter 4, 'Common Childhood Ailments'.

As a minimum I would suggest dietary changes, especially trying to trace allergies, and supplementation with *evening primrose oil*. You will need to be patient because some months of treatment is usually required.

HERBS

Taken internally

• *Clivers* • *Evening primrose oil* (also used externally) • *Heartsease* • *Red clover* • *Yellow dock*

Applied externally

• *Aloe* – use only pure, uncoloured products • *Chamomile* – the tea as a wash • *Chickweed* – as a bath or wash • *Fumitory* – as a bath or wash • *Witch hazel* – in Sorbolene or other base

FROM THE KITCHEN

• *Fenugreek* – tea or sprouts

Applied externally

• *Almond oil* – if the skin is dry, plus a few drops of *chamomile* or *hyssop oil*

DIET

Supervised water, vegetable juice or broth fast (not for children or the elderly), if possible followed by foods being introduced one at a time.

Common allergies or sensitivities to food that can trigger eczema include food colourings, additives and preservatives, milk, wheat, fruit, shellfish, eggs, soy, peanuts and chocolate.

Some practitioners suggest a course of *lactobacillus acidophilus* and *bifidobacteria* as a way of reducing food sensitivities.

Supplements

• *Vitamin C* • *Vitamin E* • *Zinc*

TISSUE SALTS OR CELLOIDS

• *Calc Phos* • *Kali Mur* • *Kali Phos*

OTHER

Homoeopathic treatment is often helpful because of the constitutional basis of eczema.

HAIR PROBLEMS

Description

Dry, brittle, split or lank hair. Alopecia is where the hair is coming out in clumps and this condition is covered in Chapter 10, 'Nervous and Immune Systems'.

Causes

Stress, faulty diet, excess sun and too many perms, bleaches or tints are some of the causes.

Treatment

HERBS

• *Burdock* – the decoction used as a rinse • *Chamomile* – infusion as a rinse for fair hair, to lighten and shine • *Horsetail* – internally • *Jojoba oil* – a small quantity massaged into the scalp • *Rosemary oil* – a small quantity massaged into the scalp daily • *Sage* – infusion as a scalp massage or as a rinse for dark hair

Women with hair problems should refer to the list of oestrogenic plants in

Chapter 6, page 113, as the problem may be hormonally based.

FROM THE KITCHEN
• *Apple cider vinegar* – dilute, as a scalp massage • *Almond, apricot* or *olive oil* – a little massaged in before shampooing, if the hair and scalp are dry

DIET
Eat a low-fat, well-balanced, wholefood diet. Include seaweed products, fish and sprouts.

Supplements
• *Vitamin A* • *Vitamin B complex* with additional *PABA*

OTHER
• *Tea tree shampoo*

INFECTIONS

Description
In the context of this book, I am discussing minor skin problems and not serious infections, some of which need to be reported to the Department of Health. If in doubt seek practitioner advice.

Causes
Viruses, bacteria or other microorganisms. Obviously, skin infections are not entirely due to microorganisms otherwise we would all get infections constantly, so we need to look at why certain people are infected. Poor nutrition, inadequate elimination or hygiene as well as physical and mental stress may also be contributing factors.

Treatment
HERBS
Antiseptic applications of essential oils for external use: • *Tea tree oil* – this is probably the most useful • *Eucalyptus* • *Lemon* • *Sandalwood* • *Thyme* and *lemon grass* oils are good antiseptics but must be diluted

because they can cause intense stinging – even to tough skins!

Taken internally
• *Burdock* • *Echinacea* • *Fenugreek* • *Garlic* • *Golden seal*

External drawing agents for poultices
• *Linseed meal* • *Slippery elm powder*

FROM THE KITCHEN
• *Cabbage* – bruised leaves externally, juice internally • *Tepid salt water* – for washing wounds

DIET
Avoid sugar and refined foods.

Supplements
• *Vitamin C* • *Zinc*

TISSUE SALTS OR CELLOIDS
• *Ferr Phos* • *Kali Mur*

INSECT BITES

Prevention
Essential oils rubbed lightly over exposed areas will often repel insects. Some examples are: • *Cajeput* • *Citronella* • *Lavender* • *Pennyroyal*

DIET
Supplement
• *Vitamin B1* – for prevention

Treatment
SOOTHING
• *St John's wort* – oil or ointment • *Nettle* – ointment • *Witch hazel* – lotion or ointment • *Vitamin E* – the pure oil used externally

FROM THE KITCHEN
• *Vinegar* – undiluted on small areas

TISSUE SALTS OR CELLOIDS
For severe cases: • *Nat Mur* • *Kali Phos* • *Silicea* • *Kali Mur* – soothing

As well as taking them internally, these tissue salt remedies may be crushed and mixed to a paste with one of the ointments mentioned above.

TO PREVENT INFECTION
- *Tea tree oil*

ITCHING AND RASHES

The fancy name for a rash is urticaria – derived from the Latin word for nettle.

Causes
Varied, including internal and external allergies or irritants, excess heat or cold, drugs, nervous or emotional upsets. As well as plants, chemical food additives may be the culprits. Some researchers say the worst additives are BHA and BHT (320 and 321) – these are ingredients in many processed foods. I suggest avoiding, or at least testing, all colourings and preservatives.

Foods that commonly irritate are: alcohol, chocolate, cheese, shellfish, eggs, coffee, oranges and other acidic fruits and chicken.

Treatment
HERBS
Taken internally
- *Alfalfa* • Herbal diuretics especially *burdock, celery, dandelion* – to help flush out irritants • *Hops* and *liquorice* – for the nervous system

Applied externally
- *Marshmallow* • *Nettle* • *St John's wort*

FROM THE KITCHEN
- *Apple* or *pear juice* • *Celery juice* • *Green bean juice* • *Parsley* – a handful a day

1 teaspoon bicarbonate of soda or Andrews Liver Salts in water may offset the effects of a sudden allergic reaction. Drinking large quantities of water may also help flush out irritating substances.

DIET
Eat rice and vegetables only for a few days in acute cases.

Supplements
- *Vitamin C* and *bioflavonoids*
- *Vitamin B12* – has helped some cases

AROMATHERAPY
- *Chamomile* • *Melissa* • *St John's wort*

NOTE **Dilute the oils in water if a large area of skin is affected. Use all external remedies with caution – they may help or make the problem worse.**

TISSUE SALTS OR CELLOIDS
- *Calc Phos* • *Kali Phos*

PREVENTIVE MEASURES
Relaxation and meditation techniques may help, especially if the cause is nervous or emotional.

I have seen cases where people are so sensitive to particular plants, such as Rhus, that they only have to pass near the tree for a physical reaction to be triggered. It may be useful to get a horticulturalist to identify possible problem plants in your yard.

NAIL PROBLEMS

Description
Nails are weak, brittle, ridged or discoloured.

Causes
Sometimes external irritants such as detergents and chemicals; also dietary inadequacies and drugs.

Treatment
HERBS
- *Chamomile* • *Horsetail*

DIET
Ensure adequate whole grains, vegetables and fruit. In Australia, lack of protein is rarely a cause but may need investigation

in vegetarians and vegans. Include seaweed products and sprouts in the diet.

Supplement
• *Organic mineral formula*

TISSUE SALTS OR CELLOIDS
• *Calc Fluor* • *Silicea*

PIMPLES

The nature and cause vary considerably with each individual. Naturopathic treatments would be individual, but some suggestions and remedies will be found in this chapter; see pages 185–7, Acne (pages 187–8), Infections (page 194) and Some Dietary Advice (page 198).

PSORIASIS

Description
A chronic disease of the skin with scaly patches that vary in appearance but which are commonly thick and silver. The lesions may be in one area only or covering almost all the body; sometimes the scales are so thick that they interfere with joint mobility. There can be itching, secondary infections and inflammation. The condition may be dormant for periods or increase in intensity with stress.

Causes
An abnormally high turnover of skin cells. It is often hereditary and may be related to fat metabolism, enzyme and hormonal functioning. Stress, some medications and infections can trigger an outbreak.

Treatment
HERBS
Taken internally
• *Barberry bark* • *Clivers* • *Efamol Marine*
• *Red clover* • *Sarsaparilla*

Applied externally
• *Chickweed* • *Liquorice* – powder mixed into Sorbolene or other base • *Evening primrose* and *fish oils*

FROM THE KITCHEN
If you can't afford the Efamol Marine use *linseed oil* (2–4 teaspoons per day) internally and a little externally.

NOTE **No other fats and oils should be eaten.**

• *Ginger* • *Globe artichoke* – can be juiced

DIET
Can start with a supervised fast (not children and the elderly). A vegetarian, wholefood diet reduces the incidence of psoriasis. Check for allergies to beer, coffee, tobacco, oranges, food additives, soft drinks, wine, cheese or nuts.

Supplements
• *Vitamin A* • *Vitamin E* • *Lecithin* • *Zinc*

TISSUE SALTS OR CELLOIDS
• *Calc Fluor* • *Silicea*

AROMATHERAPY
• *Bergamot* • *Lavender* • *Juniper oil* – can help remove the scales: test a small patch first

OTHER
• Homoeopathy.
• Avoid synthetic clothing next to skin, wear gloves when using detergents.
• Avoid soap for a trial period.
• A little sun and salt water often reduces the scaling and inflammation.

NOTE **Some pharmaceutical drugs used to treat severe psoriasis (and other skin diseases) are toxic to liver and bone marrow, may cause birth defects and more. Active levels of these drugs may persist for months, even years, after cessation of therapy.**[2]

SCARS

Description

The mark remaining after skin and other tissues have been injured. When a wound is healing, special cells are stimulated to become granulation tissue (new connective tissue), so that the injury can be knitted together. The new tissue looks different from the old skin, as it has more fibrous tissue in it, and thus a scar can be seen. If, during the healing process, the fibrous tissue overgrows, a raised scar forms. This is termed a keloid. Adhesions, a complication of scarring, are where two surfaces which should be separate are bound together by scar tissue, and this may happen after abdominal surgery.

Causes

Trauma, surgery, burns, diseases such as smallpox, and infections such as acne.

Treatment

HERBS

Taken internally

• *Aloe gel* • *Horsetail*

Applied externally

• *Aloe gel* alternating with *vitamin E oil*
• *Comfrey ointment*

These external agents should not be applied until after the initial healing has taken place, that is, when there is no possibility of infection.

DIET

Slightly increase the amount of protein in the diet.

Supplements

• *1 combined multi-vitamin and mineral* per day • *Vitamin E* • *Zinc*

TISSUE SALTS OR CELLOIDS

• *Calc Fluor* • *Silicea*

OTHER

• Acupuncture

WARTS

Description

Generally harmless but annoying small, hard lumps growing from the skin surface.

Cause

Persistent virus.

Treatment

Plantar (warts on the soles of the feet) and genital warts require practitioner treatment.

Any external treatments need to be continued for a number of weeks.

HERBS

Taken internally

• *Echinacea* • *Lemon balm* • *Thuja*

Applied externally

• *Dandelion* (the white sap from the flower stem) – apply twice daily for about three weeks • *Thuja extract* or *ointment*
• *Vitamin E oil* • *Hot chilli powder* mixed to a paste with *apple cider vinegar*

FROM THE GARDEN

• *Milkweed* • *Petty spurge*

Apply the fresh white milky substance within the stems onto the wart; this has a caustic effect over some weeks. Do not apply to the surrounding skin. This is an old-fashioned remedy, its main problem being that it causes a 'messy' wound while the wart is being eliminated.

NOTE *Caustic-like substances should not be used on the face or genital area.*

TISSUE SALTS OR CELLOIDS

• *Kali Mur* • *Nat Mur* • *Silicea*

AROMATHERAPY

• *Melissa* • *Thuja* – use both undiluted on warts, avoiding the surrounding skin

OTHER

Homoeopathy.

Treatment is often very individual – some cures have been effected by another person 'purchasing' the warts, or by using some other old wives' tales.

SOME DIETARY ADVICE

A number of skin problems have a nervous origin or are connected with allergies. In my clinical experience, for example, I find that itching skin is commonly related to coffee, oranges and grains, especially bran.

Dermatitis of the hands is often work related, either caused by emotional problems connected with the job or contact allergens. If you have recurring dermatitis on the index finger or thumb it is more likely to be related to something like insect sprays than to disliking your job or a food allergy. Although it is not always easy, try to establish the cause.

The problem of allergies is very complex and a brief introduction to the subject is given in Chapter 13, 'Food Allergies'.

AVOID

All refined, processed, packaged, canned, bottled and frozen foods, plus alcohol, tea, coffee, tobacco and salt.

MINIMAL

Fats, oils, meat, nuts and seeds.

JUICES

One or two fresh juices a day may be helpful in cleansing skin problems. Try: a mixture of juiced *celery, carrot and green bean* – with a little parsley or watercress added it desired; *apple, grape* or other fruits in season.

SPECIAL FOODS

Have 1 teaspoon *apple cider vinegar* or fresh *lemon juice* in warm water before meals; 1 tablespoon *lecithin* per day; sprouts, especially *alfalfa* and *fenugreek*.

COFFEE AND TEA SUBSTITUTES

Try herbal teas – especially *lemon grass*, but also *alfalfa, chamomile, nettle, red clover* – and *dandelion coffee, Ecco, Nature's Cuppa* and other coffee substitutes. The healthiest and cheapest drink is water (if you live in an area where the water has a high chlorine content, boil it before drinking, or let stand overnight in the refrigerator or use a water filter).

GENERAL

Include a wide variety of raw and steamed vegetables and raw fruit in your meals. Have a high-fibre diet with a range of whole grains including buckwheat, millet, oats, brown rice and rye, instead of having wheat every day. Use lentils and dried beans. Fish is a good protein choice.

If you are a vegan or vegetarian, seek professional advice to ensure you are getting adequate protein and other essential nutrients.

MAKING YOUR OWN COSMETICS

Commercial cosmetics are usually very expensive and contain many different substances – any of which might cause an allergic reaction. Here are some relatively simple and inexpensive suggestions for making your own skin products. Generally, these cause few adverse reactions and at least you know all the contents if you've found it necessary to avoid a particular ingredient.

Cleaning the face

OLIVE OIL

Olive oil removes eye makeup as well as being a cleanser. Tissue off, then wash the face with warm water. *Almond, linseed* or any edible oil may be used in the same way but don't let the oil get in your eyes.

BUTTERMILK

Buttermilk is especially refreshing. Use in the same way as you would any cleanser. Keep refrigerated.

Buttermilk is reasonably low in fats so is also a good dietary substitute for cream.

STEAM FACIAL

Make a strong tea using *chamomile flowers*, cover and let it stand a few minutes. Take the lid off and hold your face about 30 cm from the pot with a large towel over your head. Do this for 3–4 minutes; then reheat the tea and repeat. To finish, splash your face with cold water or mineral water.

Other herbs can be used for this purpose, for example *thyme, rosemary, lavender, lemon grass*. Use the leaves and flowers of these.

Face packs

These tend to draw metabolic by-products (toxins) to the skin surface. They also tone the skin and stimulate circulation. Below are some suggestions for face packs. You can improvise with similar ingredients from your kitchen.

To get the full benefit from a face pack, apply it then lie down with the feet up for 10–15 minutes; do not put the pack around the eyes but cover them with used cold tea bags or slices of cucumber.

FOR OILY SKIN

Apply just on oily patches such as around the nose and chin.
• *Almond meal* with beaten egg white.
• *Linseed meal* with apple cider vinegar or lemon juice.
• Finely ground *oatmeal* mixed to a paste with yoghurt or tepid milk.
• *Polenta* mixed into buttermilk.

FOR DRY SKIN

• Mashed *avocado*.
• *Castor oil* with some almond meal (castor oil has a 'drawing' effect).

Astringents

FOR OILY SKIN

• Diluted *lemon juice* or *apple cider vinegar* – use about 1 tablespoon to a cup of water (you can put it in a bottle and keep it refrigerated).
• *Sage, thyme* or *marjoram teas* – make as teas, cool, strain and refrigerate (they will keep for five days).

FOR DRY SKIN

• *Rosewater,* which is readily available from pharmacies and health-food stores.
• *Chamomile tea.*

Blackheads

• Massage ripe pumpkin into affected areas.
• Affected areas can be gently massaged using almond meal and a little cinnamon

mixed to a paste in the palm of the hand with water or lemon juice.

Moisturisers

Any edible oils can be used as moisturisers, with a small quantity of aromatic oil added for aroma and additional therapeutic benefit. One combination I have used successfully is:

Fixed oils
25 ml avocado
25 ml evening primrose
25 ml almond
25 ml apricot kernel
Essential oils
6 drops basil
6 drops blue chamomile
6 drops lemon grass
12 drops calendula
12 drops St John's wort

This recipe helps an ageing, wrinkled skin (what beauticians call a 'mature skin'). The problem is that it is quite greasy. I put it on first thing in the morning, have a drink and then go for my morning walk/jog. I hope that with my sunglasses on I'm unrecognisable or that anyone I meet who might recognise me will think it's sweat. The surplus can be rinsed off with warm water after about an hour.

• *Vitamin E oil* can also be used. If you can't find the pure oil, then cut open some capsules. This is especially helpful as a night-time moisturiser.

• *Sandalwood oil* – 1 teaspoon to a cup of hot water, poured over a small towel, and used as a hot compress.

GLYCERINE AND ROSEWATER

This is sold in many pharmacies and health-food stores already combined. I find the best proportion is about ⅓ glycerine to ⅔ rosewater. It can be used as a skin softener after showering. You can also use plain glycerine on the hands while they are still wet.

SORBOLENE

Sorbolene is not 'natural' but is a combination of substances that does not commonly aggravate the skin. It is often used as part of the base in cosmetics.

I use Sorbolene as a cleansing cream but it is apparently not standardised as it sometimes causes stinging, especially around the eyes. The most economical way of buying it is in a large container from a pharmacist and then blending it with some warm water to get a light, non-greasy cream.

If you wish, you can add your own herbs and oils to the cream. Experiment by mixing a few combinations in a small jar first. Some suggestions are:

• liquorice powder and a few drops of chamomile oil
• calendula herbal extract
• glycerine and rosewater, plus vitamin E oil
• jojoba and calendula oil
• ylang ylang oil and glycerine
• St John's wort oil and lavender oil.

If you are allergic to Sorbolene you can use any similar plain base for cleansing or making face, hand and body creams.

Puffy eyes

• Grate raw potato on gauze. Place over the eyes and rest with the feet up for 15 minutes.
• Cold tea bags, or slices of raw, cold cucumber, can also be used.

Gums

• Massage with a fresh sage leaf or use warm sage tea as a mouth wash.

Oatmeal or bran baths

Use as a soap substitute and for soothing irritated skin. Put 1–2 cups of oats or bran in a stocking. Let the hot tap run on to it, then cool water to blood heat before soaking in it.

Cleansing the body

1 cup Epsom salts in a hot bath (as this can make you very hot and sweaty, you might enjoy some crushed ice in a face-washer to place on your forehead).

CHAPTER 13

FOOD ALLERGIES

TYPES OF REACTIONS TO FOODS

Most healthy foods don't adversely affect people. However sometimes reactions occur to something one eats or drinks. This may be normal or abnormal. The terms allergy, sensitivity and intolerance are often used interchangeably for abnormal reactions to food.

Depending on the type of problem, some people only have a reaction to a substance when they are ill or tired, others are okay if the offending food or additive is in small quantities and not eaten regularly, while others have a bad reaction to even the tiniest portion. It is also possible that some people have a low-grade, chronic sensitivity to a particular substance that stresses the body but the only symptom may be unexplained fatigue, perhaps accompanied by excessive yawning.

NORMAL REACTIONS

1   Toxic reactions, such as vomiting or diarrhoea, when you eat poisons or infected foods.
2   Pharmacological reactions, to drugs, alcohol, caffeine and so on.

ABNORMAL OR UNUSUAL REACTIONS TO NON-TOXIC FOODS

1   Psychological: these can range from a 'pet aversion' to a major phobia.
2   Immune reactions. Your body has a specific antibody to a particular food or substance and reacts to it as though it was harmful. Some people have these same antibodies but don't get any apparent adverse reactions.
3   Non-immune reactions. A food additive, for example, may stimulate the body's release of inflammatory chemicals

such as histamine, giving you the symptoms of hayfever.

4 If you lack a particular digestive enzyme then it is not possible for you to absorb food that would normally be broken down by it. If you lack lactase you cannot digest lactose (milk sugar) and therefore dairy products – especially in large quantities – cause diarrhoea and other upsets.

5 You may have a temporary or permanent fault in the mucous membranes (linings) of the body, so that they lose their protective capacity or become abnormally permeable (leaky). Relatively large particles – which should be excreted – may get absorbed into the bloodstream and tissues causing various adverse reactions.

SYMPTOMS AND REACTIONS

Allergies may cause a range of reactions, including headaches, colic, hayfever, excess mucus, flatulence, muscular and joint problems, rashes and other skin problems, frequent infections, red and watery eyes, bad breath, candida albicans (thrush), asthmatic symptoms, tinea, fatigue, irritability, flushing, insomnia, confusion, hyperactivity, speech problems, depression and various mental and emotional disturbances. Of course, many of these symptoms may have nothing to do with allergies.

Reactions to foods are variable and the following is a selection of some actual cases.

• A six-year-old who breaks out in dramatic red, itching, lumps immediately after eating strawberries. She has no apparent reactions to any other foods.

• A thirty-four-year-old woman, medically diagnosed as having rheumatoid arthritis for two years, but the symptoms disappear if she avoids the nightshade family (potatoes, tomatoes, eggplant, capsicum, chilli, tobacco). If she eats even half a tomato, she has obvious and prolonged morning stiffness the following day. This is not the case with all arthritics but according to an American doctor, Dr Childers, about 10 per cent of arthritics have this particular allergy and he suggests avoidance of foods for three months as a trial period. My experience is that about 1 per cent of arthritics respond to nightshade avoidance – if you're that one, avoidance is well rewarded.

• A seventeen-year-old boy who had sudden and severe abdominal pains similar to acute appendicitis. A specialist diagnosed a milk allergy and when dairy products were avoided the pain quickly subsided. This boy had been drinking milk all his life and the extreme sensitivity to it apparently developed overnight, but he may have been suffering from a low-grade allergy for some time. Such sudden and dramatic developments are not common with everyday foods.

• A thirty-five-year-old woman with chronic cystitis who had been treated unsuccessfully with antibiotics for two years. She had been drinking large quantities of bottled orange juice. The cystitis symptoms completely disappeared when she changed to drinking water. In this case, it may have been a question of excess acid rather than an allergy.

• A twenty-year-old girl suffering from pimples and chronic diarrhoea – cause unknown. The diarrhoea stopped when she went on a gluten-free diet. There are now a number of books published on gluten-free cooking and health-food stores generally stock substitute foods.

• A woman in her twenties came to me following a series of allergy tests conducted by a medical practitioner. She was allergic to about sixty common foods and suffering from vertical disease, i.e. she was still functioning as a teacher but felt constantly ill from multiple symptoms. Every alternative food I gave her caused an adverse reaction – as did any supplement. She could handle white rice, lamb and lettuce but not much else. I saw her a few times, then she moved to another area and we lost touch. Eighteen months later she came to see me with her young baby. When I asked about her allergies, she replied, 'Oh, I've got more important things to think about now. I eat just about everything and have a wide variety. I've come about the baby.'

In some cases, reactions are related to quantities. For example, the tiny amounts of MSG that occur naturally in foods are seemingly tolerated quite well by almost everyone. Problems are usually caused by the synthetic crystalline MSG, which is used as a food additive, rather than natural MSG. Although industry-sponsored research finds virtually no harmful human or animal reactions to MSG, a basic computer check will give you well over a hundred references, many of which cite unfavourable reactions. You will find references to: 'monosodium glutamate-induced neurotoxicity in neonatal [new-born] rats', 'long-term developmental defects', 'permanent lesions of the hypothalamus' (an important regularity centre in the brain), 'female MSG-treated rats become more obese than males', 'dietary consumption of large quantities of MSG may represent a serious health hazard in certain individuals with pre-existing vascular disease', 'MSG – a known headache trigger', 'neonatal exposure in rats induced learning disabilities and weight abnormalities in later life', 'MSG has been found to trigger asthma' . . . G. R. Swartz, MD, toxicologist, has written a book entitled *In Bad Taste – the MSG Syndrome.*[1] His view is that MSG changes your perception of food flavours, excites the sensitivity of the taste buds and sends an electrical charge to the brain. He claims that it acts like a drug and shows all the characteristics of a drug, such as increasing tolerance to its effects.

In any event, there is no such thing as MSG deficiency, like many other chemical food additives it has not been proven to be harmless, it may cause subtle long-term reactions such as obesity, it is a known allergen to some people and therefore my advice is to avoid it. As a food additive, it is numbered 621, 622 and 623.

ARE ALLERGIES INCREASING?

Forty or fifty years ago you hardly heard of anyone reacting to commonly eaten foods. What has changed?

• Our bodies are now bombarded with literally hundreds of unnatural substances such as excess lead, pesticides, pharmaceuticals, processed foods and industrial pollutants. These are irritating our respiratory and digestive tracts. Consequently the mucous membranes become sensitive and less efficient in protecting us from irritants and harmful substances.

• Added chemicals put strain on the liver's detoxification system and a range of natural and synthetic toxins freely circulate instead of being broken down and excreted.

• Some of these chemicals are inactivated by dietary antioxidants. A poor diet doesn't give sufficient quantities of protective antioxidant nutrients.

• If you're chronically constipated or have an intestinal problem, you either don't absorb nutrients efficiently or you absorb excess toxins.

These are just a few examples to illustrate how a diet poor in nutrients but rich in man-made chemicals can add to the body's burden. It's not surprising that the immune system becomes disordered and your body loses its ability to select the harmful from the non-harmful.

SOME COMMON FOOD ALLERGENS AND SENSITIVITIES

• Milk.
• Wheat and bran – possibly including oats, barley and rye.

According to many researchers, the above are the most common food allergies. Here are some more.

• Eggs.
• Oranges – in my own clinic this is the most common allergen. However, I wonder if the real culprit is the many chemicals and dyes sprayed on citrus fruits.
• Yeast and mould foods, including cheese, mushrooms, vinegar, yoghurt, peanuts, Vegemite, Marmite, soy sauce, olives, dried fruit, fruit juices, tofu, smoked meats and most alcoholic drinks. An individual may not be allergic to all of these.
• Tomatoes.
• Chocolate.
• Coffee.
• Peanuts.
• Corn (sweetcorn and all maize products).

• Malt.
• Potatoes.
• Soya beans.
• Chemical food additives, preservatives.
• Shellfish and fish.
• White sugar.
• Smoked cured meat.
• Nuts.
• Legumes.

DETECTING FOOD ALLERGIES

Food allergies may be detected in various ways, such as blood pathology tests or putting the suspected food on the tongue and simultaneously testing muscle strength, but these tests are not always accurate. Another method is to keep a detailed diary of all foods and drinks for a week and match this to your symptoms, although this is complicated if you have many food allergies, if you get delayed reactions or if you are actually sensitive to something environmental.

I think the best method is to check tested or suspected food allergies by avoiding them to see if you improve when those particular foods are not part of your diet. Most people need professional help to establish which foods should be part of the avoidance trial. Avoidance trial periods vary from one to twelve weeks. If the particular problem is still with you at the end of that time, then you might conclude:

• you are not allergic to the foods you have gone without, or possibly you have been over-eating and your digestive system needed a rest

• you are allergic to them but there are other foods you are eating that are also upsetting you

• you have been eating the test foods without realising (for example, milk powder is in some breads and most margarines contain dairy products).

Avoidance trials have another drawback: when you give up a food – especially one you crave – for a trial period you may have quite severe and prolonged withdrawal symptoms such as a constant headache, irritability and nausea for a week or more. This is usually more pronounced with coffee and alcohol, but it is also possible with tea, sugar, milk and other foods and drinks. This may indicate an addiction.

Provocative testing is where you omit the suspect food for one week, on Day 8 have a reasonably large serving of it, then wait until the next meal. If no reaction has occurred, then have another serving and wait for at least twenty-four hours. The reactions to provocative testing could be any of these mentioned earlier in this chapter. If you have a marked reaction during a test, then this is sometimes offset by taking a glass of Andrews Liver Salts or a teaspoon of bicarbonate of soda in water.

CAUTION *If you are a severe asthmatic this type of test can precipitate an attack so it needs medical supervision.*

As you will see in Chapter 14, 'Fasting', it is not a good idea to water fast and then challenge (provocative testing) because your mucous membranes are extremely sensitive after a few days without food. In other words, after fasting the linings of your mouth, throat and digestive system can get a shock from the first few foods you eat and this may have nothing to do with allergies. If you decide to use a short fast for the purpose of allergy testing, the first foods should be in small quantities and something bland like brown rice or pears. Then you introduce all other foods one at a time, re-testing the first few foods if you had a reaction. The whole procedure will take a few months so you need to take a broad-spectrum combined multi-vitamin and mineral supplement during this period.

TREATING FOOD ALLERGIES

A relatively minor change in diet is all that is required in many cases. Any new foods, drinks, remedies or medication need to be introduced one at a time, with an interval of at least two days between introductions. Unless you have an extreme reaction, try the food again because a virus, toxin or stress may have caused the problem. Sometimes people simply dislike the taste of, say, a herbal liquid extract, but they handle the same thing in tablet form.

Anti-allergy remedies

TO HELP REPAIR INTESTINAL MUCOUS MEMBRANES
• *Aloe* • *Barberry bark* • *Golden seal*
DIGESTIVE ANTI-INFLAMMATORY HERBS
• *Ginger* • *Liquorice* • *Turmeric*
IMMUNE SYSTEM REGULATORS
• *Nettle* • *Reishi*
FOR THE RESPIRATORY SYSTEM
• *Garlic*
DIETARY SUPPLEMENTS
• *Vitamin C and bioflavonoids* • *Calcium and magnesium* • *Lactobacillus acidophilus and bifidobacteria*

On page 173 I have described a

method of using sodium ascorbate powder to protect the nasal mucous membranes – which are the first line of defence against inhaled toxins, irritants and microorganisms.

ALTERNATIVES TO COMMON FOOD ALLERGENS

Whenever you omit something from your diet you should find as many healthy substitutes as possible. You don't want to switch from an irritated body to a mal-nourished one. It takes time to adjust to different foods but don't eat things you hate – it's depressing!

Here are some examples of replacements.

Dairy foods
• Milk and yoghurt can be substituted by soy, almond, coconut or rice milks; fruit juice can be used on cereals.
• Instead of butter try tahini or nut butters; margarine is another option but most brands contain milk products so you will have to study the labels.
• To replace ice cream, you can now buy tofu ice cream or make your own from soy milk; alternatively, make or buy fruit ice blocks.
• There is no good substitute for cheese, especially if you love it, but soya cheeses are available in health-food stores and they're quite palatable grated or grilled.
• Chocolate alternatives include carob bars or buying carob powder and making your own sweets and biscuits. Chocolate is not the only 'sweet treat' – there are many different types of confectionery on the market.

Many bought biscuits, breads, cakes, dressings, sauces, sausages, gravies, hamburgers, soups, meat loaves, pies, fritters and processed foods contain butter or milk products. If the labels aren't clear, or when in doubt, ring the manufacturer. This is always interesting because some of them apparently don't know what's in their own products. A good motto is 'When in doubt, find out. If you can't find out, leave out'.

Wheat
My experience is that wheat can be the cause of migraine-type headaches. Most people eat far too much wheat and never include in their diets any of the substitutes given below. Even if you don't have a wheat allergy, I recommend using these as partial substitutes.

As well as the obvious breads, cereals, biscuits and cakes, wheat is found in the following: most pasta, thickened soups and chutneys, semolina, custards, cereals including Bran flakes, Corn flakes, Rice crispies, Fruit loops and Coco pops, farina, corn flours (unless made from maize only), batters, stuffings, ice-cream cones, sausages and similar processed meats, stock cubes and products such as rye bread – unless specifically marked 'wheat-free'.

SUBSTITUTES
• Oats, barley and rye are relations of wheat and may cause problems also. However some people with wheat intolerance can eat them safely. People with coeliac disease, which is a gluten allergy, cannot tolerate any grains and may be sensitive to millet and corn (maize). They need professional guidance.
• Rice is usually well-tolerated.
• Buckwheat is not at all related to wheat. It is actually a shrub (Fagopyrum esculentum) and the seeds may be used raw or cooked as a cereal, or you can buy

buckwheat flour, pasta and biscuits. Due to its high rutin content (3–8 per cent), buckwheat is recommended for all circulatory problems, especially those relating to weak blood vessels.

• Health-food stores stock many types of flours (linseed meal, millet, cornmeal, soy flakes or flour, quinoa, amaranth, lentil flour and so on). Basically, any starchy food can be used as a wheat substitute.

Sulphites and sulphur dioxide

Sulphur dioxide and sulphites are widely used as food additives, and are substances that commonly trigger asthmatic attacks. They are taste and colour enhancers as well as preservatives (additive numbers 220, 221, 222, 223, 224). People who have had an allergic reaction to sulphur drugs usually need to avoid this group of additives.

They are found in:

• all coloured soft drinks in glass bottles, all cordials, commercial chilled fruit juice and bottled drinks containing fruit juice (those labelled 'no preservatives' are okay)

• champagne, wine, beer, cider, alcoholic apple juice, some vinegars

• dried fruits, unless marked 'sun dried', and fruit bars (sultanas, currants, raisins and prunes are usually free of metabisulphite)

• dried vegetables, instant mashed potatoes, pickles, pre-cut and pre-peeled or commercially prepared chipped potatoes, some potato crisps and some salad dressings and sauces

• sausages and sausage mince, frankfurts, devon, brawn, uncooked fresh prawns, commercial chicken loaves and similar foods.

Although it is illegal, some fresh fruit salad from food bars and takeaways may have sulphites added. This group of additives is also illegal in fresh fish and meat but the Department of Health does catch, and fine, suppliers for using it.

Sulphites are odourless and tasteless to humans but cats are very sensitive to them. Your cat will not eat even the best cut of meat if it can smell or taste the tiniest quantity. However, if you have an asthmatic in the family you probably don't have a cat. Another problem with using a cat as a tester is that cats are notoriously temperamental – they just refuse to perform on demand. Also, you can't take your cat with you when you are eating out!

If you suspect a food supplier is using sulphites illegally, ring or write to your nearest Department of Health. Food inspectors are obviously over-burdened but if enough complaints are made about a particular outlet, an inspector will probably check it out.

Other allergens

You will have seen throughout this book and know from experience that a wide range of illnesses may be caused or triggered by many different types of foods and additives. Preservatives, especially benzoate and nitrites, artificial colourings and MSG are all likely allergens.

The Department of Health can provide you with a pamphlet listing approved food additives. Some of the additives are nutrients or non-harmful substances, such as citric acid which occurs in fruit. Many, such as sodium aluminosilicate, are suspect and add to the total body burden even though the quantity in a particular food may be quite small.

Food additives are likely to be unendingly controversial – depending on who pays for the research. Even the most enthusiastic food technologists admit that preservatives, such as nitrites, are potential hazards but to ban them completely would put a whole industry out of business. Governments allow such substances within certain limits but sometimes the set safety standards are abused. Furthermore, when you buy products such as bacon or salami, you don't know the ingredients or the additives.

My advice is not to eat or drink things that upset you and as far as practicable eat a wide variety of foods in as fresh and natural a state as possible. This will at least remove some of the dietary irritants.

CHAPTER 14

FASTING

WHAT IS FASTING?

True naturopathic fasting is total abstinence from food and should not be confused with juice diets or other restricted
eating practices. It is probably the oldest
therapy for treating illness and it can be
very effective if appropriately used and
monitored.

Treatments that have the power to heal
serious conditions also have the power to
do harm and I recommend that water
fasting is done only in a clinic where
patients can be supervised by someone
who has experience in this field.

WHO SHOULD FAST?

In my experience, those who benefit
most from fasting are people with:
• chronic gastric, digestive and intestinal
problems
• chronic viral and other infections

• severe skin conditions
• chronic joint and rheumatic problems
• fevers.

When you have an illness and lose
your appetite, it is quite safe to miss some
meals as long as you have fluid replacement; at such times you may benefit by
having juices or broths. Where there is
prolonged lack of appetite, seek professional help.

My personal experience of fasting is
based on relatively short fasts of 5–10
days. This is because, in my case, there is
no reason for a longer fast and my body
weight would not allow for it.

I have data indicating that large quantities of calcium are lost from the bones
of post-menopausal women during
fasting, and other restrictive diets. Osteoporosis is a condition that post-menopausal women are at risk of, so the risks
and benefits of water fasting need to be
assessed for individual cases.

WHAT HAPPENS WHEN YOU FAST?

This varies depending on body weight, general health and individual biochemistry. Books and articles on fasting are apparently written by the small group of people who feel mentally and physically uplifted while fasting. The majority of people feel some degree of discomfort. On the positive side, your body feels lighter and it's good to have a really flat tummy.

The following is a brief summary of common reactions.

Weight loss
One kilo per day for the first few days, then about 0.5 kilo daily. Obese people lose much more than this, and most of the weight loss is fluid.

Blood pressure
Within 4–5 days, the systolic pressure often drops 5–15 mg Hg and diastolic 5–20. This reduction is common in fasting and partly explains why people may feel dizzy, weak and faint.

For people who have above-average blood pressure, a fast might indicate that the problem could be controlled by dietary and lifestyle adjustments. A juice diet would also serve as a test for this purpose.

Temperature
Body temperature may drop from normal to 35.5°C by Day 3. You will always feel cold during a fast.

Urine
Moderate ketones are present in the urine on Day 2, then high on subsequent days, indicating that fats are being broken down to replace glucose as the main biological energy source. A small amount of protein excretion occurs throughout a fast. In some people this happens only for the first few days but high protein excretion is an indication that the fast should be broken. Excess ketones and protein in the urine can be detected by a urine test. Simply observing the colour or smell of the urine is not accurate.

You may pass 'gravel' during a fast, and experience mild kidney pain. Prolonged and repeated fasting is harmful to the kidneys and contraindicated where there is kidney disease.

Gastro-intestinal tract
TONGUE
Heavily coated throughout the fast. This happens to everyone and it has been suggested that the time to break the fast is when the tongue is clear but I don't think this is a major indicator.

STOMACH
For the first few days of a fast, great willpower is needed because you feel very hungry. The hunger disappears but if you are still hungry on Day 5, then the fast should be broken. A number of reactions can occur in the first few days, such as nausea, unpleasant taste sensations, dry and cracked lips and vomiting.

INTESTINES
In most cases as soon as you stop eating, your bowels stop functioning. I have one or two coffee enemas for the first few days (refer to Constipation, pages 81–6). Most fasting experts will disagree with this, but coffee enemas are an excellent headache cure and give you energy. If you have more than one enema a day for three days, the liver and gallbladder are

over-stimulated, which may cause excess bile excretion and dry retching.

Some people have normal bowel functioning, others have abdominal cramps and diarrhoea in the early stages of a fast.

SLEEP

Commonly I sleep only a few hours per night while fasting, although this depends on the level of daytime activity. A number of people experience vivid dreams.

ENERGY LEVELS

A basic reason for fasting is to have a complete rest – physical and mental. Some experiments have shown that people don't necessarily lose their strength while fasting, but in my experience and from observations, the majority are extremely tired and, in a long supervised fast, the only recommended exercise is short periods of walking.

Mental and emotional effects

Although mental fatigue is experienced, the mind is often quite clear. There is heightened sensitivity in nearly every way, especially sensitivity to noises. If you are in a clinic and wish to listen to music or the television, please use ear phones so as not to disturb the sensitive souls around you. Irritability is a common experience.

If you're at a health farm and talk endlessly about food to people on a fast, don't be surprised if they avoid you!

Biochemical changes

Obviously many changes take place during a fast. Scientific studies show that uric acid, cholesterol and triglyceride blood levels rise but not enough to cause gout or other problems. Blood glucose levels drop and thyroid activity is reduced. Testosterone activity decreases but oestrogens may increase.

Mucous membranes

After about three days of water fasting you start to lose cells. The first cells to go are the mucous membranes in the mouth and throat – which is why you can have sensitivity reactions to the first foods reintroduced. During long fasts (or starvation) the gums may start to bleed. This is a sign to break the fast.

Other

Particularly in the first few days, headaches are a common reaction. This happens because your body is undergoing major biochemical changes so that fats can be metabolised for energy; also you are likely to have withdrawal symptoms, not only from coffee, alcohol, etc. but also from some foods you may unknowingly be addicted to.

One of the major problems with fasting today is that all of us have pesticide residues and chemicals stored in our bodies, mainly in fatty liver tissue, and when we start to break down fats for conversion into biochemical energy these chemicals are released into our bloodstream. A number of fasting experts, with decades of experience, admit that people these days do not always react in the same way as in earlier times and they attribute this to the thousands of chemicals in our food and environment which we absorb into our bodies. Unpleasant body odours may occur.

During a fast I experience some shakiness, a little breathlessness on exertion and some joint pain. Some of these effects would be attributable to rapid weight loss and the movement of toxins (chemicals and metabolic by-products) through the system. Skin outbreaks occur in some people. Naturopaths call these types of reactions 'healing crises'.

THE PURPOSE OF A FAST

The main purposes are:
• to have a complete rest
• to treat a chronic disease or a feverish condition
• to clear toxins from the body.

This is not simply a matter of resting and cleaning the digestive tract. Over a period of years our cells accumulate metabolic waste and chemicals. During a long fast, the nucleus of cells remains the same but the overall size decreases. We are made up of billions of cells, and they can work more effectively if cellular debris is removed, and this is what is achieved during water fasting.

People often ask why some naturopaths recommend a lengthy fast for certain health problems, when it is known that people die from not eating. It is necessary to make a distinction between fasting and starvation. For example, when prisoners or protestors fast, they are doing so for the wrong physiological reasons, under poor conditions, they are physically and emotionally stressed, they often drink coffee, alcohol and fluids other than pure water, and they are never supervised by an expert in fasting. Basically, they are fasting the wrong way and for the wrong purposes from the point of view of health.

I know people who drink only water one day a week as a discipline or for spiritual reasons. From a biochemical point of view, this is a major physiological stress because at the end of Day 1 their bodies are attempting to switch to a different form of metabolism. In other words, Day 1 of a fast is a major stress day. For the sake of their health, they would be better advised to have a day on fruit and vegetables or juices.

HOW TO FAST

Although I have fasted while working this is not the way to do it. You should be in a warm, peaceful environment and resting, apart from short walks. Most importantly, you should be in a clinic with an experienced practitioner who regularly checks your bodily functions.

Your fluid intake should be restricted to pure water; the amount required is variable but you need at least 6–8 glasses per day. If you add lemon or other substances to the water this usually brings on dry retching.

Fasting is the ideal time to practise relaxation and meditation. You should avoid all scented products, have a warm shower daily, avoid sunbathing or getting chilled but have plenty of fresh air.

Starting a fast

It is usually recommended that you have a few days on fruit and vegetables, then a day on juices prior to fasting. If you feel terrible, then you are probably experiencing withdrawal symptoms.

Breaking the fast

It is very important do to this correctly, which is another reason why you need to be supervised. Once you get the taste of food after a period of abstinence, you usually feel ravenous and your taste buds and sense of smell are extremely sensitive.

Your first 'meal' should be a tiny quantity of diluted, fresh juice, which should be eaten with a spoon. The quantities should then be gradually increased and the first foods should be watery fruits and vegetables. As a guide, if you have fasted for six days, you should take three days before getting back to your normal eating patterns.

WHO SHOULD NOT FAST

• Anyone on pharmaceutical drugs.
• Women during pregnancy and lactation.
• Babies, young children and frail elderly people.
• Post-menopausal women need to weigh the risks and benefits (calcium is leached from the bones during fasting).
• Those with serious diseases such as cardiovascular, kidney and endocrine disturbances.
• Those suffering from depression or anxiety.
• People who are very weak or thin.

WHAT HAPPENS AFTER FASTING

Although I know a number of people who have been 'cured' of ailments following a long fast there are sometimes problems. After one fast, I decided to eat a peach. The whole of my mouth and throat swelled dramatically and for a few alarming minutes I could hardly breathe or talk. I've never had a reaction to peaches before. It took a while for me to pluck up courage to eat another one but I've never had any similar reaction subsequently.

Most people find that if they have broken a fast properly, they will make better food choices from then onwards, partly because they don't want to spoil the therapeutic benefits of the fast.

WHY BOTHER TO FAST?

The first reason is that some conditions do not respond to medical or standard naturopathic treatments. With conditions where there is no known cure, such as herpes and post-viral syndrome, it is especially recommended. It is very depressing to be told there is nothing to be done, so people should investigate all the possibilities rather than resigning themselves to poor health.

For certain diseases, such as AIDS, where billions of research dollars have not found a cure, it seems reasonable that supervised fasting with monitoring should be trialled on patients who are infected but who have not yet reached a completely debilitated state.

Fasting is also used to test food sensitivities, that is, by reintroducing foods one at a time. However, my own experiences indicate that people can be acutely sensitive to the first foods reintroduced.

Fasting may also be a way of getting yourself motivated to begin a healthy diet, lifestyle or weight-loss programme. Some people don't seem to be able to alter things slowly; they have to make a clean break.

Except where there are medical reasons for not fasting, I think it is an experience everyone should have at least once in a lifetime, even if it is not indicated. Apart from the self-discipline, it will teach you that you can survive for long periods without food if you really have to. There have been some particularly stupid television programmes where people have tried to survive on their own resources for a week. Unless you are trained in survival techniques, the worst thing you can do is to start eating plants that you can't positively identify as being edible. The wisest course is to find safe drinking water, stay by it, rest, avoid exposure, leave a visible sign of your position and wait for help. Normal, healthy people can do without food – but not water – for an incredibly long period without apparent long-term harmful effects.

WHERE TO FAST

Make an appointment with a natural therapies practitioner or visit a clinic in your region prior to undertaking a fast. Write down all the questions you want to ask so that you can be satisfied you are going to be in safe hands. Some people complain that it is very expensive to pay upwards of $50 a day to drink water, but you need to remember that while you are in the clinic the practitioners there are taking responsibility for your health.

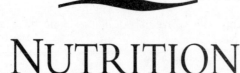

CHAPTER 15

NUTRITION

THE IMPORTANCE OF COMMON SENSE AND VARIETY

Irrespective of any advice given to you, common sense dictates that you should avoid foods which give you obvious digestive or other problems, because these may cause irritation to the digestive tract and lead to poor absorption as well as other problems. Rather than diet we should all try to develop appropriate and sensible eating habits, but this does not mean that a short period on a special or restricted diet will not be beneficial, particularly if you are ill. There are, unfortunately, certain diseases that require a specific, long-term dietary programme.

The worst feature of most diets is that you may end up eating and drinking the same things every day. Obviously, this does not apply to breast milk or to water, but the following are some important reasons for eating a variety of foods.

• Even items of food that look alike have a different range of essential nutrients, so a variety should prevent deficiencies.

• Many common foods contain tiny amounts of naturally occurring toxins and there have been well-documented cases of problems arising when people eat large amounts of one particular food over a period of time. For example, in sensitive individuals, excess cabbage can cause goitre.

• Most foods contain chemicals of one kind or another. Specific crops are attacked by particular groups of insects which are killed by a defined group of chemicals, so if you eat from a wide range of foods you are less likely to get a build-up of such chemicals.

• Food allergies and intolerances are apparently on the increase and a number of experts suggest rotation diets as a means of overcoming some of these problems.

Aim to try one new food a week. Of course, if you have a weak digestive system, don't have too many different foods in the one meal.

PROCESSED FOODS

Throughout this book I have suggested that these be avoided and the following are some of the reasons.

Refined foods

White flour, sugar, white spaghetti, cakes, ice cream, chocolate, soft drinks and all refined grains provide kilojoules but have reduced vitamin and mineral content compared to wholefoods. Refined foods also tend to increase the types of fats in the blood that are harmful when they circulate in large amounts in the bloodstream.

Refined grains are generally what is left after the outer 30 per cent of the kernel and germ is ground away. Many of the vitamins and minerals in wheat are concentrated in the part that is removed, and the following is a list of some of the losses in white flour.

Substance in wheat	Amount lost in refining (%)
Thiamin (vitamin B1)	57
Riboflavin (vitamin B2)	44
Niacin (vitamin B3)	68
Pyridoxine (vitamin B6)	98
Pantothenic acid (vitamin B5)	36
Biotin	70
Folic acid (vitamin B9)	46
Iron	66
Potassium	71
Calcium	50
Magnesium	84
Zinc	66
Phosphorus	74
Manganese	91
Fibre	87

In Australia, a nutrient enrichment programme is not mandatory for refined food producers, although a number of breakfast cereal manufacturers add back some B1, B2, B3, iron and protein and say the product is 'enriched'; however, in the light of the totality of the nutrients lost during manufacture, it might be more accurate to call such products 'deficient'.

Processed and fast foods

These invariably contain high amounts of sugar, fats, salt, colouring agents and a number of different types of preservatives.

Food additives

As explained in Chapter 13, not all additives are hazardous but I recommend avoiding those that are man-made. If you avoid processed and fast foods, you'll automatically eliminate many troublesome additives.

Dietary fats and oils

A low-fat diet is now recommended by most nutritionists throughout the world. However, one needs a small quantity of essential fatty acids: they are called essential because they need to be eaten as the body cannot make them from other substances.

If all fats are completely avoided there can be a problem in certain diets so I usually suggest the following per day: 1 teaspoon cold pressed oil or 1 tablespoon of nuts or seeds or a small piece of avocado. My reason for suggesting this minimum is that I have seen a few patients with early signs of essential fatty acid deficiencies that have been corrected by the addition of small quantities of oils to the diet.

WHY THE EMPHASIS ON WHOLE, NATURAL FOODS?

It's true that people are living longer these days in spite of their intake of processed foods and man-made chemicals, but how many people are in a state of abundant physical, mental and social wellbeing? The number of days lost from school and work, the quantities of pharmaceutical prescriptions, the high percentage of degenerative and mental illnesses in society seem to indicate that good health is relatively rare. Just look around you: how many people are cheerful and energetic?

Although Australia probably has one of the best food supplies in the world, major surveys show that a proportion of every age group is badly nourished. Here are a few examples of schoolchildren's diets in 1985.[1]

• 20 per cent of dietary kilojoules were made up of drinks, confectionery and snack foods.

• Average daily fat intake was 115 g, some having 200 g. Dietary fats made up more than 40 per cent of the daily kilojoules for one-fifth of children (the World Health Organisation recommend 15–30 per cent).

• 50 per cent were below the recommended intake for retinol (vitamin A), 10 per cent for vitamin C and 50 per cent for calcium.

In a study of inner-city children, it was found that only 20 per cent had a reasonable breakfast. American studies have shown that 10 per cent of children have higher blood pressure levels than desirable and than caffeine intake (coffee, cola drinks, chocolate) and salty foods were related to this; increasing dietary fibre reduced the risk of childhood appendicitis; and 71 per cent of children who suffered fractures had a lower bone mineral content than matched controls.

Every age group that is surveyed in Western societies reinforces the notion that affluent malnutrition is fairly common. The Department of Community Services and Health *National Dietary Survey of Adults: 1983* showed that, on average, women aged 25–34 years consumed 101 g of sugar per day, over 60 g (about 12 large teaspoons) coming from what I would classify as unhealthy foods. The average fat intake for this age group was 83 g per day. Bear in mind, too, that when researchers check people's rubbish bins or do biochemical tests, it is obvious that people completing diet diaries for surveys markedly underreport their consumption of foods such as confectionery, soft drinks and ice cream.

The survey didn't examine all the forty or so essential nutrients. Of the five vitamins and four minerals studied, significant numbers of women consumed less than the recommended daily intakes (RDI).

Essential nutrient	Percentage of 24-35-year-old women consuming less than the RDI
Vitamin A	50
Thiamin (vitamin B1)	30
Riboflavin (vitamin B2)	26
Niacin (vitamin B3)	5
Vitamin C	19
Iron	72
Calcium	64
Zinc	74
Magnesium	46

Although the RDIs are said to have a large margin of safety, they are based on the amount needed to prevent deficiency diseases rather than confer ideal health.

The quality of food eaten by child-bearing age women is not the only concern. Approximately 30 per cent of them eat too much and are overweight, while about 25 per cent are on low-kilojoule diets. Considering the quantities of nutrient-poor foods being eaten, you can appreciate that many people are badly nourished in some way.

FEEDING BABIES AND TODDLERS

Getting started

The ideal first food is breastmilk.
• It is a complete food for baby's growth.
• It is easier to digest than formula or cow's milk and results in less colic.
• It helps build the immune system and reduces sickness.
• It reduces the risk of allergies developing in later life.
• It promotes good jaw and tooth development through the sucking exercise.
• It encourages baby to satisfy the appetite without overeating.
• It creates a special closeness between mother and baby.
• It promotes loss of weight gained by the mother during pregnancy.
• It helps the uterus become smaller again.
• It is the least expensive way of feeding babies.
• It is easier and more hygienic than preparing formula.
• Cow's milk is at the end of the food chain and can be contaminated with chemical and pesticide residues of various kinds. Soy is also a common allergen and some soy milks and soy formula contain aluminium in relatively high but not hazardous quantities.

• The *Lancet* reported that breastfed babies had higher developmental scores at eighteen months than those fed formula.[2] At 7.5–8 years of age, the breastfed children had significantly higher intelligence scores – independent of education and social level of the mothers.
• Other medical studies report that breastfed babies ultimately have fewer problems with cholesterol and fat metabolism as well as cardiovascular disease.

Over a hundred years ago, O.W. Holmes wrote: 'A pair of mammary glands has the advantage over the two hemispheres of the most learned professor's brain in the art of compounding a nutritious food for infants.'

During breastfeeding, foods that disagree with the mother may also affect baby, or the baby may be intolerant to some foods she is eating; the symptom of this is usually colic. Some foods in this category are cow's milk and dairy products generally, onions, garlic, legumes, cabbage, broccoli, cauliflower and Brussels sprouts. If your baby has intermittent colic problems, write down everything you ate in the last two meals and you may be able to trace the dietary item causing the problem. However, most babies have varying degrees of colic that have nothing to do with food intolerances.

A number of pills and medicines may be unsafe for baby via breastmilk. Check with a qualified practitioner. Although a combined multi-vitamin and mineral tablet would not be harmful, there can be complications, not to mention unnecessary expense, in taking very large doses of vitamins and minerals.

Some herbal teas may help stimulate the flow of breastmilk, including aniseed, caraway and fennel. These are also helpful for flatulence and may help baby colic via breastmilk. Mild herbal teas such as peppermint and dandelion coffee would be beneficial but most medicinal herbals should be used only with practitioner supervision. Common culinary herbs are recommended except for spices such as cinnamon, cloves and nutmeg. Unless there is an allergy or colic problem, garlic is also recommended.

For the mother, I suggest a well-balanced wholefood diet, similar to that given under Pregnancy (pages 104–6). It is definitely not the time to go on a slimming diet.

Introducing solid foods

For the first year, babies' food should be very simple. Basically, give them a small portion of what you are preparing for the family. **Your taste buds have been manipulated, but babies don't know that our foods are commonly served with added sugar, salt, fat, fancy sauces, additives and taste enhancers. Keep it a secret – as long as you can!**

The general view is that around six months is a suitable age to start introducing solids. A ten-year study of over a thousand New Zealand children showed that those who were introduced to four or more types of solid foods before the age of four months had 2.9 times the risk of developing recurrent eczema compared to those not having early solid feeding. Conversely, one-sixth of exclusively breastfed Chilean children aged nine months were iron deficient.

Unfortunately, little humans (and some big ones) have a tendency to be perverse. If only we could get them to eat what we plan! However, the base or starting point should be an ideal diet. Human bodies have changed very little but in the last century in particular they have been asked to cope with hundreds of strange or unnatural substances and re-made foods.

The first taste adventure can be a tiny quantity of a single food – perhaps a few dabs on the high chair tray so the little fingers can explore and sample from familiar fingers rather than a hard spoon. Initially, foods should be smooth, creamy and one thing at a time. Ideal first solids are sweet potato, pumpkin, squash, zucchini and carrot. These should be sieved or puréed, mixed with a little breastmilk or formula but without adding salt, butter or *your* favourite taste enhancers.

Introduce new foods at two-day intervals and watch for signs such as bloating, diarrhoea, mouth or skin rashes, crankiness, watery eyes, runny nose or other allergy signs. If you suspect a particular food may have caused a problem, try it again in a few weeks because there are other causes of such reactions and you don't want to restrict future nutrition unnecessarily.

Common potatoes are okay but have a few problems. In Australia, about 25 per cent of retail stock exceeds the maximum permitted concentration of cadmium. Don't use left-over potatoes and never use them if they're green and damaged because this means they contain a high level of naturally occurring toxins. In a few words, don't give potatoes to baby every day.

Rice cereal is another suggested weaning food. You can make your own. In a blender, grind half a cup raw brown rice; store in a small airtight container. When needed cook about a quarter cup ground rice to 1 cup water, stirring constantly to prevent lumps, until the rice is creamy. Breastmilk or formula can be added as required.

Unused quantities can be used as thickening agents for something you are preparing for the family, or stored in the freezer for future use. You're probably familiar with the common method of freezing baby food: use ice-cube trays, freeze and then store the cubes in freezer bags.

Second foods to be introduced

Here are some foods suitable to be introduced between 7–9 months of age.

• Cooked, finely sieved asparagus tips, beetroot, corn, parsnip, swede, kohlrabi and fennel root (not all vegetables are suitable at this stage).

Unless you have access to, and can afford, organically grown produce, peel all vegetables and fruit to remove pesticide residues. Those which are not 'peelable' should be thoroughly washed. Much shop-bought 'fresh' food is also treated with chemicals to prevent spoilage during storage. The most recent government surveys indicate that the majority of potentially hazardous substances in our food supply are decreasing.[3] However, residue levels of organophosphate pesticides such as pirimphos methyl are increasing. These are not as nasty and long-lived as DDT-type chemicals but they are related to the 'nerve chemicals' used in warfare.

• Millet.

1 cup hulled millet (unhulled millet is almost uncookable!)

1 ¼ cups water

Bring water to the boil, add millet. Simmer gently with lid on until the water is absorbed (about 25 minutes). Don't stir. Turn off heat, leave to stand, covered, for a further 5–10 minutes. Sieve for baby.

For the rest of the family, millet is tasty served with a vegetable curry. You can also buy millet flakes, which require less cooking time.

• Ripe mashed banana.

Banana is best introduced in the second stage of foods, as if you introduce something sweetish first, you run the risk of all other foods being refused.

• Cooked apple purée.

• Ripe mashed fruit in season: kiwi fruit, paw paw, mango, peach, nectarine, plum – all without added sugar or honey.

Melon and citrus fruits may cause reactions so introduce them later.

Berries are rich in nutrients and other protective substances but the seeds may be a problem. You can sieve out the seeds for babies. For toddlers, I suggest mashing all berries so that they will not pick and eat similar-looking things in gardens and parks. Deadly nightshade berries, for example, look something like blueberries. Since many adults have problems with plant identification, I suggest that all young children be discouraged from picking their own foods. Many common garden plants are poisonous, including tomato and rhubarb leaves.

Small-stoned fruit, such as cherries and lillypilly, should not be given to children under five because the stones may cause choking.

In the USA, the Medical Association has warned that infants under one year old should not be fed honey as 30 per cent of infant botulism was related to the consumption of honey. When I rang the Australian Honey Board, they didn't disagree with this recommendation.

Third foods

Start introducing these when the baby is about 10 months old. New foods can, of course, be mixed into those that have previously passed baby's taste test.

• Cereals such as oats and barley.

• Buckwheat. As mentioned in Chapter 13, 'Food Allergies', this is a seed, not a grain and does not cause the allergy problem that wheat does. Wheat is better introduced after baby is twelve months old.

• More cooked, puréed vegetables: peas, beans, broccoli, cauliflower, leek, onion. Introduce them in small quantities as they may cause colic.

• A little softly cooked egg yolk or avocado mixed into vegetables. Egg white is harder to digest and is a common allergen, so wait a few more months before giving it.

• Poached fish. Perch is good to start with as it is soft. Check carefully with your fingers for any bones. Simmer fish gently in formula or breastmilk for about 10 minutes, then sieve and mash into the milk.

• Meat. Offal, particularly liver, is probably best avoided these days because it contains a higher proportion of chemicals than other cuts. Lean beef or lamb is suitable: mince or shred (this can be done by scraping it with a serrated knife), simmer in water until tender, then sieve or purée, using the fluid as well.

If you don't want to freeze tiny portions or your freezer becomes congested, left-over baby vegetables and meat purées may be added to casseroles, rissoles, soups, meat loaves and so on.

Foods such as raw, chopped parsley and sprouts tend to 'catch in the throat' so leave these out until the children can chew really well. You can cook a little parsley and other common culinary herbs with vegetables and then sieve together.

Teething and finger foods

• Pieces of apple or carrot tied into a handkerchief.

• Dried apple.

• Wholegrain pasta shells and spirals – cooked, of course!

• Tofu – cut into cubes and lightly roasted.

• Cooked chicken.

• Wholegrain pikelets.

• Stringless cooked green beans.

• Cheese cubes or soya cheese.

• Rusks. Some commercial rusks are high in sugars and other refined ingredients. You can make your own.

Use wholemeal bread, cutting off crusts (if you're really keen, you can make damper bread, using a variety of wholegrain flours, linseed meal, etc.).

Cut bread into strips about 1.2 cm wide and 2.5 cm thick.

Place on a baking tray, covered with another tray to keep the rusks smooth. Bake in a slow oven (140–150°C) for about 50 minutes – until they are dry and crisp. Store in an airtight container.

Rusks can be served plain or with a little Marmite, Vegemite or tahini. Better still, make your own unsweetened compôte.

1 cup dried apricots (or a mixture of dried fruit)
1 cup apple juice
Simmer in a saucepan, uncovered, for about 20 minutes or until the fluid is absorbed. Cool and mash.

Strategies for 'picky' eaters

Some children, and adults, have a small digestive capacity and it may not suit them to have three largish meals per day. After all, most adults eat something when they're hungry. Small quantities, and often, may be better for the little one, and your nervous system.

What you eat is more important than when you eat it. It might not be ideal socially, but if children want to nibble on raw vegetables while you're preparing the meal I'd let them. After all, 40 per cent of Australians are overweight and I imagine if we all had an entrée of raw vegetables and ate less of other things we'd be healthier and leaner. You might encourage this trend in your family by providing a hummous dip for raw vegetable snacks:

1 cup pre-soaked, well-cooked chickpeas
½ cup tahini (or less)
1–2 crushed cloves garlic (or chives)
¼ cup lemon juice
½ cup natural yoghurt

Blend the chickpeas in a blender with some of their cooking water. Add the other ingredients until the mixture is creamy.

• Allow a degree of choice. Generally, you don't buy foods *you* dislike. If you are serving, say, five different vegetables in a meal, you could ask the 'picky one' which three are preferred. Depending on your circumstances you might allow children to select some of their own foods when shopping. You usually have to restrict this to fresh foods, otherwise you'll have a trolley full of lollies!

• For *all* people with poor appetites, never give large servings because this tends to put them off before they start.

• Most children (and adults) resent constant reminders that a particular food is good for them. We all have foods we don't like and there isn't any virtue in being healthy but miserable. Although it's frustrating to prepare food that isn't eaten, try to make mealtimes pleasurable.

• If you have to resort to bribery, then endeavour to have the 'treat' reasonably healthy or something non-edible. There are many recipes for reasonably healthy treats, for example: fruit bars.

1¼ cups finely chopped dried fruit
½ cup water
¼ cup ground almonds or tahini
1 dessertspoon orange juice
½ cup honey
1 cup skim milk powder (or soy milk powder)
1 tablespoon wheatgerm (or carob powder)
½ cup desiccated coconut

Simmer the dried fruit in water for about 15 minutes. Remove from heat, add all the other ingredients and mix thoroughly. Spread the mixture into a lightly greased, shallow pan.

Refrigerate for about 2 hours, cut into small bars. Wrap bars in cellophone and store in fridge.

• For toddlers who love meat but refuse most vegetables, try grated or blended vegetables in rissoles, mixed through mince, in meat loaves or casseroles. Vegetables may also be somewhat disguised, for example, in pumpkin muffins, homemade damper bread and pancakes.

• Wholegrains may be cooked, blended and disguised in a thick milk or soy shake with fresh fruit, berries, ground nuts and other 'goodies'.

• Giving children a little pocket money to buy whatever they like may be preferable to having bought treats readily available at home.

I've never heard of a finicky eater starving. You can't forcefeed so there's no point in making every meal a drama. Very few people have a perfect diet, perfect children and perfect parents. Eating can be a way for older children to express their independence and be like their friends; toddlers may use mealtimes to gain attention.

If you love me don't feed me junk

Long before chocolate, chips, white sugar and Coke, our ancient ancestors hankered after taste treats but in the wild they were in short supply. In other words, you don't have to encourage a liking for sweet, fatty and salty foods. Furthermore, there's no such diseases as cola, confectionery or chip deficiency.

HEALTHIER SNACK OPTIONS

Not many children enjoy or take the time to munch on a carrot, but they may eat slices of apple with some raisins. On a hot day, you can prepare bite-sized pieces of rockmelon, watermelon or other fruit served in a broad glass with some crushed ice. In the winter, vegetable soup or hot wholemeal pikelets provide a change from wholegrain biscuits.

Use carob instead of chocolate. Here's a comparison of some of their constituents.

Per 100 g	Carob	Chocolate
Kilojoules	760	2100
Fat (g)	1.4	53
Fibre (g)	7.7	2.5
Calcium (mg)	352	78
Caffeine (mg)	0	180
Theobromine (mg) (a naturally occurring stimulant)	3	2320

As well as being sugary, fattening and stimulating, chocolate has an additional problem. All samples of dark chocolate tested in the last National Health and Medical Research Council survey, both imported and domestic, had cadmium levels above the Australian maximum permitted concentration. Cocoa samples also had cadmium concentrations above the maximum level. In most recipes carob powder can be used instead of cocoa; unsweetened carob bars are a substitute for chocolate bars.

FATS AND OILS

Babies and children do not need to go on a Pritikin-type diet. In fact, this would be disastrous because some fats and cholesterol are needed for growth and absorption of certain nutrients. That's why you don't give babies and young children skimmed dairy or reduced-fat soy products. However, this doesn't imply that they should be served bacon and fried eggs, vegetables smothered in cream, bread with lashings of butter and high-fat convenience foods. An American study showed that some four-year-old children already had the beginnings of atherosclerotic plaques in their arteries; Australian surveys indicate that 30 per cent of children are overweight. Recipes need to be adapted. Instead of frying rissoles, roll them in something such as linseed meal, polenta or millet flakes and bake in a lightly greased dish in the oven. This also saves you standing over a hot stove. To give more moisture, serve with a home-made tomato sauce as commercial sauces contain relatively high quantities of salt, sugar and other additives.

I recommend tahini and nut pastes instead of butter and margarine because these are less processed, contain more beneficial fats and a wider range of nutrients. Margarine, for example, contains a high level of trans-fatty acids, which are found in nature in tiny quantities only.

A few no nos

• Do not microwave infant formula because this changes the structure of specific amino acids (the building blocks of protein). These changes don't occur during 'normal' heating. A number of researchers have suggested that the uneven heating of food in microwave ovens may allow harmful bacteria to survive. Babies are known to be extremely sensitive to a wide range of toxins so it might be safer not to use the microwave to heat, cook or defrost foods such as meat, poultry, fish and eggs.

Defrosting generally is best done in the fridge rather than a warm room, as fridge defrosting reduces the possibility of bacterial contamination.

• Whole nuts and seeds should not be given to children under five years of age because they may cause choking, become lodged in noses or ears or be inhaled into the respiratory system and lungs. All nuts and seeds are fairly common allergens and high in kilojoules, but they are a good source of essential fatty acids, protein and other nutrients.

Peanuts have additional problems – as discussed in Chapter 9, 'Liver and Gallbladder'.

• Processed meat is best avoided. A 1990 survey of manufactured meats showed that 10 out of 36 samples failed to conform to the Food Standards Code because of excess starch, sugar, preservatives, nitrite, styrene monomer or meat content deficiency. These foods are invariably high in cholesterol, fats and salt. Nitrites are carcinogens but permitted in foods because they are effective preservatives and taste enhancers – there is no safe commercial alternative for processed meats.

In conclusion

The best advice I can give is for all the family to eat a wide range of foods in as natural a state as possible, to avoid a build-up of either naturally occurring or man-made hazards.

There is a theory that if you raise your children on healthy foods from the age of six months, this healthy eating will carry on throughout their lives. In practice it's not so easy and sometimes the best you can do is set some reasonable rules regarding the type and quantity of foods that have to be eaten. For poor eaters, I recommend giving a combined multivitamin and mineral supplement.

You need to use your own judgement about some of the information given in books and articles. For example, some children have allergies and special needs. Do the benefits of eating liver outweigh the risks of toxicity? Is it reasonable – as suggested by one author – to give a fluoride supplement to a two-week-old baby?

NUTRITION FOR THE WHOLE FAMILY

It's never too late – or too early – to improve your dietary habits, and to try to harmonise your food with your genetic equipment.

What is a natural, wholefood diet?

My definition is: food that looks and tastes like something that has grown, flown, swum, crawled or walked.

Hunting and gathering societies persisted for a few million years so they must have been quite successful. Presumably, theirs was a 'natural' lifestyle, with a reasonable range of food, adequate exercise and plenty of leisure time.

Some African people used eighty-five species of plant foods, including roots and bulbs, and had regular supplies of meat. They needed to work only six hours per day for two and a half days a week looking for food. Their diet yielded all the essential nutrients. Similar findings of good nutritional status, with only a small work-load, have been confirmed for some groups of Australian Aborigines. In North America, pre-agricultural Indians lived on grasses, seeds, fruits, berries, roots, tubers, vines, herbs, large and small mammals, migratory waterfowl, riverine birds and fish.

The average daily intake of pre-agricultural people was probably around 12 600 kilojoules. Experts estimate that on average they ate about 35 per cent meat and 65 per cent plant foods, totalling around 2250 g of food per day, that is, 790 g of meat and 1460 g of plant foods. (The proportions are not all that important because the kilojoules per gram of wild game meat roasted in an open fire would have been similar to that of wild plant foods.)

With our modern, concentrated foods, it is possible to get the same number of kilojoules from less than 1400 g. Our foods are less bulky and probably less satisfying. This may, along with pressure to be slim, partially explain the modern problems of eating disorders.

Researchers have made estimates of some of the nutrients in 'ancestral wild foods' so that we can make comparisons. My main reference book was *The Paleolithic Prescription*, S.B. Eaton et al, Harper & Row, 1988.

MEAT

Nutrients per 100 g (average)	Wild game	Domestic meat
Kilojoules	559	1619
Protein (g)	21.9	15.8
Fat (g)	4.3	29.0
Cholesterol (mg)	67.0	75.0

Not only quantity but the quality of fat differs between game and farmed meat. Wild game fat contains five times more polyunsaturated fatty acids than does fat from domestic animals. It also contains about 2.5 per cent of an essential fatty acid (eicosapentanoic acid) that may protect against atherosclerosis; domestic beef contains so little that it is hard to detect. Then, there is the problem of hormones and other substances used to fatten modern farmed animals rapidly, which remain present as residues in the meat.

VEGETABLES

Nutrients per 100 g (average)	Ancient times – wild plant foods	Today – mixed, cooked vegetables
Dietary fibre (g)	12.6	4.0
Calcium (mg)	131.0	25.0
Vitamin C (mg)	30.6	8.0
Iron (mg)	6.4	1.3
Potassium (mg)	425.0	191.0
Sodium (mg)	26.9	53.0

The majority of people today add flavourings such as fat and salt to their vegetables.

COW'S MILK AND CALCIUM

Using animals as milk providers probably began in the Sahara about 7000 BC. Prior to that time, the sole dairy product was mother's milk which was available only to infants. In spite of this, stone-age children and adults had stronger bones and teeth than modern people, according to studies of ancient human remains.

Is cow's milk good for you or the world's most overrated nutrient? Dairy products are rich in nutrients and many children would be malnourished without them. Unsweetened yoghurt is a convenient weaning food, although I would suggest introducing it after the first two groups of plain vegetables, fruits and grains because it is a common allergen.

The ability to digest dairy products depends on having the correct enzymes. Some ethnic groups, such as Thais, Fijians and Peruvians, have over 90 per cent dairy intolerance, that is, 90 per cent of them lack the digestive enzymes needed to break down dairy food, whereas Danish people have around 2 per cent. Every ethnic group has some proportion of its population unable to tolerate dairy food. One theory is that genetic adaptation of humans to cow's milk could take 10 000 years, or some 400 generations.

Some blame dairy products for just about everything – rheumatoid arthritis, diarrhoea, diabetes, multiple sclerosis, respiratory illnesses, digestive problems, heart disease, bedwetting and hyperactivity. There's even a book entitled *Don't Drink Your Milk* in which the author, Dr Oski, warns that 'during sleep the secretion of saliva is markedly decreased. Milk in the mouth is neither digested nor washed away and instead remains on the teeth and turns sour. The soured milk serves as an excellent food for the bacteria that inhibit the mouth. Decay can be so rapid that parents will report that the teeth seem to be melting away.'[4]

Cow's milk is not an essential food since it is relatively new to human nutrition and many people live long, healthy lives without it. However, it is rich in essential nutrients such as protein and calcium and, for vegetarians, it contains vitamin B12. If you can't handle dairy products, there are substitutes listed in Chapter 13, 'Food Allergies'.

Calcium

Wild vegetable foods average about 130 mg calcium per 100 g. Based on estimates of some regions 20 000 years ago, plant foods would have provided humans with about 1 800 mg of calcium per day, with another 100 mg from meat. Of course, if the people chewed on small bones, such as fowls' or rats', this would have dramatically increased their calcium intake.

The current Australian Government Recommended Intake is 800 mg for an adult female, the average intake if you can't tolerate dairy products being 707 mg. There is no need to become unduly anxious about calcium intake if you can't tolerate dairy products as there are a number of foods that are good sources of this nutrient; some are listed below.

Food	Mg of calcium per 100 g
Tahini (ground sesame seeds – high in kilojoules)	1100
Whey powder – a dessertspoon can be mixed into rice milk/ soy milk/fruit smoothies	640
Dry carob powder	350
Whole raw linseeds (these need to be ground into a 'meal')	270
Soya grits	250
Almonds (other nuts and seeds have slightly less calcium)	240
Chickpeas	150
Onions	136
Eggs	131
Tofu (whole cow's milk has about the same quantity of calcium; tofu needs to be blended into other foods or cooked to make it more appealing)	128
Broccoli	123
Raw buckwheat	114
Wheat flour	93

Foods such as torula or brewer's yeast, seaweeds and parsley are rich in calcium but the quantities eaten are generally fairly insignificant. Nearly all foods have some calcium in them. If you are concerned, consult a health practitioner before taking calcium supplements because excess of one mineral may cause depletion of another.

Many soy milks have added calcium and consequently are a good source of this mineral. Check the label. Soy milk powders can be fortified with whey powder, carob, ground nuts or seeds. Soy milks commonly contain high (but not hazardous) levels of aluminium, so if possible use organic products.

CEREALS AND BREAD

Cereals are basically the seeds of grasses. Prior to 20 000 years ago, there was little use of grindstones, mortars-and-pestles and storage pits. Generally, most groups preferred plant foods other than cereals, presumably because grass seeds are fiddly to collect, hard to chew, difficult to digest, relatively unpalatable unless broken down and cooked and only available at certain times of the year.

However, grass seeds were quite important in the traditional diets of West Africans and some Australian Aborigines while the seeds of wild grasses were a major food of southwestern American Indians before European settlement.[5] Fifty-two species of wild grass have been identified as their traditional foods, seven of which were classed as staples. Rice grass was one of the most widely used. Although these grasses were never cultivated, canals were sometimes constructed to water areas of natural growth or seeds were thrown onto muddy soils. Even this century, Indians resorted to these seeds in spring when their stores were low and new crops not yet ready for harvest.

As grasses are amongst the earliest of plants it is obvious that their seeds would have been used and, when pressure was on, the grass itself was eaten. You can easily imagine that our ancestors would have noted that soaking grass seeds in water makes them soft and that the grassy tops of some species are quite sweet to eat.

You can test this for yourself. If you soak whole organic wheat grains overnight and keep them damp for a day or two they become sweet and 'chewy'. If you sow wheat grains in a tray of soil, they shoot up very rapidly and when the grass itself is about 8 cm high it is deliciously sweet and not too hard to chew or swallow. I chop it up like chives. Older grass is unpalatable and tough.

Cereal grains such as wheat, rice and corn have been major components of our diets since the development of agriculture 10 000 years ago. These hybridised plants possibly bear little relationship to the wide variety of grass seeds eaten by our ancestors and the latter would not have been used in anything like the quantities consumed today.

If we are genetically unsuited to eating enormous quantities of cultivated grains, then the development of roller mills in the nineteenth century, leading to refined grains, was even more detrimental. Most methods of improving the palatability of refined cereals also tend to be detrimental to our health, for example, adding sugar, salt and fats. I think the sensible solution is to eat a wide variety of grain-like foods – barley, oats, rye, buckwheat, millet, quinoa, amaranth and linseed meal – as well as a wide range of legumes and other starchy but unprocessed foods.

FRUIT

Freshly picked wild plant foods are a rich source of vitamin C. The Australian green plum, for example, contains over 3000 mg of vitamin C per 100 g. The current Australian Government Recommended Intake is 30 mg!

Use your imagination, and recipe books, to encourage the family to eat fruit by preparing it in bite-size pieces or mixing it with other foods. Here is a fruit 'ice cream' substitute.

*4 tablespoons plain, unsweetened yoghurt
or silken tofu*

*4 tablespoons mashed mango, peach, ripe
plum, paw paw or berries (for babies and
infants sieve berries – eating the skin
and seeds yourself!) or puréed, cooked
fruit such as apple and blackcurrant or
cooked, dried fruit*

1 ripe banana

Put yoghurt in freezer for about 1½ hours – until half-frozen. Refrigerate the fruit except banana.

Combine the half-frozen yoghurt with the refrigerated fruit and the ripe banana. Mash thoroughly or blend, then freeze for about 1½ hours. Then whisk with a fork or blend to break up any ice crystals. Return to the freezer until firm.

Alternatively, you can make this ice cream into a firm ice block, or simply blend the ingredients together to make a topping over, say, slices of pears or cold rice pudding. A rice pudding cooked with soy milk, a little almond meal and served with blended strawberries, banana and yoghurt is quite tasty and is a meal in itself for toddlers.

FATS

Fats and oils tend to make foods more palatable. A small quantity of fats is essential for human health.

Our earliest ancestors apparently had a fairly low fat intake as wild game contains about one-seventh the fat of modern farm animals. These ancient people scavenged for marrow-rich bones and cracked them open with stones. The limb bone of an adult wildebeest is a rich source of marrow, made up of 94 per cent fat and providing around 12 000 kilojoules of energy. In a number of ancient cultures, the fatty parts of animals were the most sought after.

This desire for fatty, dense foods would have been fairly difficult to satisfy in the wild, except by Eskimos. Nuts and witchetty grubs (in Australia) were also highly prized.

Today it's unfortunately too easy for us to get fats and oils. Instead of using them excessively in cooking, try adding herbs and spices for flavouring.

THE HUMAN 'SWEET TOOTH'

Paintings found in Spain dated 10 000–12 000 years ago show a woman climbing a tree to obtain honey. She is surrounded by bees. Pygmies in tropical rainforests and Nepalese mountain folk risk their lives to get honey. These are testimonies to the strength of the human sweet tooth and the natural difficulty of satisfying it. In the wild, sugar craving is hard to indulge.

Sugar is a 'natural part of life' but the refined product is new to human nutrition and particularly detrimental to some people. Eskimos, for example, once lived on a diet of fat and protein with very little carbohydrate. Their metabolic requirement for glucose came from protein. Sucrose in their present diet is thought to be responsible for the persistent diarrhoea and gastroenteritis that commonly occurs in Eskimo infants during the post-weaning period. Another example is diabetes among American Indians: it was non-existent until the recent introduction of dietary sucrose. In some areas, American Indians now have more than a 40 per cent incidence of diabetes. American Indians, like Australian Aborigines, evolved to cope with feast and famine times, plus plenty of physical activity, and they haven't been able to make the rapid change to a completely sedentary existence with a regular, over-supply of food. Their bodies become bulky and lazy, instead of thrifty and active.

In most western countries, up to 20 per cent of our kilojoules are derived from refined sugar. 'Sweet' should be a treat rather than a major part of our diet.

FIBRE

The estimated intake of fibre by our pre-agricultural ancestors is 130–150 g per day, most of it being soluble fibre from vegetables and fruit, which is considered to lower cholesterol levels. The average Australian intake is 20 g, most of which is unsoluble fibre from grains.

SEAFOOD

Surprisingly, analysis of remains around ancient living sites shows that aquatic foods – fish and shellfish – were not commonly eaten until about 25 000 years ago. This may partially explain why seafood often occurs on allergy lists.

Although fish is a highly recommended protein food, all our oceans are polluted in varying degrees. Seafood from coastal areas picks up industrial and domestic pollutants, large ocean fish accumulate toxins because they are at the end of the food chain and there is an ever-increasing use of preservatives. I suspect that some of the problems people have from eating fish are toxic rather than allergic.

SODIUM AND POTASSIUM

The figures speak for themselves.

| | Average daily intake (mg) | |
	Hunter-gatherers	Modern man
Sodium	700	2300–6900 (In northern Japan it may exceed 20 000)
Potassium	7000	1500–4600

DRINKS

After breastmilk, the ultimate health drink is water. Getting people to drink it is difficult. The most popular drinks for children are those containing sugars of various kinds and caffeine. So it's not surprising that as they get older they switch to alcohol and coffee – they are habituated to drinking things that give them a 'hit'. You don't even know what you're getting inside bottles of fizzy drinks as colas and similar products don't give full details on labels.

Fruit juices are a better alternative but they should be restricted. Here are some reasons.

• As a weaning food, fruit juice encourages a sweet tooth and may damage emerging teeth. If babies and infants are given juices they should be extremely diluted and not something to be sucked on constantly. Orange and pineapple juice, in particular, are too acidic for tiny and delicate stomachs. Sugar doesn't change the acidity but masks it.

• Juices are relatively expensive and wasteful. They contain very little fibre. The fibrous part of fruit is rich in protective substances such as bioflavonoids and pectin. Pectin, for example, absorbs toxins, helps lower cholesterol, soothes and protects the digestive tract.

• They are less 'filling' than whole fruit and contain more kilojoules. A medium orange has 290 kilojoules while a medium glass of orange juice has 305 kilojoules. Try chilled (not frozen) segments of thinly peeled oranges as a snack.

For those who refuse to drink water, try adding a few cubes of pure, frozen juice to water for flavouring, with a few thin slices of orange, perhaps topped with several sprigs of fresh mint leaves.

ALCOHOL

Of some fifty hunter-gatherer groups studied this century, none had 'invented' alcoholic drinks. Mead, a fermented drink made from honey, and other types of alcohol, were all introduced by outsiders.

It's not surprising that some of the remaining hunter-gathering societies apparently prefer the rigorous uncertainties on the marginal lands we have 'given back' to them rather than what we like to call 'civilisation'.

Nutrients in general

Stone-age diets would have provided an adequate intake of most nutrients. Exceptions include iodine deficiency in a few inland mountain areas.

The actual cuisine of our ancestors is somewhat speculative but we know that their larders were not stocked with any of the most popular items purchased today.

The biggest selling items in Australian supermarkets[6]

1	Coca-Cola, 375 ml
2	Coca-Cola, 1 litre
3	Coca-Cola, 2 litre
4	Diet Coke, 375 ml
5	Cherry Ripe
6	Nestlé's condensed milk
7	Tally Ho cigarette papers
8	Mars Bar
9	Kit-Kat
10	Crunchie Bar
11	Eta 5-Star margarine, salt-reduced
12	Heinz baked beans
13	Double-Circle canned beetroot
14	Diet Coke, 1 litre
15	Bushell's tea
16	Cadbury's Dairy Milk chocolate
17	Pepsi Cola, 375 ml
18	Coca-Cola, 1.5 litre
19	Kellogg's Corn flakes
20	Maggi two-minute chicken noodles
21	Generic brand lemon drink
22	Panadol tablets, 24-pack
23	Meadow Lea margarine
24	Generic brand lemonade
25	Mrs MacGregor's margarine

Dr W. A. Price, in *Nutrition and Physical Degeneration*, describes how many 'primitive races' share our health problems when they adopt our conception of nutrition. He describes a traditional-living Eskimo woman who had twenty-six children and no dental caries; her husband could carry 45 kg in each hand and 45 kg in his teeth for a considerable distance.

Although people today are generally not as hardy, human bodies have changed very little over the last few million years and we are genetically poorly equipped to handle the lifestyle we have developed: children munching on lollies as they watch television; women striving to work long hours on low-kilojoule diets with high expectations regarding personal appearance; people battling for hours a day in congested transport systems, then sitting at work for long periods of time; constant availability of taste treats; increasing levels of atmospheric and food chemicals and so on.

Of course, it is only in the last century that the majority of people have been assured of a regular and varied food supply. Farming, manufacturing and technology have given us this benefit.

You might have romantic notions about the great bison herds that took two days to pass by and flocks of birds literally darkening the sky. However, they are now too many people on the planet for us to revert to hunting and gathering, as this requires something like 2 square kilometres of fertile land per person. However, after around 2 500 000 years of human existence, you'd think that we would have worked out a healthier way of feeding ourselves than our present diet.

VEGETARIANISM

According to scientific researchers, very few groups of pre-agricultural people were completely vegetarian. However, the range of nutrients in plant foods may be more in harmony with our genetic design than most of the animal foods people eat today.

The first international congress on vegetarian nutrition was held in the USA in 1987, the papers being published in the *American Journal of Clinical Nutrition*.[7] There is plenty of evidence showing that vegetarians have less obesity, atonic constipation, lung cancer, alcoholism, hypertension, coronary artery disease and type II diabetes than omnivorous eaters. There is also evidence that vegetarians have less breast cancer, diverticular disease, colon cancer, calcium kidney stones, gallstones, osteoporosis, dental erosion and dental caries. There are, additionally, sound global economic, environmental and ethical reasons for vegetarianism.

Healthy vegetarian nutrition is bulky and satisfying (once you get used to it!). It is not healthy to eat a standard Australian diet and simply omit the meat. I suggest you make dietary changes slowly. It takes time to learn about new foods and your digestive system has to make adjustments.

Your individual biochemical system also has to adapt. For example, when you eat meat, your body has a good iron supply but without meat your biochemistry takes a while to learn to be more thrifty. Protein should not be a problem but I generally recommend eating a variety of plant foods that are rich in protein as well as following food-combining principles. *Diet for a Small Planet* by Frances Moore Lappé is one of the best books for explaining how to use food combining to get complete protein meals.

With the exception of restrictive vegan regimes (no dairy foods or eggs), most vegetarian diets meet the requirements for childhood growth, development and disease prevention.

Vitamin B12 may be a problem for vegans and some vegetarians. Aside from tiny amounts in dairy foods and eggs, there are only a few plant foods that contain this essential vitamin: tempeh (a soy bean fermented product), mushrooms and possibly some seaweeds such as wakame, kombu and arame. However, my experience is that there's a limit to how much of these you can eat. Miso may also provide a little but is high in salt.

You may be able to store up to twenty years' supply of vitamin B12 in your body. The mystery is that some people are vegans all their lives and never show any signs of vitamin B12 deficiency. Do they cheat a little by having an occasional meat treat? Since this vitamin is produced in all our intestines, perhaps a thrifty body is able to re-cycle and absorb it? Perhaps some individuals can convert the B12 analogues in plant foods or metabolise their own in some way? Vegans who are healthy and energetic need not worry but I recommend routine supplementation for pregnant and lactating vegans and for vegan children.

For many people it's easier, and probably just as healthy, to include fish and small amounts of lean meat in the diet, using a wide variety of beans, grains, lentils, chickpeas and similar foods as meat extenders.

WEIGHT REDUCTION

There's no such thing as a magic diet, that is, one that will satisfy everyone's needs and allow one to be reed-slim without effort. A number of tables and theories exist which set out how many kilojoules you can eat and still maintain your ideal weight, but after some years of self-experimentation and clinical experience, I know that such systems apply only to some people. Trying to eat a little when you love eating is like trying to sleep if you are an insomniac; the harder you try the worse the problem becomes.

People inherit different genes and have different metabolisms, which means that they utilise nutrients somewhat differently. Aside from philosophical considerations, your primary aim should be to reach your optimal health. However, in the real world, physical appearance is important for most of us. It attracts mates, helps you get work, brings prestige and so on. Here, therefore, are some guidelines to help you lose weight.

TWENTY-EIGHT TIPS FOR WEIGHT LOSS

1   Exercise is probably more important than dieting. If you exercise sufficiently, you should be able to eat as much as you like (not necessarily what you like). In my experience, it is not sufficient to go for a brisk walk, slow jog or similar, for twenty minutes three or four times a week *if* you are sedentary the rest of the time. You probably need something like fifteen hours of physical activity per week, but it doesn't have to be athletic workouts. Reasonably energetic housework (not light dusting), gardening and similar household activities keep your joints mobile and burn up kilojoules. Bush-walking is an ideal weekend activity for office workers.

2   There are foods you can eat in almost any quantity, so consider them as snacks or part of a meal.

1 cup of the following contains 170 kilojoules or less:

alfalfa and bean sprouts	lettuce
	mushrooms
brussels sprouts	onions
cabbage	parsley
carrots	radishes
celery	spinach
cucumber	squash
green string beans	silver beet
	zucchini
leeks	

The following also contain about 170 kilojoules:

1 small apple	1 kiwi fruit
2 apricots	1 nectarine
¾ cup strawberries	1 small orange
	1 peach
½ grapefruit	

There are also a number of different types of low-kilojoule, wholegrain biscuits on the market. Read the labels carefully.

3   When you are on a lowish kilojoule eating programme, it is especially important to make every mouthful nutrient-rich. Each day you should eat vegetables, fruit, cereals/starches and protein but minimal fats, refined sugars and salt.

4   My main recommendation is: **get to love vegetables and eat a wide variety of them.** Eat at least five cups of vegetables a day. Why vegetables? Almost everyone agrees that they're good for you. They're relatively high in potassium, which may be beneficial if you tend to retain fluid. Starchy vegetables such as peas, potatoes and corn are somewhat higher in kilojoules than others but they are filling, provide energy and are less fattening than foods such as cake, chocolate, pizza and Cheezals. When I'm hungry, I grill a couple of thinly sliced potatoes, using less than a teaspoon of oil, and flavour them with low-salt tamari or shoyu.

• Learn how to make vegetables more appealing without adding unnecessary kilojoules. Use low-fat salad dressings, lots of herbs, seasonings such as chilli, ginger and curry.

• Make snacks and entrées comprising raw, sliced vegetables sprinkled with herbs and lemon juice. Keep them in the fridge so you always have something healthy to nibble.

• Although raw vegetables are generally healthier and give more oral satisfaction than cooked, some are notoriously difficult to digest. Broccoli, cauliflower and green beans are much better slightly cooked. Left-overs may be used cold in salads.

• Vegetable soup makes an excellent low-kilojoule snack in the winter.

• Lightly steamed vegetables with added herbs, and soya cheese grated on top and grilled, makes a tasty, quick meal.

• Start stir-fried vegetables in a teaspoon of oil, with some grated ginger root or mustard seeds, then lightly cook some onion before adding the rest of the vegetables and a little water.

• Thicken casseroles with bean sprouts.

5   Don't skip meals. Always have breakfast or at least a large early morning snack. Your brain uses energy while you sleep. Your metabolism also needs an energy boost.

6   Avoid eating most of your kilojoules late at night. It should be the other way around.

7   No fruit juices. These are low in fibre but relatively high in kilojoules and sugar. The pectin and other fibre in fruit is of great benefit to your gastrointestinal system and this is reduced or lost when you juice fruit. Whole fruit is better for you, is more filling, contains more nutrients and is less fattening. Losing weight is more successful if you fill up on vegetables rather than fruit so I usually suggest a maximum of four pieces of fruit per day.

8   Except for an occasional treat, don't eat any refined foods.

9   Artificial sweeteners are best avoided. There are many reports of adverse effects, suspected carcinogenic action and dubious benefits.

10 Allow yourself a daily treat, not necessarily something sweet. If you like alcohol have an occasional glass of wine; other treats might be a small handful of nuts or some tasty cheese. Aside from food, what alternatives are there to reward or console yourself?

11 It's usually better for weight loss not to snack between meals because if you eat

something between meals this doesn't necessarily make you less hungry three hours later. However, if you become very hungry you rarely make good food choices because your body wants a 'quick hit'. Always have low-kilojoule snacks nearby in case they're needed, i.e. fresh fruit, bite-sized vegies, soup, low-kilojoule biscuits or low-fat yoghurt.

12 My weight-loss programmes always include three main meals with a small serving of some form of low-fat protein with each meal, for example:
• a grain with fat-reduced soy milk for breakfast
• egg, fish, tempeh or cottage cheese for lunch
• grilled meat, beans/legumes or soya cheese for dinner.

13 Diets that give you meals in packets are no good because they don't teach you about shopping or buying different types of foods and they often reduce 'normal socialising'.

14 Don't add salt to food or eat obviously salty foods, except for the occasional treat. Use alternative seasonings or a little salt-reduced soy sauce such as tamari and shoyu.

15 Avoid alcohol. One drink contains around 500 kilojoules without contributing any protein, vitamins and minerals. You could have a few glasses a week as part of your 'treat package'.

16 Reduce to a minimum all obviously fatty foods. If you're really serious, use only 1–2 teaspoons of oil or butter per day. All oils, butter and margarine have a similar kilojoule count – about 145 kilojoules in each teaspoon. It takes a long time to lose your taste for butter, cream and oily foods. Fats are, unfortunately, satisfying to the taste buds and give a feeling of fullness, but, like many of our

primordial instincts, a degree of control is required. Next time you're in a large shopping centre, have a look around. In 99 per cent of cases, it's the overweight folk who are munching on things like chips and ice cream as they stroll or loll around.

17 Cereals should be unsweetened and have no added nuts, coconut, salt, fat and only a little dried fruit.

Wholegrain cereals such as two Weetbix or ⅔ cup cooked oats contain about the same quantity of kilojoules as a rasher of grilled bacon. Cereals provide energy and warmth and should be part of your diet.

18 If you try to avoid starchy foods altogether you will probably get food cravings. Most wholegrain breads contain about 290 kilojoules per slice so you can see that two slices of bread per day are not going to increase weight. It is the spreads and fillings that contribute the high kilojoules. Choose from a variety of grains, as mentioned in various chapters in this book. You might like to make your own damper bread with barley and millet flour, or have buckwheat pancakes.

In vegetable salads or curried vegetables, include about ½ cup brown rice or lentils to make the meal more filling.

19 Grilled low-fat meat and fish, other than shellfish, are suggestions for weight watchers.

For vegetarians, low-fat cottage cheese, tofu, eggs and combinations of grains, beans and legumes are suggested. Nuts and seeds are good sources of protein but, unfortunately, they are expensive and very fattening, as mentioned earlier. Buckwheat may be substituted for nuts in biscuit recipes.

I rarely restrict eggs as they are such a valuable source of nutrients, although meat-eaters with cholesterol and cardiac problems might be advised to use the whites only. My advice to vegetarians is to eat 3–4 eggs per week.

Recommended protein intake is becoming somewhat lower each year and many international experts are now talking of a 'safe level of protein intake' without being able to set upper limits. The Australian Government Recommended Intake is 45 g per day for an adult female and 55 g for males. It's very easy to get these levels – even for vegetarians.

20 You should include beans and other legumes in your daily diet. Half a cup of cooked beans contains about 380 kilojoules. For example, use split peas in soups, savoury rice with lentils, chickpeas with curried vegetables and Mexican-style dishes. These foods are high in nutrients including protein and fibre, low in fat and very cheap. I always suggest cooking legumes much longer than indicated in most recipe books. If you add chilli, it improves the taste and helps with absorption. Try combining kidney beans with brown rice, or rice with soya grits. These types of foods can be used as meat substitutes, and also instead of nuts in nut loaves, etc.

21 If you're lowering your food intake, it's important to ensure that your metabolic rate (energy) does not decrease. You may need to revise your eating plan or take one of the supplements suggested later in this chapter. Being tired, cold and cranky are indicators of low metabolism. Warm drinks and soups seem more filling than cold foods.

22 Some people don't realise how much they are eating. For seven days, make a list of everything you eat and how much exercise you get. You may be able to see for yourself where adjustments need to be made. If you make your list on the left-hand side of each page, you could make your own suggestions opposite each item that needs improving. Alternatively, take the list to a health practitioner.

23 **One of the worst things you can do is dislike yourself because you've broken some of the health rules. You break these sorts of rules because you're a normal human being. Don't use this as an excuse for giving up exercise and healthy food.**

24 Use all the help you can get. Relaxation and meditation techniques help some people to make lifestyle changes. Give yourself other rewards – music, clothes, exotic fruit, perfume, good books and good company.

25 Weigh yourself only once a week – or not at all. If you're overweight you'll feel more comfortable when the programme starts to work.

26 Be patient with yourself. It takes time to change your habits. Most people tend to think that **their** habits are okay. If you're overweight, there's every possibility that the way you've been eating and your lifestyle doesn't suit you. Increasing your energy may be a better way to focus to start with.

27 I don't recommend that you weigh foods or attempt to count every kilojoule but you need to know, approximately, what your kilojoule intake is. For example, I had a patient who regularly snacked on nuts but didn't realise that a cup of unsalted nuts is around 3000 kilojoules. You may need to buy a book such as *Nutrition Almanac* or *The Australian Calorie Counter*. With practice, you will get to know the approximate kilojoule values of foods without having to check.

28 I also suggest that you buy or borrow

some low-fat recipe books to get ideas on making food substitutions. For example, instead of butter or sugary jams on bread or toast, you can use tomato and grilled soya cheese, savoury lentils, mashed banana or your own jam recipe:

1 cup dried apricots
1 cup apple juice
a few sultanas

Simmer together in a saucepan, uncovered, for about 15–20 minutes. Cool, then blend or mash.

WHY MOST DIETS DON'T WORK

1 They may be too restrictive and nutritional essentials are not being met, with the result that you don't function optimally.
2 Taste buds and social needs are not satisfied.
3 As a general rule, when you lose, say 5 kg, you are losing:
1 kg water
2 kg muscle
2 kg fat.
When you put on weight again, you gain:
1 kg water
1 kg muscle
3 kg fat.
When you lose weight very rapidly, you are losing protein and water. When you lose protein, you are losing cells. When you lose excess cells, you start to compromise intestinal and immune functioning.
4 Low-kilojoule diets need careful planning to provide adequate protein to avoid muscle loss and other health problems.
5 Low energy and low carbohydrate diets lower your metabolism so that

ultimately you are eating less simply to maintain your current weight.
6 Mono diets and fasting are not recommended for weight loss for the above reasons; they also tend to increase the incidence of food sensitivities.

In other words, unless slimming diets are carefully planned to give appropriate and sufficient nutrients, they can be guaranteed to make you fat for life.

There is some evidence that obesity is genetic. Even in the absence of a metabolic disorder, certain people have a tendency to store energy as fat tissue and this has been confirmed by studies of identical twins who have been reared apart.[8] In other words, it's extremely difficult for some people to lose weight, while others simply need to cut out a little food and marginally increase physical activity. Of course, we may take on our parents' lifestyle habits as well as their genes.

SUPPLEMENTS

On a lowish kilojoule diet, it is wise to take a combined multi-vitamin and mineral supplement.

If you are hungry all the time, eat a snack of vegetables or fruit and drink one or two glasses of water plus Spirulina. (Spirulina is derived from freshwater algae and acts as an appetite suppressant for some people. It is rich in essential nutients but, like seaweeds, it has natural tendency to pick up heavy metals such as arsenic. If you're worried about possible heavy metal contamination ask your supplier about the levels of contamination or buy an organic product.) My experience with natural appetite suppressants is that their effects tend to wear off after a few months, so have periodic breaks or use a different product.

FOR FATIGUE
• *Zell oxygen* • *Kelp tablets* – not the powder • *Ginseng*
FOR FLUID RETENTION
• *Celery seed tablets* or *extract* • *Dandelion*
TO BOOST METABOLISM
• Hot *chilli* – in food (to taste) or 2 capsules per day • *Turmeric* – 1 teaspoon per day
OTHER
To maintain very efficient protein utilis-ation, I recommend a dessertspoon of *protein powder* with breakfast – especially for vegetarians. The supplement I use is hydrolysed lactalbumin and rice protein concentrate. It can be sprinkled on cereal or blended with fruit, water, low-fat soy milk and a little rice bran. This makes a filling, low-kilojoule meal.

BEING THE RIGHT WEIGHT

We're all different, but in modern, devel-oped societies, it's unfortunate if you happen to be a large person with a rela-tively slow metabolism.

Only about 5 per cent of the popula-tion seem to conform, naturally, to the so-called physical ideal. No amount of dieting, exercising, cosmetic surgery, laser treatment, daily trips to the beautician or 'miracle creams' will turn an average person into 'model of the year'.

On the other hand, it isn't sensible to simply say, 'What the hell, like me as I am' and spend your days lolling around looking at television, stuffing yourself with food and drinking heaps of alcohol.

Most people don't need scales, a chart or a practitioner to tell them they're over-weight. They simply feel uncomfortable and, worst of all, they're usually tired. Because you put on weight relatively slowly, you don't appreciate what a drain it is on your energy. I usually illustrate this by giving the patient a bag of pota-toes to hold and telling them to imagine they have to carry it all day. Your excess bodyweight is not as obvious as a bag of potatoes but just as burdensome. You should also be aware of the risks of obesity – increased susceptibility to heart problems, diabetes and so on.

Being underweight or having signifi-cant fluctuations in weight is also risky. An American survey of 4710 people found that low body weight was associ-ated with a high death rate, except for females between the ages of 55–64 years of age. Another study of 2107 men found that the risk of death from all causes was lowest in the group with no weight change. Death from heart disease was 26 per cent higher in those who gained or lost weight significantly over a twenty-five-year period. One researcher has stated that constant fluctuations in body weight may be more hazardous than smoking cigarettes.[9] Very thin females have a higher incidence of osteoporosis and they're not as cuddly.

This is just a brief guide to sensible dieting; it is worth repeating that any diet that does not cover a wide range of foods and that does not provide you with plenty of energy is not worthwhile.

I know some adult females who weigh less than 50 kg but who are not taut and trim. You can be slim and still have a poor ratio of fat to muscle. Others are firm and shapely, and usually less wrin-kled than the rest of us, even though they may be somewhat heavier than average.

The question is: do **you** really want or need to lose weight? With food, as many other things, you have to find the path between senseless austerity, unreasonable vanity and harmful self-indulgence.

CHAPTER 16

RECOMMENDED HERBS

The long history of herbs has proved their value in restoring health, with very few side-effects and without being habit-forming. Scientific research over the last century has confirmed many ancient beliefs about the medicinal value of herbs.

Over the years I have collected thousands of research papers relating to herbs, as well as doing a three-year, full-time training course, attending post-grad-uate seminars and running a clinic.

The herbs listed in this chapter are those I consider to be safe for the general public to use and I have tried to keep the information concise and clear. In spite of objections by practitioners, self treatment is the most common of all therapies, but if your symptoms do not 'go away' then you should visit a qualified person so that a joint effort can be made to find and treat the underlying problem.

Safety of herbs

In all my research I have not found one clear case of toxicity from taking common herbal teas; that is not to say that there are not instances of allergic reaction, because certain individuals can be highly sensitive to plants, including some of the common foods. It is inter-esting to note that some of the criticisms of herbs over the last 10–15 years cite the same cases again and again, for example, where a thirty-five-year-old woman suf-fered a serious shock reaction after drink-ing chamomile tea. In Europe, in particular, millions of people drink cham-omile tea and it would be surprising if there were not some cases of allergic reac-tion. The other possibility is that the tea may have been made from one of the many little daisy flowers that resemble chamomile but which are not edible. Another often-cited case is where an elderly couple consumed foxglove leaves thinking they were comfrey.

The authors of many of the articles criticising herbs have never used them and are so biased that the examples they cite, such as hemlock and deadly nightshade, are simply poisonous plants rather than medicinal herbs. Then there is the question of dosage. It may be that a particular herb has a recommended dose, based on centuries of use, of around 2 ml three times a day. Of course 100 ml could be harmful, but this does not mean the usual dosage is dangerous.

The scientific approach is to isolate and synthesise the active principle from plants and this is how drugs such as digoxin, which is a component of the foxglove plant, were derived. The basic problem of these 'herbal critics' is that much of their information is founded on one isolated component of a plant rather than all of the constituents. When you consider, for example, that a particular alkaloid is only one of hundreds of constituents in a plant and that it is usually less than 1 per cent of the total plant, you will appreciate that the whole plant, as used in herbal medicine, does not have the same type of result as a single constituent.

To illustrate this, ephedrine, extracted from the plant *Ephedra sinica*, will increase blood pressure if prescribed as a drug, but in the whole plant there are other alkaloids which prevent a rise in blood pressure.

In fact there are nutritive, therapeutically active and naturally occurring toxins in all the foods we eat, so if one were to ban all those foods which had specific known toxins, then we would have to eliminate almost everything from our diet except simple foods such as refined sugar. Some of our foods contain similar groups of compounds to poisonous plants and specific parts of some edible plants may be very toxic. The common potato is a good illustration of this because it is in the Solanaceae (nightshade) family; although deadly nightshade is poisonous it does not follow that potatoes are, although people should not eat those that are green and sprouting. If one were going to test the level of alkaloids in potatoes to establish a harmful quantity, it wouldn't make sense to test the leaves and then declare that all potatoes are poisonous.

This is exactly the type of 'evidence' that was used to condemn comfrey. I have made a particular study of comfrey over many years and followed up some reports of poisoning. There is not one case of comfrey harming any human from the reports I have investigated, and this has been verified by liver tests on forty long-term users of comfrey, some of them having eaten comfrey leaves every day for over twenty years.

In some instances comfrey was blamed when another plant had been used by mistake. In one case – that of a man whose death was attributed to comfrey which was widely reported in the press – not one person apart from myself visited the community where the person had lived to find out what he had been eating. The death was certainly not due to comfrey as it wasn't growing there at the time, and Statutory Declarations by the people he was living with completely refute the possibility of comfrey causing the problem. It really is a case of 'a herb in search of a victim'. I am not advocating the regular eating of comfrey leaves and suggest that people eat a variety of foods. Comfrey is hardly a popular food and only small quantities are used in herbal remedies; further, it has known healing properties – that's why one of its constituents is used by pharmaceutical companies. For a herbalist, there's no plant that can replace comfrey. It is also an excellent garden mulch and useful as animal fodder.

In any event, the discussion of comfrey is now somewhat belated, as the Australian government has classified products for internal use made from dried comfrey as poisonous, although fresh leaves have a much higher alkaloid content. Peanuts and comfrey probably have equally toxic components. Why is comfrey on the Poisons Schedule but not peanuts? Who knows. Perhaps scientists and government officials enjoy eating peanuts, in spite of their liver-damaging aflatoxins, whereas to them comfrey is weird. Perhaps the government doesn't want to put the peanut industry out of business? Perhaps the peanut lobby is stronger than the herbal lobby?

Another criticism made is that herbal remedies are not 'standard'. This is quite true, because all plants' constituents vary depending on where they are grown, the season, soil fertility and so on. That is why professional herbalists use a conservative dose within a specified range.

The most sensible argument for herbalism is that the results have been verified by hundreds of years' experience, which is far more important than studies in laboratories, or on animals that do not metabolise and excrete substances in the same way as humans.

It is interesting that some of the early herbalists related their therapies to the 'vital force'. In the last few years Kirlian photography, biophysics and electromagnetic field experiments have given some respectability to the notion that plants,

animals and people may indeed have a life force, or a subtle energy system, that plays an important role in our wellbeing. In other words, some herbalists believe that plants possess an energising or healing factor that cannot be scientifically determined.

Herbal remedies

Throughout the book I have given a fairly wide range of herbal remedies for each health problem. Not all of them will be in your local stores or nurseries and some will be included within capsulated or tablet combinations. The aim of this chapter is to give you some details to help you choose remedies that are most likely to be beneficial in your particular case, bearing in mind that your main health problem is probably associated with other difficulties.

NOTE *Very few herbs are recommended during pregnancy, although they have considerably fewer adverse effects than pharmaceuticals. If you require help while pregnant it is better to see a professional herbalist than self treat.*

No two plant species are alike, and each contains hundreds of different components. You would expect that every herb would be capable of producing a range of different effects, and this is so, which is why the same herb can be used to treat widely differing ailments.

Some of the herbs on my recommended list are available to the public only as part of commercial mixtures and combinations. My clinical experience is that an appropriate herbal combination formula usually gives a better therapeutic result than a single remedy, even though the total dose is the same in both cases. Don't be afraid to use a commercial combination remedy as long as some of the herbs in it relate to your particular problem. The disadvantage of a formula is that if you have an allergic reaction you won't know which herb caused it.

Herbal remedies are becoming increasingly available in pharmacies and health-food stores. Tablets, capsules and fluids may be in varying strengths. The dosages I have given are based on traditional manufacturing methods. The best advice is to follow the instructions on the label.

HERBS

Agrimony *(Agrimonia eupatoria)*
CULTIVATION
Grows well in Australia.
PART USED
Above-ground parts.
THERAPEUTIC USE
Helpful for a number of gastro-intestinal problems such as weak digestion, intestinal inflammation and diarrhoea. Used by many herbalists for sluggish liver, gall-bladder and urinary problems.
HOW IT IS USED
Infusions and herbal extracts.
DOSE
Infusion: 50 ml three times a day (or one cup of the weak tea sipped before meals). Herbal extract: 2 ml three times daily.

Alfalfa *(Medicago sativa)*
Also known as lucerne.
CULTIVATION
Commonly grown.
PART USED
Seeds, or above-ground parts.

THERAPEUTIC USE
Alkalising effect, which makes it useful for digestive problems such as gastritis and ulcers, and for bladder irritations. It is rich in vitamins and minerals and is a support treatment for arthritis, high cholesterol and high triglyceride levels in blood and atherosclerosis. It has nutritive and oestrogenic properties. It may help increase the flow of breast milk and decrease menopausal flushing.
HOW IT IS USED
Herbal extract, infusion, tablets, sprouted seeds. A decoction of the seeds is also recommended.
DOSE
Extract: 5 ml three times daily.
Infusion: may be drunk freely. As it is not very palatable as a tea, it is suggested that when used in this way it can be combined with peppermint or caraway.
Sprouts: 1 cup daily for menopausal-age women.
Decoction of seeds: 20 g to 500 ml water. This amount to be drunk daily. Can be flavoured with other herbs, lemon or taken cold with fruit juice. This strong dose is not meant for long-term use.

CAUTIONS **Never use agricultural (crop) seeds for teas, sprouts or decoctions as these have been treated with fungicides and other chemicals.**

Alfalfa contains weak plant oestrogens so may be inappropriate in very large doses in some cases.

It has been reported that alfalfa (and legumes) contain a constituent that may aggravate SLE and rheumatoid arthritis.

Aloe *(Aloe vera)*

CULTIVATION

Grows well in Australia except in heavy rainfall and very cold regions. Aloe likes to grow in light soils and is a good container plant.

PART USED

The gel inside the leaves (the lower, mature leaves are more therapeutic than young leaves). Also juice. You can either buy a commercial juice or blend the freshly harvested gel from inside the leaves.

THERAPEUTIC USE

Helpful externally in nearly all skin conditions, especially wounds, scalds and household burns. Internally has helped a number of chronic conditions, including gastro-intestinal weakness and irritation. Large doses have a laxative effect.

HOW IT IS USED

Taken internally: the pure gel is suggested for a range of conditions such as irritable bowel syndrome, dyspepsia, arthritis and allergies.

Applied externally: the gel or internal part of the fresh leaves is very useful for cracked lips, sores, fungal infections, sunburn, sore gums, scarring and many skin problems.

The juice makes an effective mouth wash for ulcers and may be used as nasal drops for blocked or inflamed noses, but it needs to be diluted in tepid, slightly salty water.

NOTE **The therapeutic effect of fresh gel lasts only a few days after harvesting. Commercial products are stabilised.**

DOSE

Gel products internally: start with 2 teaspoons twice daily in unsweetened fruit or vegetable juice. Build up to 25 ml twice daily, reducing the dose if the stools become loose. Treatment is generally long term, i.e. for months.

Angelica *(Angelica archangelica)*

CULTIVATION

Grows well in Australia (a tall, attractive plant). In warm climates, filtered sun is best.

PART USED

Leaf, stem and root.

THERAPEUTIC USE

Used mainly as a culinary and digestive aid; also for coughs and other bronchial conditions, including tightness of the chest.

Some herbalists recommend it as a circulatory tonic, for psoriasis and other skin problems. Angelica relaxes smooth muscles, i.e. in blood vessels and mucous membranes (the body's linings), which explains its suitability as support treatment for angina and hypertension.

The Asian variety of angelica (dong quai) is best prescribed in formulas for menstrual problems, especially period pain. It also contains plant oestrogens.

HOW IT IS USED

The fresh or dried leaves are used externally as a poultice or compress; or internally as an infusion. The young stems are used as a decoction or cooked with apple or rhubarb. Some people chop a little of the fine stems into salads. The root is used as a decoction, which can be taken with warm apple juice and a little cinnamon or cloves. It has an unusual and pleasant aroma.

CAUTION **Large quantities can affect blood sugar levels.**

DOSE
Infusion or decoction: 30 ml three times daily.
Extract or tincture: 2 ml three times daily.

Aniseed *(Pimpinella anisum)*
CULTIVATION
Will grow in Australia. (Not to be confused with Chinese or star aniseed which is also used therapeutically.)
PART USED
Seeds. The above-ground parts can also be used in salads and cooking.
THERAPEUTIC USE
An excellent anti-flatulent; also helpful in coughs and colds. Helpful at menopause and to increase the flow of breast milk, because it contains weak plant oestrogens.

The infusion, or a few drops of aniseed oil in water, may be used as a mouthwash or gargle.

CAUTION **Aniseed oil is toxic internally in large doses. Not recommended internally for young children and babies. For adults maximum use two or three drops three times daily for three weeks.**

HOW IT IS USED
Infusion of the crushed or powdered seeds.

In cooking, put 1 teaspoon crushed seeds inside a tea ball. If you place the filled ball in the food you are cooking you will get the flavour without the bits of seeds. You can use this procedure for all herbs that are not finely powdered. If you grow aniseed, you can use the chopped stems and leaves in salads and cooked meals.
DOSE
Infusion: 1 teaspoon crushed seeds to a cup of hot water. For small children and babies this should be further diluted and taken in small doses as required.

Arnica *(Arnica montana)*
CULTIVATION
Not commonly grown in Australia.
PART USED
Flowers.
THERAPEUTIC USE
A useful external agent for speeding up the healing of bruises, sprains and swelling after injury.
HOW IT IS USED
Ointment, diluted herbal extract.
DOSE
Not to be taken internally in herbal form; however, arnica is a common homoeopathic remedy.
Extract: 1 part extract to 20 parts water, used as compress.

CAUTIONS **Not to be applied on broken skin.**

Not to be used internally.

Arrowroot *(Maranta arundinacea)*
CULTIVATION
Will grow in Australia.
PART USED
Starch from the rhizome (underground parts).
THERAPEUTIC USE
Nourishing and soothing to the digestive system.
DOSE
1 tablespoon mixed to a paste with cold water, then add 500 ml liquid – apple or pear juice, soy milk, rice or barley water. Drink the 500 ml throughout the day during periods of convalescence or digestive upsets.

Barberry bark *(Berberis vulgaris)*

CULTIVATION
Not commonly grown in Australia.

PART USED
Bark from root and stem.

THERAPEUTIC USE
A digestive and organ tonic, especially to the liver, gallbladder and kidneys. Often recommended for constipation, skin eruptions and infections. It has antibacterial and antiprotozoal actions so may be useful for treating chronic infections such as diarrhoea.

HOW IT IS USED
Extracts, tincture, tablet complexes, decoction – very bitter.

DOSE
Extract and tincture: 2 ml three times daily.
Decoction: 50 ml three times daily (the bitter taste must be disguised).

Basil, holy or sacred *(Ocimum sanctum)*

CULTIVATION
A perennial that grows all year round in warm climates.

PART USED
Leaves.

THERAPEUTIC USE
A traditional tonic as well as a remedy for nausea, cough and fever. Recent studies show that it enhances the immune system.

DOSE
As Sweet Basil, below.

Basil, sweet *(Ocimum basilicum)*

CULTIVATION
The common culinary herb. An annual, growing only in the warm seasons.

PART USED
Leaves.

THERAPEUTIC USE
Colic, poor digestion, flatulence, nausea, fatigue, insomnia, anxiety, headaches and coughs. The fresh juice can be used as drops for inflammatory ear conditions and as a mouth freshener, or for treating thrush.

HOW IT IS USED
All varieties of basil may be used freely in cooking and salads. Also juice.

DOSE
A medicinal tea can be made from both varieties of basil using a small handful chopped fresh leaves to about 1 litre water. This would represent the quantity to be taken in one day. For dried leaves use 1 dessertspoon of the herb. Dried basil leaves won't be therapeutic unless they have retained their colour and characteristic odour – this applies to all herbs.

Bayberry *(Myrica cerifera)*

CULTIVATION
Bayberry is not commonly grown in Australia.

PART USED
Bark of the root.

THERAPEUTIC USE
An astringent and general circulatory tonic. Commonly recommended for colitis, diarrhoea and for problems related to excess mucus, such as congested throats.

NOTE **Astringents are drying, excessive use can irritate.**

I recommend adding glycerine to all herbal gargles.

HOW IT IS USED
Extract, decoction.

DOSE

Extract: 20 drops three times daily.
Decoction: 30 ml three times daily – as a tea or gargle.

Bergamot (Oswego tea/ beebalm) *(Monarda didyma)*

CULTIVATION

Some varieties cultivated as ornamentals for their colour and aroma (one of the mint family).

PART USED

Above-ground parts.

THERAPEUTIC USE

Mainly used as a tea for stimulating the digestion and for menstrual pain. Helpful for flatulence, nausea and also as a diuretic and kidney stimulant.

HOW IT IS USED

As a tea and small amounts of leaves in salads. Bergamot is used to flavour Earl Grey tea.

DOSE

Infusion: 1–2 teaspoons per cup.

Bilberry *(Vaccinium myrtillus)*

CULTIVATION

Grown in Australia but, like many berries, it needs cold winters to bear fruit.

PART USED

Ripe berries.

THERAPEUTIC USE

Recommended for the prevention and treatment of eye disorders, for strengthening weak blood vessels and as support therapy in urinary tract infections. Bilberry should benefit inflamed joint problems and conditions such as weak gums because it stabilises collagen (connective tissue). It also helps prevent blood stickiness and is suggested as part of the treatment of cardiovascular disorders. One

study has shown that it relieves painful periods.

HOW IT IS USED

Extract, fruit.

DOSE

Fluid extracts are usually prescribed at around 5 ml per day. Ripe berries can be eaten freely except that excessive quantities may cause gastric upsets. All blue–purple berries, including cranberries and blueberries, are particularly rich in flavonoids and carotenoids. They function as antioxidants and are good for the eyes, blood vessels and urinary tract.

Black cohosh *(Cimicifuga racemosa)*

CULTIVATION

Not commonly grown in Australia.

PART USED

Underground parts.

THERAPEUTIC USE

Traditionally prescribed for rheumatic complaints because of the salicylic acid content. Generally classed as a uterine tonic and used to treat painful periods – particularly if associated with agitation. It reduces blood pressure in some cases and can be effective for menopausal flushing.

HOW IT IS USED

Extract, tincture, tablets.

DOSE

Extract and tincture: 1 ml three times daily.

Boneset *(Eupatorium perfoliatum)*

CULTIVATION

Not commonly grown in Australia.

PART USED

Above-ground parts.

THERAPEUTIC USE

Traditionally used for body aches and pains, especially those affecting the bones.

Useful in respiratory problems and particularly recommended during influenza.

HOW IT IS USED
Infusion, tincture.

DOSE
Infusion: 30 ml three times daily.
Tincture: 2 ml three times daily.

Burdock *(Arctium lappa)*

CULTIVATION
Grows readily in Australia.

PART USED
Underground parts (the leaves can also be used for poultices).

THERAPEUTIC USE
A 'blood cleanser' and diuretic, particularly recommended for skin problems. Also a gentle stimulant to the stomach and gallbladder, with mild antibacterial properties. Helpful for fluid retention.

HOW IT IS USED
Herbalists generally use extracts or tinctures. Sometimes included in tablet combinations. Also decoction of the dried root.

DOSE
Extract and tincture: 2–5 ml three times daily.
Decoction: 150 ml three times daily.

Cabbage, white *(Brassica oleracea)*

CULTIVATION
Commonly grown vegetable.

PART USED
Organically grown, outside leaves are most therapeutic.

THERAPEUTIC USE
Healing and antiseptic properties, internally and externally. Recommended for a variety of swellings and injuries, including engorged breasts.

HOW IT IS USED
Juice (a juicer is required to make this) or poultice.

Make poultice from washed, outside leaves. Remove main stems, flatten with a rolling pin to soften, then place in layers over the wound. Lightly bandage. Change the poultice twice daily. If the wound becomes inflamed, don't use the poultice constantly.

If the wound is very sensitive, dip the leaves in hot water first, cool, and place over gauze which has been soaked in almond oil or pure olive oil.

DOSE
Applied externally – for sores and injuries: dab on the undiluted juice.

Taken internally – for gastric ulcers and intestinal inflammation: 1 tablespoon juice to start, gradually increasing to one cup or more per day. May be diluted with carrot juice to improve the taste.

NOTE *In rare cases, regular ingestion of large amounts of cabbage has depressed the function of the thyroid.*

Calendula *(Calendula officinalis)*
Also known as common or pot marigold.

NOTE *Do not confuse with other similar-looking yellow or orange 'daisy' flowers.*

CULTIVATION
Grows well in Australia.

PART USED
Flower petals.

THERAPEUTIC USE
Especially recommended for external use for a range of wounds and skin conditions including sebaceous cysts and cold sores.

Useful as a cold compress or ointment for varicose veins. It has antiseptic, anti-inflammatory and anti-fungal properties and is especially effective for post-menopausal, dry skins.

It has an oestrogenic effect; is used for menopausal symptoms and some cases of amenorrhoea. Herbalists also prescribe it for gastritis, enlarged lymph nodes and as a healer to the digestive tract.

HOW IT IS USED

Externally as an ointment (for sores can be mixed to a paste with a little calcium ascorbate powder), wash, bath or compress (make as strong infusion and let it cool before applying).

The fluid extract may be used as a skin softener and works well mixed into Sorbolene or other base.

Taken internally as extract, tincture or infusion.

DOSE

Extract or tincture: 20 drops twice daily. Infusion: 1–2 teaspoons petals to a cup of water twice daily. A stronger infusion makes an excellent gargle for a sore throat and a mouthwash for ulcers.

NOTE **The internal dose is very low.**

Caraway *(Carum carvi)*

CULTIVATION

Grows well in Australia.

PART USED

Seeds.

THERAPEUTIC USE

A common culinary herb, useful for flavouring some herbal decoctions and for digestive problems such as colic and flatulence. A good additive for herbal teas during respiratory problems or for colic.

HOW IT IS USED

Dried seeds or powder.

DOSE

Small quantities of powder or crushed seeds added to food or drinks.

Cardamon *(Ellataria cardamomum)*

CULTIVATION

Not commonly grown in Australia.

PART USED

Seeds. A common culinary spice.

THERAPEUTIC USE

Nausea and flatulence.

HOW IT IS USED

The seeds should be crushed (I put them in a clean cloth and use a hammer or blend them). If they are not crushed the therapeutic properties are not readily extracted.

DOSE

2–3 crushed seeds in a cup of herbal tea. (For culinary use, I generally combine 1–2 teaspoons of various seeds and dried herbs and place them in a tea ball which stays in the dish or pot during cooking.)

Catnip *(Nepeta cataria)*

Catmint is a different species. Your cat will love you and smell delicious if you harvest a handful of fresh catnip leaves, crush them between your hands and rub the bruised leaves all over its body.

CULTIVATION

Grows well in Australia.

PARTS USED

Above-ground parts.

THERAPEUTIC USE

Has a wide range of uses for humans including digestive weaknesses, flatulence, coughs and colds, insomnia, headaches and is especially recommended as a nervine for irritable children. It promotes sweating.

Said to help cranky and sick cats. My cat enjoys lying in it in the garden and will eat it with relish, but only the tiny new shoots and only if hand fed. It is beneficial in toys and herbal pillows for both children and cats – to settle them down.

HOW IT IS USED
Extract, infusion, footbath, herbal pillow.

DOSE
Extract: 2 ml three times daily.
Infusion: 1 cup 3–4 times daily.

Celery *(Apium graveolens)*

CULTIVATION
A commonly grown vegetable.

PART USED
Above-ground parts juiced. Root grated. The seeds are more therapeutic and they are very strong. Commercial herbal remedies are made from the seeds. You will notice that the dose is low.

THERAPEUTIC USE
Commonly used for joint and muscle problems, hypertension, arthritis, gout, fluid retention and bladder irritations, mainly due to its diuretic effect. The juice as a gargle is helpful for sore, husky throats, due to its antiseptic and anti-fungal effect.

HOW IT IS USED
The whole plant can be juiced. Seeds used in tablets and herbal extracts. Celery root can lower blood cholesterol levels.

DOSE
Juice: 1–2 glasses per day for 2–4 weeks (can be combined with carrot or wheat-grass and a little parsley); a lesser amount long term.
Root: ½ cup per day grated into food.
Extract: 15 drops three times daily.

NOTE For problems such as arthritis, celery seed products need to be taken over a period of months.

Centaury *(Centaurium erythrea)*

CULTIVATION
Will grow in Australia.

PARTS USED
Above-ground parts.

THERAPEUTIC USE
A bitter herb that stimulates the gastric juices and helps increase appetite. A mild tonic to the liver and gallbladder.

HOW IT IS USED
Herbal extract, infusion.

DOSE
Extract: 2 ml three times daily.
Infusion: 50 ml three times daily.

NOTE Centaury is best taken about 30 minutes before a meal. This applies to all bitter-tasting herbs prescribed for digestive weakness.

Chamomile, Roman or German *(Anthemis nobilis, Chamomilla recutita)*

CULTIVATION
Both species are easy to grow in Australia and both have similar properties. The German chamomile is somewhat stronger.

NOTE The little daisy flowers can easily be confused with other plants. The leaves have an apple-like odour.

PART USED
Flowerheads.

THERAPEUTIC USE

Especially recommended for gastric irritations and nervous problems. Has anti-inflammatory, sedative and anti-spasmodic properties that make it useful for a wide range of conditions. It is often helpful for menstrual pain, insomnia and irritable children. May also be used as a steam inhalation for chest congestion, such as mild asthmatic symptoms.

HOW IT IS USED

Commonly used as a tea. More palatable with added ginger root or with lemon. Also as tinctures, extracts, tablets, infusions, footbaths and herbal pillows.

A cold infusion may be used as a rinse for fair hair.

Chamomilla is a commonly prescribed homoeopathic remedy for irritable, teething children. I have never had reactions with it in this form.

DOSE

Extract and tincture: 2 ml three times daily.

Infusion: 2–3 cups of weak infusion may be taken per day. A stronger, cooled infusion can be used as a gargle for sore throats and a mouthwash for inflamed gums.

CAUTION *There have been a few reports of strong allergic reactions to this herb.*

Chaste tree *(Vitex agnus-castus)*
CULTIVATION
A small tree that grows in Australia.
PART USED
Ripe berries (seeds).
THERAPEUTIC USE
For premenstrual tension (especially where depression is a symptom),

amenorrhoea and irregular menstrual bleeding – but you must have a gynaecological check first. In a controlled study, 70 per cent of acne sufferers, both male and female, showed an improvement in their condition taking chaste tree. Used to reduce menopausal flushing.

In the old days, it was used to dampen sexual urges, i.e. to keep one chaste. However, there is no good evidence that it worked then – or now.

NOTE *This herb is not appropriate for children.*

HOW IT IS USED
Infusion, extract.
DOSE
Infusion: 1 cup of weak tea per day.
Extract: 30 drops a day.

NOTES *Dose is very low.*

There are a few reports of chaste tree causing headaches.

Chickweed *(Stellaria media)*
CULTIVATION
A common garden weed.

NOTE *Do not confuse with the spurges and other weeds.*

PART USED
Above-ground parts.
THERAPEUTIC USE
Mainly recommended as an external agent for skin diseases, eruptions, itching, rashes and minor injuries.
HOW IT IS USED
Ointment – I recommend non-greasy products.

The fresh plant is also used as a poultice, or a strong infusion as a compress or bath.

Chilli, hot *(Capscium annum, minimum* or *frutescens)*

Also incorrectly called cayenne.

CULTIVATION

Chilli can be grown from seeds or seedlings in most areas of Australia. It is best treated as an annual and grown in the warm seasons.

PART USED

Ripe fruits.

NOTE **Some ornamental varieties are not edible.**

THERAPEUTIC USE

An important circulatory, digestive and general stimulant. Recent research shows that it is an antioxidant, lowers blood cholesterol levels, thins the blood and may help weight-loss programmes. Chilli is quite antiseptic, loosens mucus in the throat and lungs and has pain-relieving qualities – aside from the heat being diverting. Surprisingly, it has been used successfully to treat gastric ulcers, but this needs practitioner supervision.

HOW IT IS USED

Tincture, capsules, fresh, dried or powdered fruits.

When applied externally the powder may be mixed into something like Sorbolene. For joint and muscle pain you can add a little wintergreen oil to enhance the analgesic, counter-irritant effect. Always do a small test patch first in case of an allergic reaction.

DOSE

Tincture: 5 drops three times daily in a large glass of water, juice or herbal tea.

Powder: ¼ teaspoon mixed to a paste, with ½ glass warm water added (can be added to herbal teas, apple juice or tomato juice). To be sipped slowly after meals.

CAUTION **Chilli may irritate inflamed or sensitive gastro-intestinal conditions. Very large quantities are harmful.**

Cinnamon *(Cinnamomum zeylanicum)*

CULTIVATION

Cultivated in tropical regions.

PART USED

Inner bark.

THERAPEUTIC USE

Helpful in tiny doses for flatulence, nausea and colds. Used mainly as a flavouring herb.

HOW IT IS USED

Extract, sticks, powder.

DOSE

A small piece of stick added to a herbal tea.

Extract: 5 drops three times daily.

CAUTION **Cinnamon is toxic in large quantities.**

Clivers *(Galium aparine)*

Also known as cleavers, goosegrass.

CULTIVATION

Clivers is found wild in some parts of Australia.

PART USED

Above-ground parts.

THERAPEUTIC USE

A 'blood cleanser', diuretic and lymphatic tonic; commonly used for kidney and bladder problems. Also prescribed for swollen glands.

HOW IT IS USED
Herbalists generally use herbal extracts. Also used as fresh juice, eaten like spinach and taken as an infusion.

DOSE
Juice: 5–10 ml three times daily.
Infusion: 50–100 ml three times daily.
Extract: 2 ml three times daily.

Cloves *(Eugenia caryophyllus,* syn. *Syzygium aromaticum)*

CULTIVATION
Grown in tropical regions.

PART USED
Unexpanded dried buds.

THERAPEUTIC USE
A mild circulatory stimulant, a refreshing mouthwash and gargle, with antiseptic and pain-killing properties. Small amounts are helpful for gastric wind, diarrhoea, nausea and poor digestion. A small quantity may be added to herbal teas.

HOW IT IS USED
Herbal extract, infusion, oil and powder.

DOSE
Extract: ¼ teaspoon added to a herbal gargle formula.
Powder: small amounts for culinary use or in warm water as a gargle and mouthwash.
Infusion: One bud added to herbal teas.
Oil: for symptomatic treatment of toothache use directly on the tooth, using cotton wool.

CAUTION *As with all volatile oils, clove oil should be used with care and never for young children.*
1–2 drops may be diluted in water and used internally for a few days.

Comfrey *(Symphytum officinale)*

CULTIVATION
Grows well in Australia.

NOTE *Comfrey is listed as an internal poison by the Australian Department of Health. For external application only.*

PART USED
Root and leaves.

THERAPEUTIC USE
A long history of use as a healing agent. May be helpful for the relief of gout, neuralgia. Useful as an anti-fungal agent, and for a range of skin diseases including dermatitis.

HOW IT IS USED
A decoction of the root or an infusion of the leaves used as a bath, compress, lotion or douche. Also ointment and poultice.

Corn silk *(Zea mays)*

CULTIVATION
Common vegetable crop.

PART USED
Silky part (styles and stigmas).

THERAPEUTIC USE
A non-irritant diuretic with soothing, anti-fungal and anti-inflammatory properties. Traditionally used for urinary tract infections, vaginal irritations and benign prostate enlargement – as support therapy. Contains allantoin, which has healing properties.

HOW IT IS USED
An infusion may be made from the fresh silky part of the common garden corn. Also extract, tincture and tablets.

DOSE
Infusion: 150 ml three or four times daily.
Extract and tincture: 5 ml three times daily.

Cowslip *(Primula veris)*

CULTIVATION
Grows in Australia.

PART USED
Flowers.

THERAPEUTIC USE
For anxiety, restlessness, irritability, insomnia, headaches.

HOW IT IS USED
Infusion of the dried flowers; extract.

DOSE
Extract: 20 drops three times daily, or 3 ml after dinner for insomnia.

Cramp bark *(Viburnum opulus)*

CULTIVATION
Grows in most areas of Australia.

PART USED
Bark.

THERAPEUTIC USE
Often prescribed for muscle cramps, painful conditions of the female reproductive system and joints. It can give good results for internal problems such as colic, irritable bowel, spasms and nervous tension generally.

HOW IT IS USED
Extracts and tablets.

DOSE
Extract: 2 ml three times daily.

Dandelion *(Taraxacum officinale)*

CULTIVATION
Grows wild.

NOTE **Do not use from polluted roadsides. Dandelion is difficult to identify as many plants look similar.**

PART USED
The root is used in herbal medicine.
The leaves are very rich in potassium and Vitamin A, so add a few to your salads – chop very finely as they have a bitter taste.

THERAPEUTIC USE
A non-toxic, restorative, liver remedy. A mild laxative and gallbladder tonic. Has a diuretic effect and is a mild pancreas tonic, which makes it useful in the treatment of hypoglycaemia. Also an adjunct to the treatment of kidney and gallbladder stones.

HOW IT IS USED
Extract, tincture, decoction, dried powdered root and tablet complexes. The root may be cut, roasted, powdered and used as a coffee substitute. (It is hard to grind down so if you use pieces of the root it is more economical to soak them in water before making up the decoction).

DOSE
Extract and tincture: 5 ml three times daily.
Dandelion coffee: 3 cups per day.
Fresh root juice: 1 teaspoon three times daily.

NOTE **The flower stem is toxic.**

Devil's claw *(Harpogophytum procumbens)*

CULTIVATION
Not grown in Australia.

PART USED
Tuber.

THERAPEUTIC USE
An anti-rheumatic herb recommended for painful conditions of joints and muscles because of its anti-inflammatory and diuretic qualities.

HOW IT IS USED
Extract, tincture, tablets and capsules.

DOSE
Extract: 5 drops three times daily.
Tincture: 15 drops three times daily.

Dill *(Anethum graveolens)*
CULTIVATION
Grows in Australia.
PART USED
Seeds are strongest and most medicinal, but the leaves and young stems may be used in salads and in cooking.
THERAPEUTIC USE
Flatulence and colic, particularly in babies. May help the flow of breast milk.
HOW IT IS USED
Infusion of crushed seeds or distilled dill water. Culinary herb.
DOSE
Infusion: 1 teaspoon crushed seeds to 1 cup water three times daily before meals.

NOTE **Dose for babies: 1–2 teaspoons of the infusion in water.**

Echinacea *(Echinacea angustifolia* and *purpurea)*
Also known as purple coneflower.
CULTIVATION
Will grow in Australia.
PART USED
Underground parts.
THERAPEUTIC USE
Helps purify the blood and lymph systems. Has antiseptic, antibiotic, antifungal properties. It's an organ tonic, helps preserve connective tissue, improves immune functioning and is an adjunct in the treatment of arthritis.
HOW IT IS USED
Extract, tincture, decoction, capsules and tablets. For skin infections, the extract can be used externally.

DOSE
Extract and tincture: 20 drops three times daily.
Decoction: 5 g to 200 ml water; 20 ml three times daily.

Elder *(Sambucus nigra)*
CULTIVATION
Grows easily in Australia.
PART USED
Flowers.
THERAPEUTIC USE
Traditionally used for mild fevers, coughs and colds. It is helpful as a decongestant in influenza and all mucous membrane problems related to the sinuses, nose and throat. Commonly used as a tea and is a pleasant addition to respiratory remedies. Combines well with yarrow and peppermint.
HOW IT IS USED
Infusion – to help promote sweating – and herbal extract.
DOSE
Infusion: 60 ml three times daily.
Extract: 3 ml three times daily.

Eucalyptus *(Eucalyptus globulus* and other species)
CULTIVATION
Native to Australia.
PART USED
Leaves and volatile oil extracted from them.
THERAPEUTIC USE
In the old days the leaves were boiled in a pot, without the lid, as an air freshener and mild antiseptic. A leaf may be added to a pot of tea.

The distilled oil is commonly used as a chest rub, an antiseptic inhalation and gargle to help clear airway passages in respiratory disorders affecting the nose and throat. It can be added to massage oils or diluted with water to wash wounds. The oil may be applied undiluted on small areas, pimples, etc.

HOW IT IS USED
Oil.

DOSE
2–4 drops in ½ cup warm water as a gargle or in hot water as an inhalation.
1 teaspoon to ½ cup warm water to wash wounds.

CAUTION *The oil is too strong to be used internally.*

Evening primrose oil
(Oenothera biennis)
PART USED
Oil extracted from seeds.

NOTE *This plant is not commonly grown in Australia and readers should not confuse it with other plants also called evening primrose.*
   Although it is generally considered to be an internal remedy, there have been cases of success using it externally, even after the internal use did not have any effect.

THERAPEUTIC USE
Helpful in many cases of acne, atopic eczema or dermatitis, PMT and hyper-activity, due to the action of the essential fatty acids on prostaglandins. May assist in rheumatoid arthritis, multiple sclerosis and cardiovascular disease. Also useful externally for dry skin conditions.

HOW IT IS USED
Capsules or oil.

DOSE
Up to 6 capsules per day or 1 ml oil twice daily. Treatment is long-term – use for 2–3 months, then if it has helped continue with a low maintenance dose of 1 capsule per day.

Eyebright *(Euphrasia officinalis)*
CULTIVATION
Eyebright is not commonly grown in Australia.

PART USED
Above-ground parts.

THERAPEUTIC USE
An anti-catarrhal and anti-inflammatory herb with an antiseptic action, useful in treating colds, sinusitis, earache and sore throat. Traditionally used for minor eye irritations and infections such as conjunctivitis.

HOW IT IS USED
Infusion, tincture and herbal extract.

CAUTION *These methods of treating the eyes are not sterile. Any remedy for the eyes needs to be made fresh each time. Equipment needs to be cleaned in boiling water before use.*

DOSE
Infusion: 50 ml three times daily.
   The standard infusion strength may be used externally as a cold compress for red, swollen eyes. As an eye wash, you need to make the infusion with ½ teaspoon per ½ cup boiling water; stand covered until tepid and strain carefully before use. If only one eye is affected, take care not to infect the other.
Extract or tincture: taken internally, 3 ml three times daily.
   As eye drops or an eye bath, 2 drops of extract to 10 ml boiled, cooled water or saline solution. It is easier and more hygienic to use an eyedropper rather than an eye bath.

Fennel, wild and sweet

(Foeniculum vulgare and *dulce)*
Florence fennel is the variety with the enlarged edible base.

CULTIVATION

Wild fennel grows as a weed in large areas of Australia. The sweet fennel is easy to grow as a vegetable.

NOTE *Do not collect from polluted areas and roadsides because it may have been sprayed with toxic weedicides or be contaminated with lead.*

PART USED

Seeds are most therapeutic. The young stems and leaves are also used in salads and in cooking. The fresh green seeds are delicious in a salad or as a mouth freshener.

THERAPEUTIC USE

An anti-flatulent which also contains weak plant oestrogens. May be helpful to improve the flow of breast milk. It is a mild herb, especially recommended for flatulence, digestive problems related to nervous agitation and infant colic.

HOW IT IS USED

Extract, infusion, volatile oil.

DOSE

Extract: 20 drops three times daily.
Infusion: 1 teaspoon crushed seeds per cup, three times daily. Babies 1 teaspoon to 1 tablespoon of the infusion 3–5 times daily.
Volatile oil: 2–4 drops in ½ cup tepid water sipped after meals.

NOTE *The oil is not to be given to babies.*

Fenugreek *(Trigonella foenum-graecum)*

CULTIVATION

Cultivated in Australia.

PART USED

Ripe seeds.

THERAPEUTIC USE

May be used as a drawing agent externally – as a poultice or plaster (see Chapter 1, 'Using the Remedies'). Internally a digestive tonic and respiratory decongestant. May be helpful for stimulating the flow of breast milk. Some herbalists recommend it for its cleansing and flushing properties, including where there is congested blood flow.

Fenugreek powder can lower blood glucose levels – making it an option for non-insulin-dependent diabetes or as a preventive treatment for those with a family history of diabetes. Fenugreek also has a cholesterol-lowering effect.

HOW IT IS USED

Commonly available in tablets, powder or dried seeds. Also extract and tincture. The seeds can be sprouted.

NOTE *When using fenugreek regularly, you will have a mild, curry-like body odour.*

DOSE

Extract or tincture: 2 ml three times daily.
Decoction: 50 ml three times daily.
Infusion: to taste.
Powder: as a diabetes preventive measure, 1–2 tablespoons every second day, mixed into food.

Feverfew *(Tanacetum parthenium,* syn. *Chrysanthemum parthenium)*

CULTIVATION

Grows readily in Australia.

PART USED
Leaves.

CAUTION *The flowers are never used internally.*

THERAPEUTIC USE
Nervousness, migraine, fevers, painful periods, arthritis.

HOW IT IS USED
Infusion, tincture, extract and capsules.

DOSE
Infusion: 20 ml daily.
Tincture and extract: 10 drops daily.
Fresh leaf: 1 leaf daily.
Capsules: 1 per day.

As a rule, the treatment for long-term problems takes many months and there is no benefit from taking higher doses. Once relief is achieved, the dose should be reduced as low as possible, some people finding that a few drops per week is enough for a maintenance programme.

NOTE *After some months on the treatment, there have been occasional reports of side effects such as mouth ulcers, sore tongue or abdominal upsets. Should this happen, discontinue treatment.*

Others have experienced beneficial side effects, such as better sleep, improved digestion and reduction of pain.

Fumitory *(Fumaria officinalis)*
CULTIVATION
Grows as a weed in Australia.

PART USED
Above-ground parts.

THERAPEUTIC USE
A mild tonic, especially for organ sluggishness and skin eruptions.

HOW IT IS USED
Fresh or dried aerial parts as an infusion or decoction; also used as an external lotion.

DOSE
Infusion and decoction internally: 50 ml three times daily.
Externally: 1 handful steeped in 500 ml boiling water; cool and strain before using.

Garlic *(Allium sativum)*
CULTIVATION
Easy to grow but slow to mature.

PART USED
Bulb.

THERAPEUTIC USE
Helpful in a wide range of conditions due to its anti-bacterial and mucus solvent effect. Also considered to be an adjunct in the treatment of high blood pressure, high cholesterol and heavy metal toxicity.

As well as being a good remedy for most respiratory problems, garlic is anti-inflammatory, anti-fungal, anti-viral, anti-oxidant and anti-clotting (blood). It may assist in the treatment of diabetes, various kinds of toxicities, post-viral syndrome and cardiovascular disease.

NOTE *The fresh plant may cause blisters externally.*

HOW IT IS USED
The fresh cloves are cooked as part of the diet. Also used as powder, tablets and capsules.

DOSE
Up to 6 capsules or 2 cloves per day to help combat infection. The powder sprinkled on the feet often helps tinea (athlete's foot).

CAUTIONS *Not suitable for babies and small children unless specifically formulated for them. Some people are allergic to it internally. Don't take on an empty stomach.*

Raw garlic and garlic oil should be used sparingly as some research shows that, aside from allergies, these can irritate the digestive tract.

RECIPES

For using garlic for respiratory infections.

1 *1 teaspoon finely chopped garlic*
1 teaspoon finely chopped ginger root
2 teaspoons seedless raisins
1–2 tablespoons lemon juice
Simmer all for 15 minutes in 1 cup of water.

Sip warm, ½ cup at a time. It tastes quite pleasant, although the smell is somewhat strong, but this can be improved by placing a small sprig of fresh peppermint on top. A little honey can be added and there are many optional add-tions, such as aniseeds and thyme. To be effective the garlic, ginger and lemon must remain. A larger quantity can be made and kept in the fridge.

2 Dr Christopher's Oxymel recipe
250 ml vinegar
7 g caraway seeds, crushed
7 g fennel seeds, crushed
40 g garlic cloves, finely sliced
300 g honey
Simmer fennel, caraway and garlic in vinegar for 15 minutes. Then strain liquid (press out of solid material) and add honey. Boil until it has the con-sistency of syrup. Cool, bottle and keep in fridge.

Take about 2 tablespoons 3–4 times daily or use as a gargle.

Gentian *(Gentiana lutea)*

CULTIVATION
Will grow in Australia.

PART USED
Dried, underground parts.

THERAPEUTIC USE
A strong, bitter-tasting tonic, benefiting the whole of the digestive tract. Increases salivary flow, stomach secretions and bile flow. Useful as a herbal aperitif.

HOW IT IS USED
Tincture, capsules, tablets. The tincture is unpalatable but most effective, so it can be made as a predinner drink as follows.

Use a long glass. Cut small thin slices of half a lemon, including the peel. Add some mint leaves (or slices of orange). Add 2 ml tincture of gentian. Top up with mineral or plain water and a sprig of mint.

As a stimulant to the appetite and digestion, sip slowly about a half-hour before meals. Other herbs can be used for flavouring but don't add sweeteners.

DOSE
Tincture: 2 ml twice daily before meals – it's a bit hard to take before breakfast!

Ginger *(Zingiber officinale)*

CULTIVATION
Grows readily from root (rhizome) cut-tings in warm climates.

PART USED
Underground root (rhizome).
I find fresh ginger more effective unless the powder is very fresh and aromatic.

THERAPEUTIC
A circulatory and digestive stimulant, especially useful for nausea, motion sick-ness and flatulence. Consistent use helps lower blood pressure and acts as an anti-inflammatory for arthritis. In addition ginger reduces blood stickiness, lowers blood and liver cholesterol, is a mild heart

tonic and has antibiotic properties. Professional herbalists often include it in remedies because it functions as a 'carrier'.

HOW IT IS USED

Tincture, infusion, tablets, decoction of the fresh root, powder.

To make decoction: add 1 dessertspoon finely chopped root to 500 ml water. Bring to boil, let simmer 15 minutes. Cool and strain. This is especially useful for nausea and travel sickness.

DOSE

Decoction: 1 dessertspoon five or six times daily or as required.

Tincture: 5 drops three times daily.

The root or small quantities of powder may be added to herbal teas.

Medicinal dose: 1 teaspoon powder or 2 teaspoons fresh per day added to food.

CAUTION **Some unconfirmed reports indicate that ginger may produce undesirable side effects if used in large quantities during late pregnancy.**

Ginkgo/Maidenhair tree
(Ginkgo biloba)

CULTIVATION

An interesting deciduous tree that grows in most areas of Australia except tropical regions.

PART USED

The green leaves are used, remedies being prepared by a special extraction process.

CAUTIONS **The fruits are toxic.**

There have not been any studies of remedies using unprocessed leaves. Use professionally prepared remedies.

THERAPEUTIC USE

Improves blood circulation, which is why it has a reputation for helping brain function in the elderly, for treating memory loss, aiding stroke and heart attack recovery and relieving headaches, leg cramps, tinnitus and a wide range of disorders where there is restricted blood flow. It has antioxidant properties and assists the functioning of nervous tissue.

HOW IT IS USED

Extracts, tablets and capsules.

DOSE

Extract: 20 drops three times daily.

Tablets and capsules: as manufacturer's recommendations.

Ginseng, Asian (Panax ginseng) and Siberian (Eleutherococcus senticosus)

CULTIVATION

Not grown in Australia.

PART USED

Root.

THERAPEUTIC USE

Asian: general tonic, especially recommended in old age and debility; for mental and nervous exhaustion, stress, depression, insomnia and memory loss. It is generally restorative, a blood thinner, helps the immune system and protects against premature ageing. (Unfortunately, nothing can make you young again – if that's what you're after.)

Although considered to be a 'male' herb, it can reduce menopausal flushing. Some researchers say that it is neither oestrogenic nor testosteronal but balances the body's hormones.

Siberian: nerve and muscle tonic, antioxidant. One of my menopausal patients accidentally purchased Siberian ginseng instead of the Asian species and found that this also markedly reduced her 'flushing'.

Ginseng has been called 'the world's best anti-stress tonic'. Both types of ginseng are adaptogenic, i.e. they help the adrenal glands, increase stress hormones and enhance hormonal activity depending on the needs of the body. In other words, your sense of wellbeing is increased.

HOW IT IS USED
Various tablets, fluid essences and extracts.

DOSE
According to manufacturers' instructions.

CAUTIONS **In some people it worsens insomnia if taken late in the day.**

A few reports of ginseng-abuse syndrome have surfaced. Stick to the recommended dose and perhaps have breaks off the remedy.

Globe artichoke *(Cynara scolymus)*

CULTIVATION
Native to North Africa – a thistle-like plant that grows in most temperate and sub-tropical areas.

Jerusalem artichoke (*Helianthus tuberosus*), which is grown for its edible root, is not known to have specific therapeutic qualities.

PART USED
Fresh choke, leaves and root.

THERAPEUTIC USE
Herbalists consider it to be a valuable remedy for jaundice and liver insufficiency, anaemia and liver damage caused by poisons. Stimulates and aids digestion; anti-dyspeptic. Considered to be a preventive against atherosclerosis. Also

recommended for its diuretic effect in eliminating uric acid (gout).

HOW IT IS USED
Fresh choke eaten as a delicacy. The blanched cooked leaf stalks may be cooked as a vegetable. The root and leaves may be juiced or made into a tincture or extract.

DOSE
To my knowledge there is no official dosage. I would suggest 20 ml of juice three times daily or 3 ml per day of an extract.

Golden seal *(Hydrastis canadensis)*

CULTIVATION
Not commonly grown in Australia.

PART USED
Underground parts.

THERAPEUTIC USE
A digestive and general tonic with antiseptic, antibiotic and antimicrobial properties. Commonly used by herbalists for skin conditions. A tonic for people with low blood pressure. Useful in the treatment of chronic, infectious diarrhoea and glandular fever.

CAUTION **Not recommended during pregnancy or with hypertension.**

Should never be taken in combination with liquorice.

HOW IT IS USED
Herbalists generally use tinctures. These are effective but the strong, bitter taste may be too much. Some may need to use tablets or capsules. Golden seal combines effectively with a little hot chilli.

DOSE
Tincture: 2 ml three times daily.
Decoction: 10 ml three times daily.

Gotu kola *(Centella asiatica)*

CULTIVATION

Grows as a weed in some areas of Australia.

NOTE *Needs careful identification because it may be confused with similar, violet-like leafed plants.*

PART USED

Leaves.

THERAPEUTIC USE

A traditional nerve and memory tonic, helpful in some inflammatory skin disorders. Asian herbalists often include it in formulae for strengthening the lungs. In India it is used externally for treating skin wounds. Modern research indicates that it improves the circulation to connective tissue, which explains its recent popularity as an arthritis remedy.

HOW IT IS USED

Leaves, extracts, tinctures.

DOSE

1–2 fresh leaves per day.
Extracts and tinctures: 2 ml twice daily.

Hawthorn *(Crataegus oxyacanthoides, laevigata and monogyna)*

CULTIVATION

Grows wild in some cool, temperate areas of Australia.

PART USED

Ripe berries (dried) and young spring leaves.

THERAPEUTIC USE

Has a historical use for treating heart and circulatory disorders. Overseas studies have backed up its use for lowering blood pressure and dilating peripheral blood vessels. As with most herbs, the action depends on all the constituents working together, and not a particular isolated constituent. It helps increase capillary membrane strength. I suggest it be used for mildly raised blood pressure in conjunction with a circulatory stimulant such as ginger or chilli, as well as a relaxant like scullcap or chamomile.

Hawthorn has antioxidant properties which specifically stabilise collagen and is recommended as part of the treatment of angina and atherosclerosis. It also reduces menopausal flushing.

HOW IT IS USED

The crushed or powdered dried fruits or leaves as an infusion. Fluid extracts, tinctures or capsules are not usually available in retail outlets.

DOSE

Infusion: 5 g per day or in a formula as follows:

> 1 tablespoon dried chamomile flowers
> 1 tablespoon dried hawthorn berries
> 1 tablespoon ginger root

All three are dried and crushed. Combine together. Make as an infusion, 1 teaspoon per cup. Take 2 cups per day.

CAUTION *Do not use hawthorn without practitioner advice if you are taking pharmaceutical drugs.*

Heartsease *(Viola tricolor)*

Also known as wild pansy.

CULTIVATION

Grows well in temperate Australia.

PART USED

Above-ground parts.

THERAPEUTIC USE

Has anti-inflammatory and diuretic properties and is recommended for skin eruptions. Herbalists often use it in eczema formulae and sometimes for coughs.

HOW IT IS USED

Extract, infusion. Products are not generally available from retail outlets but professional herbalists have them in their dispensaries.

DOSE

Extract: 2 ml three times a day.
Infusion: 1 teaspoon dried or 2 teaspoons freshly chopped leaves to 1 cup water, three times daily.

Hops *(Humulus lupulus)*

CULTIVATION

Grown as a cash crop.

PART USED

Strobiles (flower-like head).

THERAPEUTIC USE

Contains bitter principles that make it helpful as a general digestive tonic. Commonly recommended as a mild sedative for treating insomnia, painful periods, nervous coughing and irritable bowel syndrome. Has oestrogenic properties.

NOTES *Generally not recommended in depression.*

Beer does not possess the above-mentioned therapeutic properties.

HOW IT IS USED

Extract, tincture, infusion, herbal pillow.

DOSE

Extract and tincture: 20 drops three times daily or 3 ml after dinner, for insomnia.
Infusion: 30 ml three times daily.

Horse chestnut *(Aesculus hippocastanum)*

CULTIVATION

Grown in cool temperate climates.

PART USED

Ripe fruit after it has fallen from the tree.

CAUTION *The outer covering of the fruit is toxic – so are the green fruits. Not to be confused with sweet chestnut.*

THERAPEUTIC USE

Traditionally used for varicose veins and haemorrhoids because of its beneficial action on blood vessels and its anti-inflammatory properties. It has been used successfully in treating lumbago and sports injuries. May be useful for repetitive strain injury and related conditions.

HOW IT IS USED

Extract, tablets. The extract is not commonly available from retail outlets but most herbalists stock it.

DOSE

Extract: 20 drops three times daily.

Horseradish *(Cochlearia armoracia)*

CULTIVATION

Grows well in Australia.

THERAPEUTIC USE

An effective decongestant, antiseptic, circulatory and digestive stimulant, particularly recommended for blocked sinuses and nasal passages. It is warming and stimulating generally and has some antibiotic action. In Europe it is sometimes used externally as a counter-irritant for painful and congested conditions but it is not used on broken skin and may cause blisters!

CAUTIONS *Always take with or after meals as it can irritate the stomach. Not recommended for children.*

Horseradish may be slighly depressing to the thyroid but this is unlikely at medicinal doses.

HOW IT IS USED
Tablets and the fresh or dried root.

DOSE
Root: ½ teaspoon grated with food.
Tablets: 2 after each meal for 1–2 days, then 1 after each meal or according to the the manufacturer's instructions.

Horsetail *(Equisetum arvense)*
CULTIVATION
Grows in Australia.
PART USED
Stems.
THERAPEUTIC USE
Traditionally used to strengthen hair and nails, mainly because of the silica content. Has mild antiseptic, anti-haemorrhagic and astringent properties. Is often recommended in arthritic, urinary and circulatory problems, including bedwetting, benign prostate enlargement, chronic diarrhoea and for healing old wounds.
HOW IT IS USED
Infusion, extracts, tablets (usually sold under the Latin name).
DOSE
Extract: 2 ml three times a day.
Infusion: 50 ml three times a day.
Tablets: as manufacturer's instructions.

Hyssop *(Hyssopus officinalis)*
CULTIVATION
Grows well in Australia.
PARTS USED
Above-ground parts.
THERAPEUTIC USE
Has mild sedative, bitter and anti-viral properties; its main use is for a range of respiratory conditions such as head colds, sore throats and coughs.
HOW IT IS USED
Infusion, herbal extract and tincture.

DOSE
Infusion: 50 ml three times daily.
Extract or tincture: 3 ml three times daily.

Juniper *(Juniperus communis)*
CULTIVATION
Relatively easy to grow in Australia.
PART USED
Ripe berries.
THERAPEUTIC USE
Commonly used as a urinary antiseptic. Also for gout and rheumatic conditions. It is useful as a diuretic and is often included in naturopathic treatments for fluid retention.

CAUTION **Not to be used during pregnancy, where there is kidney disease or longer than 6–8 weeks without a break.**

HOW IT IS USED
Infusion of crushed seeds, extract and tincture.
DOSE
Infusion: 50 ml three times daily.
Extract and tincture: 2 ml three times daily.

Lavender *(Lavandula officinalis* and *angustifolia)*
CULTIVATION
Grows well in Australia.
PART USED
Leaves and flowers.
THERAPEUTIC USE
The dried flowers are used in herbal sedative pillows for insomnia, nervous and respiratory problems. The fresh or dried flowers and leaves can also be used as hand and footbaths to relieve aching joints and muscles.

The oil may be used undiluted on

small areas to relieve pain and tension, for example, on the back of the neck for headaches or diluted in a massage oil and rubbed into joints and muscles. The oil also has mild antiseptic and sedative properties and may be used diluted in water as a skin wash, or used in the bath as a relaxant.

CAUTION *Not for internal use except a tiny quantity of flowers or leaves as suggested in some recipes.*

Lemon

Lemon is not a herb – as you well know. I have included it because it is therapeutic and if used with herbal teas (infusions) and decoctions it helps to draw out the active constituents in the plants.

Lemon may be used in a number of ways to help skin, digestive and respiratory conditions, and a few of these are given below.

FOR COUGHS AND COLDS

Put a whole lemon in a hot oven; when it starts to split remove it and spoon out the juice. I think the juice of a baked lemon has a better flavour than fresh lemon juice.

FRESH LEMON JUICE

Add some to herbal extracts and tinctures as well as to herbal teas as a taste enhancer. Lemon is a particularly useful therapeutic additive when you are treating digestive problems and infections.

2 teaspoons in hot water first thing each day can be helpful for constipation and digestion. The fresh juice may also be used liberally over salads to aid the digestion. If you squeeze a little over steamed vegetables you don't miss a reduction in salt.

If you're watching your weight, one way to make raw vegetables more palatable and digestible is to slice them very finely (you can use raw beetroot, swedes, zucchini as well as carrots, celery, etc.); put them in a plastic container with some fresh herbs, such as mint, thyme, chives and oregano, then squeeze over liberal amounts of lemon juice. This keeps the vegetables fresh, lessens discoloration and provides low-kilojoule snacks throughout the day.

Diluted lemon juice is good for restoring the acid balance to the skin but it is drying. It may be applied undiluted on pimples and sores as an antiseptic and drying agent.

LEMON PEEL

Grated lemon peel may be added to soups and casseroles.

HALF A LEMON

Discoloured or smelly hands, for example from handling fish or onion, may be rubbed with half a lemon.

It is also good for sore feet and insomnia – rub over the feet, especially the soles, after a hot foot bath.

Lemon balm *(Melissa officinalis)*

Also known as balm.

CULTIVATION

Grows vigorously in most parts of Australia.

PART USED

Leaves.

THERAPEUTIC USE

A mild sedative which is particularly recommended for nervous digestive disorders. It promotes sweating, helps to relax blood vessels and functions as a mild nerve tonic. Recent research shows that it possesses antiviral activity and it is recommended as an external remedy for herpes.

HOW IT IS USED

Extract, infusion, tablets, foot bath. A little juice or undiluted extract can be applied to herpes lesions. The extract can also be made into an ointment.

DOSE

Extract: 2 ml three times daily.
Infusion: 60 ml three times daily.

Lemon grass (Cymbopogon citratus)

CULTIVATION

Grows readily in most soils and climates; also in containers.

PART USED

Leaves – fresh or dried.

THERAPEUTIC USE

A mild 'blood cleanser', especially helpful for pimples and mild skin irritations and infections.

Suggested as a support in the treatment of hypertension and fluid retention.

If your cat will munch on the leaves you will find it good for 'feline halitosis' (bad breath) and it makes the coat shine.

HOW IT IS USED

Commonly used as a tea. The thickened lower stem is used in cooking – very finely chopped. Also as a facial steam treatment.

Available in tablet form.

DOSE

Tea: 2–3 cups per day. An iced tea can be served with some fruit juice.

Linden (Tilia europaea and other species)

Also known as lime flowers.

CULTIVATION

Grows in Australia.

PART USED

Flowers and bracts.

THERAPEUTIC USE

A general sedative, mild diuretic and sweat promoter. Often used as support therapy in hypertension, atherosclerosis, circulatory disorders and migraine. Helpful for colds, flu and insomnia but don't have more than a small cup of tea after dinner.

HOW IT IS USED

Infusion, tincture, extract.

DOSE

Infusion: may be drunk freely as a herbal tea.
Extract and tincture: 2 ml three times daily.

Linseed (Linum usitatissimum)

Also known as flaxseed.

PART USED

Ripe seeds.

CULTIVATION

Grows in Australia.

THERAPEUTIC USE

A mild laxative due to its capacity to swell; useful as a nutritive and also soothing to respiratory and digestive irritations. Has a drawing and soothing effect when used externally as a poultice.

Along with a number of other foods, some researchers suggest it as a cancer preventive. Linseed oil is a good source of omega-3 fatty acids, which are now considered to be very beneficial to the heart and circulation.

HOW IT IS USED

Decoction, seeds or meal. The linseed meal may be added to porridge or used in any cooked cereal. It can be used in cooking in the same way as flour, as an additive to biscuits, bread, rissoles and so on. The seeds are fairly unpalatable and hard to chew.

To make a decoction: add 1 table-spoon seeds to 500 ml water, bring to boil, simmer for 20 minutes then cool and strain.

DOSE
Decoction to soothe a cough or an irri-tated digestive system: 100 ml three times daily.

Liquorice *(Glycyrrhiza glabra)*
CULTIVATION
Will grow in Australia.
PART USED
Peeled root.
THERAPEUTIC USE
A soothing, anti-inflammatory agent with mild expectorant, immune-enhancing, antioxidant, antiviral and laxative prop-erties. Useful as an adrenal tonic and for peptic ulcers.

Herbalists class it as a natural cortisone. Liquorice contains plant oestrogens.

CAUTIONS **In some people liquorice may cause fluid retention, hypertension and potassium loss. Studies have shown that even relatively small amounts of confectionery can cause loss of potassium if eaten regularly.**

Incompatible with some asthmatic and cardiac pharmaceutical drugs.

Liquorice remedies should never be combined with golden seal.

HOW IT IS USED
Extract, decoction, infusion, powder, tablets.

The powder (finely ground) mixed into Sorbolene or other base is an effec-tive skin softener and anti-irritant.

NOTE **The confectionery is not recommended as a therapeutic agent.**

DOSE
Extract: 2 ml three times daily.
Decoction: 50 ml three times daily.

Marjoram *(Origanum marjorana)*
CULTIVATION
Commonly grown in Australia.

NOTE **This is the sweet marjoram, not the common oregano.**

PART USED
Leaves, soft stems and flowers.
THERAPEUTIC USE
Apart from its culinary use, it is a mild sedative with some antiseptic action. In the context of this book, it is recom-mended as a hot foot bath, which helps decongest the head, making it also useful for headaches, anxiety and insomnia as well as coughs and colds.
HOW IT IS USED
Infusion: as a tea or for gargles and foot baths. The oil is popular as an external treatment in aromatherapy.
DOSE
Infusion: ½ teaspoon per cup to be used as a tea; 1 teaspoon per ½ cup as a tepid gargle; 1–2 tablespoons as a hot foot bath (this amount is for dried marjoram; use much more of the fresh herb).

Marshmallow *(Althaea officinalis)*
CULTIVATION
Grows well in Australia.
PART USED
Root and leaves.
THERAPEUTIC USE
A soothing and healing action, used inter-nally particularly for irritations of the

digestive system. Also for the urinary tract and coughs. A common herbal ointment.

HOW IT IS USED

Most internal benefit is obtained from decoctions of the powdered root, which is steeped in cold water and not heated, or a tea made from the leaf, rather than fluid extracts. It's also available in tablet form.

DOSE

Infusion (leaves): 100 ml three times daily.

Decoction (roots): 50 ml three times daily.

Maté (Ilex paraguariensis)

Also known as Paraguay tea.

PART USED

Leaves.

CULTIVATION

Not grown in Australia.

THERAPEUTIC USE

Stimulant to the central nervous system, also used as a pick-me-up. Recommended for headaches and depression, especially with fatigue. Also used as an anti-rheumatic.

HOW IT IS USED

Infusion.

DOSE

In South America it is a commonly used herbal tea but many herbalists here are reluctant to recommend it because it contains caffeine and large amounts of tannin. I suggest that it could be used for a few weeks, having one or two cups in the early part of the day.

Meadowsweet (Filipendula ulmaria, syn. Spiraea ulmaria)

Also known as queen-of-the-meadow.

CULTIVATION

Grows well in Australia.

PART USED

Above-ground parts.

THERAPEUTIC USE

A general digestive, relaxant and intestinal remedy, helpful in mild fevers. Also useful for inflamed joint and muscle problems due to salicylate constituents.

HOW IT IS USED

Extract, infusion, cold compress for external swellings and inflammation. Sometimes included in tablet complexes.

DOSE

Infusion: 3–4 cups a day. A very strong infusion, cooled, may be used as an external compress to ease pain and inflammation.

Extract: 2–4 ml three times daily.

Milk thistle or variegated thistle (Silybum marianum)

CULTIVATION

Classifed as a noxious weed in some parts of Australia.

PART USED

Ripe seeds – they're difficult to harvest.

THERAPEUTIC USE

A well-researched liver protectant and anti-oxidant. Helps protect against toxic damage and a useful restorative for most liver and gallbladder diseases. In some cases it has been successful in treating psoriasis and other chronic skin disorders.

HOW IT IS USED

Although extracts and tinctures are available, these are preserved with alcohol. I recommend tablets or powders for treating liver problems.

DOSE

10 g powdered seeds simmered in three glasses of water, plus a dessertspoon of apple cider vinegar or lemon juice. Take this throughout the day, flavouring with a little pear or apple juice if necessary for palatability.

Motherwort *(Leonurus cardiaca)*

CULTIVATION
Grows in Australia.

PART USED
Above-ground parts.

THERAPEUTIC USE
Nervousness, palpitations, insomnia, angina, period pain, cramps, arthritic conditions. It is also used for treating irregular menstrual cycles, fibroids, hypertension and menopausal symptoms. It may help reduce blood stickiness.

HOW IT IS USED
Infusion, extract, tincture, tablet complexes.

DOSE
Infusion: 50 ml three times daily.
Extract and tincture: 2 ml three times daily.

Mustard, black *(Brassica nigra)*

The black mustard seeds produce much stronger powder than pale-coloured ones, although the powders are all yellow.

CULTIVATION
Grows in Australia.

PART USED
Dried, powdered seeds.

THERAPEUTIC USE
Apart from its use as a culinary herb to stimulate digestion and circulation, the powdered mustard used externally is a drawing agent, working by reddening and irritating the skin. The aim is to stimulate the circulation and to 'draw' irritating substances to the surface of the skin.

HOW IT IS USED
As a plaster or foot bath (refer Chapter 1 'Using the Remedies').

DOSE
1 teaspoon in a foot bath for a head cold, or varying amounts for plasters depending on the area to be covered.

Myrrh *(Commiphora myrrha* var. *Molmol)*

CULTIVATION
Usually grown in the Middle East.

PART USED
Gum.

THERAPEUTIC USE
A strong antiseptic, anti-catarrhal astringent especially recommended for mouth and throat conditions. Also helpful for weak gums and bad breath.

HOW IT IS USED
Powdered gum, tincture and sometimes included in herbal toothpastes. The powder is not generally available at retail outlets.

DOSE
Tincture: 1 ml three times daily internally.
As a mouth wash and gargle: 2 ml tincture in ½ cup warm water (or in a tea made from sage or cloves) and a teaspoon of glycerine.

Nettle, stinging *(Urtica dioca)*

CULTIVATION
Grows wild. It makes an excellent garden mulch or compost additive.

PART USED
Above-ground parts.

NOTE **Use gloves when collecting!**

THERAPEUTIC USE
Helpful in a range of problems relating to poor circulation, fluid retention, rheumatic conditions, gout and skin conditions, especially where there is itching. An astringent and diuretic. May be used to treat hayfever. Recent research shows that that it has beneficial effects on the immune system and it can lower blood glucose levels.

NOTE *Although used as an anti-allergen, it sometimes causes a reaction – like any other plant.*

HOW IT IS USED
Ointment, fresh juice, tablets, extract, infusion. Also as a vegetable: the sting is neutralised when it is cooked, juiced or dried. Rich in nutrients but tastes horrible.

DOSE
Fresh juice: 10 ml three times daily.
Infusion: 50 ml three times daily.
Extract: 2 ml three times daily.

Oak bark *(Quercus robur)*

CULTIVATION
Grows in Australia.

PART USED
Inner bark.

THERAPEUTIC USE
An astringent, so it has a tonifying effect on the skin and gastro-intestinal linings.
Sometimes may be constipating. Used for diarrhoea, gastritis, colitis. Also useful as a gargle for sore throats and as a foot bath for excess foot perspiration.

CAUTION *Large doses may be too drying and cause irritation.*

HOW IT IS USED
Extract, decoction.

DOSE
Extract: 20 drops three times daily.
Decoction: 20 ml three times daily.

Oats *(Avena sativa)*

CULTIVATION
Grown in Australia.

PART USED
Whole oats including the outside parts or whole rolled endosperm.

THERAPEUTIC USE
Nervous exhaustion, depression, general weakness and debility. Helpful in convalescence. May help reduce the craving for cigarette smoking and other drugs.

HOW IT IS USED
Broth, decoction, extract, tincture.
To make broth: 20 g oat flakes in 1 litre water, boil gently for 30 minutes then strain.
To make decoction: boil 500 g whole oats and 60 ml glycerine in 1.5 litres water for 30 minutes, then strain.

DOSE
Broth: 3 cups per day.
Decoction: 60 ml three times daily.
Extract and tincture: 2 ml three times daily.

CAUTIONS *Overdosing of the concentrated extract can cause excitability – as happens with horses!*

Generally not tolerated by those with gluten sensitivity.

Parsley *(Petroselinum crispum)*

CULTIVATION
Commonly grown as a culinary herb. The seeds are slow to germinate.

PART USED
The seed is stronger and more therapeutic than the leaves and stems; the root is also used medicinally.

THERAPEUTIC USE
Helpful for flatulence, digestive weakness, bad breath, during menopause, for fluid retention and arthritis. Rich in vitamins and minerals, particularly iron, potassium and calcium. Parsley contains weak plant oestrogens.

HOW IT IS USED
Small quantity of juiced leaves, crushed

seeds or grated root. Tablets. Leaves are used in cooking and salads or chewed as a mouth freshener.

DOSE
The maximum dose is a handful a day – either fresh or juiced – or 1 dessertspoon seeds or root.

CAUTION **Only minimal amounts of parsley should be used during pregnancy.**

Passion flower (Passiflora incarnata)

CULTIVATION
Will grow in Australia.

NOTE **This is not the edible fruit species.**

PART USED
Above-ground parts.

THERAPEUTIC USE
Irritability, insomnia, palpitations, nervous stomach, period pain, hypertension.

HOW IT IS USED
Extract, tincture, tablets.

DOSE
Extract and tincture: 5–10 drops 3 times daily or 30 drops after dinner for insomnia.

CAUTION **This herb does not agree with everyone.**

Peppermint (Mentha piperita)

NOTE **Spearmint has similar properties and usage.**

CULTIVATION
Grows readily.

PART USED
Leaves.

THEAPEUTIC USE
Useful in nausea and flatulence. It also has a mild diaphoretic effect (that is, it promotes perspiration) and gives symptomatic relief in head colds. Helpful as a mouthwash.

HOW IT IS USED
Culinary – the fresh leaves chopped into a salad or mixed into natural yoghurt. The infusion and oil as a mouthwash, gargle or inhalation, or a few drops of oil on your toothpaste.

CAUTIONS **The oil is toxic internally in large doses.**

No volatile oil should be given internally to pregnant women or children, although a few drops of peppermint oil gently massaged into the abdomen may relieve infants' colic.

DOSE
An infusion of the dried or fresh leaves may be drunk freely.
Essential oil: 2 drops in ½ cup tepid water before meals for flatulence, or 2–3 times daily as a mouthwash or gargle. For an inhalation, use hot water.

For problems in the lower part of the abdomen, such as spastic colon, you can try enteric-coated casules (Mintec) available from pharmacies.

Psyllium (Plantago psyllium and ovata)

Two species with similar properties.

CULTIVATION
Not commonly grown in Australia.

PART USED
Dried ripe seeds.

THERAPEUTIC USE
A bulk-swelling, intestinal lubricant used for chronic constipation, irritable bowel syndrome and colitis. Helps lower cholesterol.

NOTE *Laxatives, herbal or otherwise, should be used as a short-term remedy. Appropriate diet, exercise and adequate fluid intake must be considered. An attempt should be made to establish the cause of any intestinal problem.*

HOW IT IS USED
Infusion of the crushed seeds or powder.
DOSE
Seeds: 1–2 teaspoons crushed seeds soaked in 1 cup warm water for about 4 hours. Strain and drink before bed.
Powder: 1 tablespoon 1–2 times daily, taken with a large glass of fluid.

Raspberry leaf *(Rubus idaeus)*
Also known as red raspberry.
CULTIVATION
Grows in Australia.
PART USED
Leaves.
THERAPEUTIC USE
As astringent, used for gastric upsets, nausea and diarrhoea. It may be used in tablet form throughout pregnancy, especially for 'morning sickness' and as a general uterine tonic.
HOW IT IS USED
Extract, infusion, tablets.
DOSE
Extract: 3 ml three times daily.
Infusion: 1 cup three times daily. Flavour with lemon or peppermint leaves.
Tablets: as manufacturer's instructions

except use half the dose if taking during pregnancy.

Red clover *(Trifolium pratense)*
CULTIVATION
Grows wild.

CAUTION *It is difficult to identify this species. Some clovers are toxic.*

PART USED
Flowerheads.
THERAPEUTIC USE
Used for a wide range of skin problems. Also helpful as an expectorant and as a poultice. Contains weak plant oestrogens.
HOW IT IS USED
Infusion, extract, tincture, sprouts.
DOSE
Extract: 1–2 ml three times daily.
Infusion: 50 ml three times daily.

Reishi *(Ganoderma lucidum)*
CULTIVATION
Not grown in Australia, to my knowledge. A type of mushroom.
PART USED
Above-ground parts.
THERAPEUTIC USE
For over 5000 years it has been used as a tonic in China. An effective adaptogen (protects the body from stress-related illness) and is useful in treating a range of disorders including infections, chronic fatigue syndrome and hypertension. It is said to thin the blood and act like an anti-histamine so it may help some cases of hayfever, asthma and chronic allergies.
   Shiitake *(Lentinus edodes)* is another therapeutic mushroom. Both enhance immune function and have a reputation as tumour inhibitors.

HOW IT IS USED
Dried products are soaked and then added to foods such as stir-fry dishes. Tablets.
DOSE
1–2 mushrooms a day, or a small handful in cooking two or three times a week.

Rosehips *(Rosa canina)*
Also known as wild dog rose.
CULTIVATION
Grows wild in parts of Australia.
PART USED
Ripe fruits.
THERAPEUTIC USE
Has astringent and nutritive properties. The tablets may be helpful in diarrhoea, gastric upsets and as a vitamin C supplement.
HOW IT IS USED
Infusion of the crushed fruits or tablets.
DOSE
The infusion may be drunk freely but much of the vitamin C is lost in the heat. The infusion is more palatable with a piece of cinnamon stick, lemon or honey added.

Rosemary *(Rosmarinus officinalis)*
CULTIVATION
Grows easily in temperate Australia.
PART USED
Leaves and flowers.
THERAPEUTIC USE
The traditional 'memory' herb, which is also used by herbalists for stimulating the gallbladder as well as for a range of digestive disorders. Classed as a nerve tonic. The essential oil is useful externally for hair and scalp problems. A few drops of oil in a foot bath or in a full bath is quite refreshing to the nervous system and the muscles. It is also recommended externally for joint and muscle problems.

HOW IT IS USED
Infusion and extract internally, the essential oil externally. Foot, hand or full body baths – using either the essential oil or a strong infusion.
DOSE
Infusion: internally as a weak tea – 50 ml three times daily (not long term).
Extract: 20 drops twice daily for a few days or weeks.
Fresh leaves: 1 small, new shoot chewed daily – for the memory.
Dried leaves and flowers: in cooking and in herbal pillows.
Oil: drops massaged into the scalp or rubbed into aching muscles and joints. If used on large areas, dilute with massage oil.

NOTE *Do not use the oil internally.*

Sage *(Salvia officinalis)*
CULTIVATION
Grows in Australia.
PART USED
Leaves.
THERAPEUTIC USE
Has antiseptic and astringent properties, which is why the infusion is recommended for diarrhoea and as a gargle and mouthwash. Helpful for hot flushes in menopause largely because of its oestrogenic and anti-perspirant effect. Traditionally used to aid memory and concentration. Also recommended for excessive breast milk during weaning. Sage oil is good for the hair and scalp.
HOW IT IS USED
Infusion: as a cold tea for menopausal flushes and excess perspiration; as a tepid gargle for a sore throat. Also extract, and as a common culinary herb.

To make a cold infusion: soak 30 g dried leaves overnight in juice of 1–2 lemons and 500 ml tepid water. Strain and refrigerate. Can be flavoured with apple or pear juice.

To make a hot infusion: 1 teaspoon dried leaves to 1 cup boiling water. Cool and strain if using as a gargle or mouthwash.

DOSE
Cold infusion: 80–100 ml three times daily. This high dose should not be taken for more than six to eight weeks.
Extract: 2 ml three times daily.

CAUTION *Excesive use can be drying to the mucous membranes (the body's internal linings).*

St John's wort *(Hypericum perforatum)*

CULTIVATION
Classed as a noxious weed in some Australian states.

PART USED
Flowers and leaves.

THERAPEUTIC USE
Has astringent, anti-inflammatory antibiotic, antiviral and mild analgesic properties which is why it is often recommended as an external healing agent for injuries and irritations. Internally it is used as a sedative and antiviral.

Traditionally used for menopausal nervousness, insomnia, arthritis, neuralgia-type pains and skin rashes. It may help cases of mild depression.

HOW IT IS USED
Infusion, ointment, extract, tincture, oil, tablets.

DOSE
Infusion: 50 ml three times daily.

NOTE *Infusion not to be used long-term unless there are breaks between. In animals it can cause photosensitivity (skin reactions to light).*

Extract and tincture: 2 ml three times daily.

NOTE *The oil is never taken internally. It is usually used undiluted on skin lesions.*

Sandalwood *(Santalum album)*

CULTIVATION
A native of India, not commonly grown in Australia.

PART USED
Essential oil extracted from wood.

THERAPEUTIC USE
Aromatic, antiseptic and external healing agent. The aroma has a sedating effect.

HOW IT IS USED
Essential oil products. Small quantities are useful internally for infections, particularly in the urinary tract. May be dabbed on small areas of the skin in undiluted form, or applied with warm compresses for dry skin. For oily skin use undiluted.

Dilute with other oils for massage.

DOSE
2 drops three times a day in water or honey. It is more effective for the urinary tract to take these drops in a capsule – you can buy empty capsules from pharmacists.

CAUTION *This internal dose can be used for a maximum period of 4 weeks but is not recommended in this form for children.*

Sarsaparilla *(Smilax officinalis)*

CULTIVATION
Not commonly grown in Australia.

PART USED
Dried underground parts.

THERAPEUTIC USE
Traditionally classed as a 'blood cleanser'; recommended for psoriasis, skin disorders of various kinds and arthritic conditions. Has tonic effects and contains various plant hormones but their biological effect is not yet known. Probably oestrogenic.

HOW IT IS USED
Extract, tincture, tablets and dried root.

DOSE
Decoction: 100 ml three times daily.
Extract: 3 ml three times daily.

Saw palmetto/sabal *(Serenoa serrulata)*

CULTIVATION
Not commonly grown in Australia.

PART USED
Ripe fruits.

THERAPEUTIC USE
For benign prostate swellings, urinary tract infections and menopausal symptoms. Contains oestrogenic substances.

HOW IT IS USED
Extract, tincture, tablets.

DOSE
Extract: 20 drops three times daily.
Tincture: 3 ml three times daily.

Scullcap *(Scutellaria lateriflora)*

CULTIVATION
Can be grown in Australia.

PART USED
Above-ground parts.

THERAPEUTIC USE
Headaches, palpitations and other nervous heart conditions, painful periods, mental 'fuzziness', insomnia, muscle aches and pains.

HOW IT IS USED
Infusion, extract, tincture, tablet complexes.

DOSE
Infusion: 30 ml three times daily.
Extract and tincture: 2 ml three times daily.

Senna *(Cassia acutifolia)*

CULTIVATION
Cultivated in India and the Middle East.

PARTS USED
Pods and leaves.

THERAPEUTIC USE
Laxative. Constipation is best treated through the diet, exercise and fluid intake rather than by taking laxatives. A professional consultation may be required to establish the cause of the problem.

HOW IT IS USED
Extract, infusion of pods or leaves, tablets.

DOSE
Pods: 6–12 pods soaked in 1 cup warm water for 4–6 hours together with ½ teaspoon ginger root or crushed cardamon seeds. Strain and drink before bed.
Infusion: 1 teaspoon leaves together with 1 teaspoon peppermint leaves in 1 cup hot water, stand for 5 minutes. Strain before drinking.
Extract: 3 ml before bed, taken with ½ cup peppermint tea.

The additives prevent griping.

CAUTION **Senna should be used short term.**

Shepherd's purse *(Capsella bursa-pastoris)*
CULTIVATION
Grows as a weed in pastures, lawns, semi-cultivated areas, roadsides, etc.

NOTE *Don't harvest from high traffic areas.*

PART USED
Above-ground parts.
THERAPEUTIC USE
An astringent (tonifying and drying effects) with mild antiseptic properties. Commonly used for urinary tract problems but also for diarrhoea, varicose veins, haemorrhoids and menstrual irregularities.
HOW IT IS USED
Extract, infusion, tablet complexes. The leaves may be used as a vegetable – in hard times!
DOSE
Extract: 1–2 ml three times daily.
Infusion: 30–60 ml three times daily.

Slippery elm *(Ulmus fulva)*
CULTIVATION
Not commonly grown in Australia.
PART USED
Powdered inner bark.
THERAPEUTIC USE
Mainly used for its soothing effects on the stomach and intestines. A poultice of the powder is useful as a drawing agent for boils, splinters, etc. and, combined with linseed meal, for coughs.
HOW IT IS USED
Powder, tablets. As an internal remedy, slippery elm powder is obviously more soothing than tablets, especially for coughs and problems in the oesophagus and stomach. However, use tablets if you don't like the taste and texture of the powder.

DOSE
Powder: for gastric upsets, nausea, diarrhoea, coughs, 1 teaspoon in ½ glass warm water before meals or between meals; for constipation, 1–2 tablespoons once or twice daily with a wholegrain breakfast cereal or with fruit and yoghurt plus plenty of fluid.

Sweet violet *(Viola odorata)*
CULTIVATION
Commonly grown in Australia.
PART USED
Leaves.
THEAPEUTIC USE
An internal and external cleanser, recommended for intermittent use only. Useful in some rheumatic conditions; also for coughs and colds.
HOW IT IS USED
Gargle, lotion, poultice or juice for skin problems, douche, infusion, extract.
DOSE
Infusion: 1 dessertspoon chopped fresh leaves to 200 ml boiling water, stand covered overnight. Take 50 ml 4 times daily for 1–4 weeks once a year.
This infusion can be used also as an external lotion or douche.
Extract: 20 drops three times daily for four weeks.

Tea tree oil *(Melaleuca alternifolia)*
CULTIVATION
Native to Australia.
PART USED
Essential oil extracted from leaves.
THERAPEUTIC USE
An anti-fungal, antiseptic and germicide for a range of external infections.
HOW IT IS USED
May be applied directly on small areas such as pimples, minor wounds and insect

stings. Use diluted on sensitive skins and large areas.

As a gargle, mouthwash or douche, use 2–3 drops to a cup of warm water. It is also recommended as a chest rub or a few drops in a cup of hot water as an inhalation.

Useful as a household disinfectant.

CAUTION **This oil is concentrated (see 'Cautions' on pages 7–8.)**

Thuja *(Thuja occidentalis)*
CULTIVATION
Will grow in Australia (tree in the conifer family).
PART USED
Young twigs.
THERAPEUTIC USE
Prescribed professionally in extract form for some female and respiratory problems.

Externally thuja is mainly used for its irritant effect and is commonly recommended for warts. It has antiviral activity.
HOW IT IS USED
Ointment. Fluid extract or oil applied undiluted on warts. Practitioners use the extract internally – in tiny doses – and homoeopathically.

Thyme *(Thymus vulgaris)*
Also known as common thyme.
CULTIVATION
Commonly cultivated as a culinary herb.
PART USED
Leaves and flowers.
THERAPEUTIC USE
Has astringent, drying qualities, with antiseptic, anti-fungal and antibiotic effects. Useful as a hot, weak infusion (flavoured with lemon juice and a little honey) for coughs, colds and infections of the digestive and urinary systems. A stronger,

cooled infusion with added glycerine makes an effective gargle and mouthwash.

Thyme extract has been used successfully to prevent bedwetting.

For sores and wounds on small areas of the body, thyme oil may be used but it is extremely strong and needs to be diluted in almond oil, Sorbolene or water. Do a test patch first!
HOW IT IS USED
May be used fresh or a tea made from the dried leaves. Use the leaves freely in cooking, salads, garlic bread etc.

Also available as extract and sometimes in tablet complexes for colds and infections.
DOSE
1 cup weak infusion 3 times daily – use 1 dessertspoon fresh leaves or ⅓ teaspoon powder per cup.
Extract: 20 drops three times daily.

NOTES **Drying to the skin and mucous membranes.**

For dried herbs to be therapeutic they should retain their original colour and smell. Old, grey bits and pieces of plants are what herbalists call 'exhausted'.

Turmeric *(Curcuma longa)*
CULTIVATION
Grows in tropical climates.
PART USED
Underground part (rhizome).
THERAPEUTIC USE
Centuries of use for treating liver and gallbladder problems. An effective digestive tonic, with verified anti-inflammatory and antioxidant properties. Suggested as support therapy for arthritis,

gastric ulcers, reducing blood cholesterol and blood stickiness.

Recent studies show that it possesses anti-tumour, anti-fungal and antibiotic action. It may be used as an external healing agent.

HOW IT IS USED
Powder – in food and tablets.

It's also a colouring for rice and other foods (additive no. 100).

DOSE
Powder: 1 teaspoon a day for a therapeutic effect. It's quite hard to take this quantity because of the strong, bitter taste but it mixes into foods reasonably well. At least use it freely as a culinary spice. A little powder can be mixed into Tea tree oil to make an external healing paste.

NOTE **Turmeric externally stains the skin (temporarily) and clothes (permanently).**

Valerian *(Valeriana officinalis)*
CULTIVATION
Easy to grow in Australia.
PART USED
Underground parts.
THERAPEUTIC USE
Generally for muscle, organ and nervous tension. Specifically for insomnia, anxiety, excitability, cramps, period pain and headaches.

NOTE **Occasionally individual adverse reactions. (I once prescribed it for a cranky insomniac. She rang me at 3 a.m. to say her insomnia was worse!)**

Do not over-dose. Consider it as a short-term remedy.

HOW IT IS USED
Infusion (unpalatable but helped by the addition of lemon and honey), tablets. Because of the infusion's taste, I usually recommend tablets.
DOSE
Infusion: 20–60 ml per day.
Tincture: 5 ml per day.
Extract: 3 ml per day.

These quantities may be taken in three divided doses throughout the day or in one dose after the evening meal.

Vervain *(Verbena officinalis)*
CULTIVATION
Grows readily in most parts of Australia.

NOTE **There are non-medicinal species of vervain.**

PART USED
Above-ground parts.
THERAPEUTIC USE
A mild digestive tonic, used to quieten nervous dispositions and to reduce muscle tension. Suggested for nervous coughing, headaches and insomnia. A strong infusion is a good mouthwash for infected gums.
HOW IT IS USED
Herbalists use extracts and tinctures. Tea is available.
DOSE
Extract: 2–3 ml three times daily.
Infusion: 50 ml three times daily.

White horehound *(Marrubium vulgare)*
CULTIVATION
Grows well in Australia.
PART USED
Leaves and flowers.

THERAPEUTIC USE
Mildly tonifying to the digestive system but mainly recommended for coughs, particularly bronchitis where there is a non-productive cough. It helps increase mucus secretions and relax the bronchioles.

HOW IT IS USED
Decoctions, extract.

Decoctions need to be made with ten per cent lemon juice or apple cider vinegar. To a 500 ml decoction, you can add 2–4 teaspoons of honey or glycerine.

DOSE
Extract: 2 ml three times daily.
Decoction: 60 ml three times daily.

Wild lettuce *(Lactuca virosa)*

CULTIVATION
Not commonly grown in Australia.

PART USED
Leaves.

THERAPEUTIC USE
Insomnia, excitability, irritable cough and organ pains.

HOW IT IS USED
Tablets, extract.

DOSE
Extract: 2 ml three times daily, or 3 ml after dinner and 3 ml before bed.

Wild yam *(Dioscorea villosa)*

CULTIVATION
Not commonly grown in Australia.

PART USED
Underground parts.

THERAPEUTIC USE
An anti-cramp, anti-inflammatory remedy. Commonly prescribed for joint and muscle problems and colic. Improves digestion and the body's fat metabolism. Probably oestrogenic but its hormonal effects in humans is not yet known.

HOW IT IS USED
Extract, decoction.

DOSE
Extract: 2–3 ml three times daily.
Decoction: 50 ml three times daily.

Willow *(Salix alba)*

CULTIVATION
Grows in Australia (the roots are invasive).

PART USED
Dried bark.

THERAPEUTIC USE
Formerly used to treat fevers due to its salicin (a compound related to aspirin) content. Suggested for the symptomatic relief of arthritis and other painful conditions of the joints and muscles.

HOW IT IS USED
Decoction, extract or tablets.

DOSE
Decoction: 20 ml three times daily.
Extract: 2 ml three times daily.

---

*CAUTION **Because of the salicin content, doses in excess of the recommended level could cause gastric irritation. Always take after meals.***

Wintergreen *(Gaultheria procumbens)*

CULTIVATION
Not commonly grown in Australia.

PART USED
Essential oil distilled from the leaves.

THERAPEUTIC USE
The oil is commonly used in linaments for its warming and analgesic action. It is used in arthritis and rheumatic conditions for its counter-irritant effect, that is, it reddens the skin in the locality of the pain. It is helpful for use in strains and

sports injuries, after the initial treatments have been applied.

CAUTIONS *The oil must not be used internally.*

The oil may produce a slight rash that will soon disappear. This needs to be distinguished from an allergic reaction, such as prolonged rash, swelling or itching, which indicates that it is not suitable for everyone. It is better diluted with a massage oil for sensitive skins.

Witch hazel *(Hamamelis virginicus)*
CULTIVATION
Not commonly grown in Australia.
PART USED
Bark, sometimes the leaves.
THERAPEUTIC USE
An anti-inflammatory and astringent with a tonifying effect but with a tendency to dry the skin.
HOW IT IS USED
Externally the ointment is particularly helpful for haemorrhoids. Commercial extracts are useful as compresses and lotions for bruising and swelling, especially following applications of crushed ice. Also recommended for oily skin conditions and weak capillaries.

The fluid extract is an effective dermatitis remedy when mixed into Sorbolene, or any non-irritating base.

Wood betony *(Betonica officinalis)*
Also known as betony.
CULTIVATION
Can be grown in Australia.
PART USED
Above-ground parts.

THERAPEUTIC USE
Headaches, especially those connected with poor liver function and digestive disorders; also suggested for palpitations, anxiety, insomnia, nerve pains, rheumatic disorders.
HOW IT IS USED
Infusion, extract, tincture.
DOSE
Infusion: 50 ml three times daily.
Extract and tincture: 30 drops three times daily.

Yarrow *(Achillea millefolium)*

NOTE *There are many other species of yarrow that look similar but are not used medicinally.*

CULTIVATION
Grows readily in Australia. All species tend to 'take over' in the garden.
PART USED
Above-ground parts.
THERAPEUTIC USE
This is a versatile herb with anti-inflammatory, astringent and antiseptic properties. It is recommended for fevers, high blood pressure, haemorrhoids, menstrual and bladder problems. Sometimes used as a tonic. Achilles is said to have used the leaves to heal his warriors' wounds.
HOW IT IS USED
Infusion, extract, tincture. Usually mixed with herbs such as peppermint to cover the unpleasant taste.
DOSE
Infusion: 50 ml three times daily.
Extract and tincture: 20 drops three times daily.

NOTE *Occasional allergic reactions have been reported.*

Yellow dock *(Rumex crispus)*

CULTIVATION
Grows wild in Australia.

PART USED
Underground parts.

THERAPEUTIC USE
A bitter tonic for the liver and gallbladder. This herb has a laxative effect. Traditionally used for skin problems.

HOW IT IS USED
Decoction of the dried root. Also tincture, extract, tablet complexes.

DOSE
Decoction: 30–50 ml three times daily.
Extract and tincture: 1–2 ml three times daily.

Yucca *(Yucca schidigen)*

CULTIVATION
Native to south-west USA and Mexico. Grown in Australia as a specimen horticultural plant.

PART USED
Usually the root. Some books refer to other species and other parts of the plant.

THERAPEUTIC USE
An American herbalist, Dr Bingham, considers that 'it is non-toxic and useful to prevent and correct disorders which may have their origin in the gastro-intestinal tract, particularly high blood pressure, high blood triglycerides and high blood cholesterol levels. It is particularly beneficial to patients with arthritis who suffer from these somatic disorders'. I also suggest it for fluid retention.

HOW IT IS USED
Available in Australia in tablets or capsules.

DOSE
According to manufacturer's instructions.

NEW HERBS NOW BECOMING AVAILABLE IN AUSTRALIA

Astragalus *(Astragalus membranaceus)*

A traditional Chinese herb that is useful for fatigue and to strengthen the immune system.

Cat's claw *(Uncaria tomentosa)*

This South American herb is recommended for digestive problems and diseases that relate to malfunctioning of the immune system and inflammation, including rheumatoid arthritis, and as a support therapy for cancer patients.

Pau d'arco *(Tabeuia impetiginosa or avellandedae)*

Another important South American herb that is helpful for digestive disorders and common respiratory problems as well as support treatment for candida and herpes. It is also recommended for chronic fatigue and as support therapy for immune-related disorders.

REFERENCES

Chapter 2
1 *Nature*, 1988; 333: 816–8.
2 *Lancet*, 1986; 2: 881–6.
3 *British Journal of Clinical Pharmacology*, 1978; 6: 391–5.
4 *British Medical Journal*, 1991: 302; 316–21.
5 Deck, Josef, *Principles of Iris Diagnosis*, 1982.
6 *Medical Journal of Australia*, 1981; 2: 676–9.
7 Stalker, D. and Blymour, C., ed. *Examining Holistic Medicine*, Prometheus Books, Buffalo, NY, 1985.
8 *Australian Family Physician*, 1980; 9: 309–18.

Chapter 3
1 *Nutrition and Health*, 1991; 7: 89–100.
2 *British Medical Journal*, 1989; 299: 365–6.
3 *Lancet*, 1991; 338: 899–902.
4 *British Journal of Clinical Pharmacology*, 1990; 9: 453–9.

5 *Lancet*, 1984; 2: 1171–4.
6 *British Medical Journal*, 1987; 295: 1238.
7 *Journal of Rheumatology*, 1989; 16: 1.
8 *Australian Prescriber*, 1991; 14: 3.
9 *Archives of Internal Medicine*, 1992; 152: 615–32.
10 *General Practitioner*, 1992; 24: 21.
11 *British Journal of Phytotherapy*, 1991; 2: 17.
12 *Journal of Applied Nutrition*, 1976; 28: 34–47.
13 *Journal of Alternative and Complementary Medicine*, 1990; 8: 23.

Chapter 4
1 *British Medical Journal*, 1987; 295: 700–2.
2 *Psychology Today*, 1986; 20: 6.
3 *International Clinical Nutrition Review*, 1989; 9: 185–8.
4 *New England Journal of Medicine*, 1992; 326: 501–6.

5 *New Scientist*, 1991, 131: 9.
6 *British Medical Journal*, 1991; 302: 1116-8.
7 *British Medical Journal*, 1991; 303: 1426-31.
8 *Lancet*, 1988; 2: 334-5.
9 *British Medical Journal*, 1991; 303: 1450-2.

Chapter 5

1 *Gastroenterology*, 1991; 101: 84-8.
2 *Human Nutrition: Applied Nutrition*, 1985; 38A: 469-73.
3 *Lancet*, 1990; 336: 1096-7.
4 *Lancet*, 1992; 340: 69-72.
5 *Scandinavian Journal of Gastroenterology* 1991; 26: 747-50.

Chapter 6

1 *Nutrition and Health*, 1991; 7: 69-88.
2 *American Journal of Clinical Nutrition*, 1992; 55: 891-5.
3 *British Medical Journal*, 1986; 293: 583-4.
4 *Journal of Clinical Dentistry*, 1991; 248: 75-6.
5 *Lancet*, 1991; 337: 300.

Chapter 7

1 *Gerontologist*, 1974; 14: 13.
2 *International Clinical Nutrition Review*, 1991; 11: 134-9.
3 *Lancet*, 1990; 336: 129-33.
4 *Indian Journal of Medical Sciences*, 1986; 40: 149-52.
5 *Lancet*, 1992; 339: 1168-9.
6 *Journal of the American Medical Association*, 1991; 266: 1225-9.

7 *British Medical Journal*, 1984; 289: 1021-2.
8 *Journal of the American Medical Association*, 1992; 267: 1776.
9 *British Medical Journal*, 1992; 304: 75-8.

Chapter 8

1 *New England Journal of Medicine*, 1991; 324: 1599.
2 *British Journal of General Practice*, 1992, 42: 138-9.
3 *Townsend Letter for Doctors*, Feb/March 1991; 107-110.
4 *New England Journal of Medicine*, 1991; 325: 1303-4.

Chapter 9

1 *Journal of the Royal Society of Medicine*, 1987; 80: 76-7.
2 *British Medical Journal*, 1984; 288: 133.
3 *Australian Prescriber*, 1991; 14: 75.
4 *1990 Australian Market Basket Survey*, National Health and Medical Research Council, AGPS, Canberra.
5 *Science*, 1987; 236: 271.

Chapter 10

1 *Health and Disease in Tribal Societies*, Ciba Foundation Symposium 49, Elsevier, London, 1977.
2 *International Clinical Nutrition Review*, 1989; 9: 137-43.
3 *Townsend Letter for Doctors*, July 1991; 546-7.
4 *Lancet*, 1991; 337: 331-2.
5 *Journal of Ethnopharmacology*, 1990; 29: 267-73.

Chapter 11

1 *Lancet*, 1989; 2: 1039.
2 *Journal of Internal Medical Research*, 1992; 20: 234-46.
3 *Lancet*, 1986; 2: 881-6.
4 *Lancet*, 1990; 335: 1381-3.

Chapter 12

1 *Medical Journal of Australia*, 1990; 153: 455-8.
2 *The Prescriber*, 1988; 11: 83-4.

Chapter 13

1 Swartz, G.R., MD, *In Bad Taste – the MSG Syndrome*, New American Library, New York, 1988.

Chapter 15

1 *National Dietary Survey of Schoolchildren (aged 10–15 years), 1985*, Department of Community Services and Health, AGPS, Canberra.
2 *Lancet*, 1992; 339: 261-4.
3 *1990 Market Basket Survey*, National Health and Medical Research Council.
4 Oski & Phillips, *Don't Drink Your Milk*, Pythagorean Press, New York, 1988.
5 *Economic Botany*, 1984; 38: 52-63.
6 *Time*, 1992; 7:55.
7 *American Journal of Clinical Nutrition*, 1988: 4; supplement.
8 *New England Journal of Medicine*, 1990; 322: 1477-87.
9 *New England Journal of Medicine*, 1991; 324: 839-44.

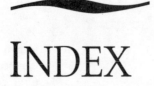

INDEX

Note This index is a listing of the main topics only. For example, a particular herb may be mentioned under a number of different illnesses but is listed in the index only when that herb is a separate topic or has unusual or special significance. In other words, the index is linked primarily to health problems rather than the remedies.